Healing
Herbs

THE ESSENTIAL GUIDE

Healing Herbs

THE ESSENTIAL GUIDE

H. WINTER GRIFFITH, M.D.

Technical Consultant

Cynthia Thomson, Ph.D., R.D.

Clinical Nutrition Research Specialist, Arizona Cancer Center
University of Arizona Prevention Center

FISHER
er
BOOKS™

Publishers: *Fred W. Fisher,*
   Helen V. Fisher & Howard W. Fisher
Managing Editor: *Sarah Trotta*
Editors: *Meg Morris, Melanie Mallon*
Consulting Editors: *Brian Engstrom,*
   Jean Anderson
Index: *Michelle B. Graye*
Production: *Randy Schultz, Ann Olsen*
Cover Photo: ©*Digital Vision/Wonderfile*
Cover: *Gary D. Smith,*
   Performance Design

Published by Fisher Books, LLC
5225 W. Massingale Road
Tucson, Arizona 85743-8416
(520) 744-6110

Library of Congress
Cataloging-in-Publication Data

Griffith, H. Winter (Henry Winter), 1926-
   Healing herbs : the essential guide /
   H. Winter Griffith ; technical consultant,
   Cynthia Thomson.
      p. cm.
   Includes bibliographical references
   and index.
   ISBN 1-55561-231-8
   1. Materia medica, Vegetable—Dictionaries.
   I. Title.

RS164.G679 2000
615'.32'03—dc21
                                    99-053878

Printed in U.S.A.
10 9 8 7 6 5 4 3 2 1

Contents

About the Author

H. Winter Griffith, M.D., received his medical degree from Emory University in 1953 and spent more than 20 years in private practice. At Florida State University, he established a basic medical science program and also directed the family practice residency program at Tallahassee Memorial Hospital. After moving to the Southwest, he became associate professor of Family and Community Medicine at the University of Arizona College of Medicine. He devoted most of his time to writing medical-information books for general readers.

Dedication

To each of you who wishes to be informed enough to become the most important member of your own healthcare team.

About Medicinal Herbs

A popular backlash currently exists against conventional medicine as it is practiced today. The medical profession has brought some negative feelings upon itself. Part of this backlash takes the form of returning to "natural" medicine—specifically to any of the 2,500 herbs that have been used throughout history for medicinal purposes. People self-prescribe these plant materials and believe they are saving time and money by not consulting their physician. Because medicinal herbs are natural and generally unregulated, many people believe they are without hazards. This is not true!

For centuries, people have collected herbs to use for medicinal purposes. Although some are experienced in their use, most base their use of herbs on anecdotal experience rather than scientific study. Some of the most useful medicines, such as digitalis, rauwolfia (used for mental illness and hypertension), cromlyn (used for preventing asthma attacks) and curare (a muscle relaxant), have all come from herbal "folk remedies."

Herbs are a potentially invaluable treatment for many ills but will need to undergo standardized scientific study before they are generally accepted for clinical use.

Many medicinal herbs have pharmacological properties that we know are useful. But at the same time they may be harmful or toxic. Medicinal herbs are available in many forms, but most have not been scrutinized for safety and effectiveness by the U.S. Food and Drug Administration (FDA). It is also important to point out that the most experienced prescribers of herbs are trained Traditional Chinese Medicine (TCM) practitioners who seldom prescribe a single herb but instead claim therapeutic benefits based on herbal combinations.

People have turned to medicinal herbs, believing they are "natural," safe, effective and wonderful. However, experience has taught us any effective medicine can also have uncomfortable side effects, adverse reactions and dangerous potential toxicity, just as many pharmaceuticals do.

Active ingredients of medicinal herbs vary greatly, whether you personally collect plant drugs or buy them. Variable factors include

- Conditions under which the plant was grown (soil conditions, temperature, season)
- Degree of maturity of the plant when it was collected
- Type of drying process
- Type and duration of storage

In conventional medicine, these variables are controlled by manufacturing procedures or government tests or assays to standardize the amount of the active principle and therefore the predictable safety and effectiveness of the material. None of these safeguards currently exist for medicinal herbs except on a voluntary, manufacturer-specific basis.

The Placebo

The *placebo effect* has long been held as an advantage of using medicinal herbs. Many scientists and researchers claim most herbs do not really help people. It is the placebo effect of using these herbs that really heals. The word *placebo* comes from a Latin predecessor meaning "to please" or "to serve." Under a strict interpretation of the term as it is now used, a placebo medication has no pharmacologically or biologically active ingredients. Another interpretation asserts that small

amounts could not affect the body, but large amounts of the same substance may.

For centuries, healers have helped people who were ill, no matter what the illness. Many ancient healers used remedies that have no pharmacological effects in the body, but these remedies were not always useless. They frequently proved to be very effective.

Modern studies conclusively prove all remedies help relieve symptoms in some people. In the early 1900s, many patients and physicians believed placebo therapy was quackery. Today, we know this to be untrue. Placebos *can* mimic the effect of almost any active drug. Placebo effects are real and can be a powerful adjuvant to conventional treatments.

How does the placebo effect work? We don't know for certain, but there are different theories.

Endorphins—chemicals normally present in the brain—can be activated by exercise, stress, mental exercises and imaging. Once endorphins have been activated, they kill pain the same way narcotics kill pain. Placebo treatment can trigger the production of endorphins and hormones in the body, such as cortisone and adrenaline. This can affect the way we behave, the way we feel, the way we think. If the placebo can cause production of these chemicals, this may relieve symptoms of many disorders.

Harder to explain is the part that "power of suggestion" may play in the effectiveness of any remedy, whether it is a powerful drug, a supplement, an herb or a placebo. The gentle touch of the healer, the taste and smell of the product, the packaging, the cost—all are factors that have been studied and found to play a part in the placebo effect.

Understanding Common Terms

When you read about medicinal herbs, you will run across the following common terms. They refer to ways in which medicinal herbs can be useful.

Compress—Cloth is soaked in a cool liquid form of an herb, wrung out and applied directly to skin.

Decoction—The herb is boiled 10 to 15 minutes, then allowed to steep.

Extract—A solution resulting from soaking the herb in cold water for 24 hours.

Fomentation—Cloth is soaked in a hot liquid form of an herb, wrung out and applied directly to skin.

Infusion—Tea is prepared by steeping herb in hot water. Infusions can be made from any part of a plant.

Ointment—The powdered form of an herb is mixed with any soft-based salve, such as lanolin, wax or lard.

Poultice—The herb applied to a moistened cloth, then applied directly to skin.

Powder—The useful part of the herb is ground into a powder.

Syrup—The herb is added to brown sugar dissolved in boiling water, then boiled and strained.

Tincture—The powdered herb is added to a 50/50 solution of alcohol and water.

Points to Remember

Precautions apply to all herbal medications. Read the checklist on page 10. Also keep the following in mind:

- Children under age 2 should *not* be given herbal medications.
- Pregnant and lactating women should avoid herbal medicines because of potential damage to the fetus or breastfeeding child.
- Collecting medicinal herbs for yourself is unwise, unless you have received a great deal of training. Correctly identifying plants and knowing how to select, preserve and use them properly requires a great deal of knowledge and judgment.

Labeling

Currently, herbal and other supplements are regulated under the Dietary Supplement Act of 1994. This act states that labels can only display information related to the structure and function of the herb and not directly link it to prevention or treatment of disease. The burden of proving false claims or harm remains with the FDA.

In 1998, the FDA Modernization Act of 1997 took effect. According to this law, manufacturers are now permitted to use claims if such claims are based on current, published, authoritative statements from the National Institutes of Health (NIH), Center for Disease Control and Prevention (CDC), the Surgeon General, the Food and Safety Inspection Service and the Agricultural Research Service within the Department of Agriculture.

Guide to Medicinal-Herb Charts

The medicinal-herb information in this book is organized in condensed, easy-to-read charts. Each medicinal herb is described on a 1- to 2-page chart, as shown in the sample chart on the next page. Charts are arranged alphabetically by the most common name. If you cannot find a name, look for alternate names in the Index or ask your health-product or herbal-medication retailer for alternative names.

A—Popular name

Each chart is titled by the most popular name. When there is more than one popular name, alternative names are shown in parentheses. If an herb has several possible names, you'll find the least common listed under *Basic Information.* The Index contains a reference to each name listed. Popular names may vary in different parts of the world.

B—Biological name (genus and species)

This section identifies the medicinal herb by genus and species.

These Latin names are commonly used by biologists and plant scientists. They are included to help you make a positive identification. Note: Some herbs have more than one biological name and some include so many species, just the genus is listed.

C—Parts used for medicinal purposes

Here you'll find what parts of the herb are used to supply the expected effects. Roots, leaves, bark and flowers are commonly used portions of the plant. Sometimes the entire plant is used.

D—Chemicals this herb contains

Chemicals and family names of chemically related groups are listed in this section. Chemically related groups include saponins, tannins, volatile oils and others.

E—Known Effects

This section lists identified chemical actions of the medicinal herb being discussed. These

Sample Chart

A — ## Astragalus (Huang-Qi, Milk Vetch)

Basic Information

B — Biological name (genus and species):
Astragalus membranaceous

C — Parts used for medicinal purposes:
Root

D — Chemicals this herb contains:
- Asparagine
- Astragalosides
- Calcyosin
- Formononetin
- Kumatakenin
- Sterols

Known Effects

E —
- Stimulates and protects the immune system
- Produces spontaneous sweating

F — **Miscellaneous information:**
Available as tea, fluid extract, capsules and dried root.

Possible Additional Effects

G —
- May reduce fatigue/weakness
- Potential cold and flu treatment
- May increase stamina
- Potential treatment for immune-deficiency problems (AIDS, cancer)
- May reduce symptoms of chronic fatigue syndrome
- May improve appetite
- May alleviate diarrhea

Warnings and Precautions

H — **Don't take if you:**
- Are pregnant, think you may be pregnant or plan pregnancy in the near future
- Are currently feverish

Consult your doctor if you: — **I**
- Take this herb for any medical problem that doesn't improve in 2 weeks (There may be safer, more effective treatments.)
- Take any medicinal drugs or herbs including aspirin, laxatives, cold and cough remedies, antacids, vitamins, minerals, amino acids, supplements, other prescription or nonprescription drugs

Pregnancy: — **J**
Use only on the advice of your physician.

Breastfeeding: — **K**
Use only on the advice of your physician.

Infants and children: — **L**
Treating infants or children under 2 with any herbal preparation is hazardous.

Others: — **M**
None.

Storage: — **N**
- Store in cool, dry area away from direct light, but don't freeze.
- Store safely out of reach of children.
- Don't store in bathroom medicine cabinet. Heat and moisture may change the action of the herb.

Safe dosage: — **O**
Consult your doctor for the appropriate dose for your condition.

Toxicity — **P**
Comparative-toxicity rating is not available from standard references.

Adverse Reactions, Side Effects or Overdose Symptoms — **Q**

None are expected.

effects have been identified and validated by scientists and researchers through various studies. Some effects may be beneficial; others are harmful.

F–Miscellaneous information

This section contains information that doesn't fit into other information blocks on the chart. If no additional information exists, this section will be missing.

G–Possible Additional Effects

This list contains symptoms or medical problems this drug has been *reported* to treat or improve. These claims may be accurate, but they haven't been proved with well-controlled studies.

H–Don't take if you

Here you'll find circumstances under which the use of this herb or supplement may not be safe. In formal medical literature, these circumstances are listed as *absolute contraindications.*

I–Consult your doctor if you

This section lists conditions in which this herb should be used with caution. In formal medical literature, these circumstances are called *relative contraindications.* Using an herb under these circumstances may require special consideration by you and your doctor. The guiding rule: *The potential benefit must outweigh the possible risk!*

J–Pregnancy

The more we learn about effective medications, including herbal medications, the more healthcare workers fear the possible effects of any medicinal product on an unborn child. This fear holds for *all* chemicals that cause changes in the body. That herbal medicines occur naturally does not free them from possibly causing harm. *The best rule to follow is don't take anything during pregnancy if you can avoid it!*

K–Breastfeeding

Although a breastfeeding infant is not as likely to be harmed as an unborn fetus, be cautious. If you take a medicine or an herb during the time you breastfeed, do so *only* under professional supervision.

L–Infants and children

Treating infants and children under 2 years old with any herbal preparation is hazardous. Dosages, uses and effects of an herb cannot be gauged easily with a young child. Do not use medicinal herbs to treat a problem your child may have without first discussing it thoroughly with your doctor.

M–Others

Warnings and precautions appear here if they don't fit into other categories.

N–Storage

This section advises you on how to store herbs to best preserve them. It also includes a crucial reminder: *Always store any herb safely away from children!*

O–Safe dosage

Safe dosages of herbs have not been documented by procedures outlined by the FDA. For these, it is impossible to list a "safe" dosage and have it carry any significance. People who have had experience with herbs are usually qualified to predict safe doses if they know the person's age, medical history and some important facts about his or her current health.

Many reputable distributors of herb products have recommendations for ranges of safety, but these may vary a great deal from manufacturer to manufacturer, according to age and purity of the product. The most important fact to understand is the more you ingest over a long period of time, the more likely a toxic reaction will occur. Most available herbs and supplements are safe when taken in small doses for short periods of time. Never fall into the trap of thinking "if a little is good, more is better."

P–Toxicity

This section includes a general, average toxicity rating for each medicinal herb.

Q–Adverse Reactions, Side Effects or Overdose Symptoms

Adverse reactions or side effects are symptoms that may occur when you ingest any substance, whether it is food, medicine, vitamin, mineral, herb or supplement. These are effects on the body other than the desired effect for which you take them. The term *adverse reaction* means the effects can cause hazards that outweigh benefits.

The term *side effect* may include an expected, perhaps unavoidable, effect of a medicinal herb. For example, a side effect of horseradish may be nausea. This symptom is harmless although sometimes uncomfortable and has nothing to do with the intended use.

If you suspect an overdose, whether symptoms are present or not, follow instructions in this section.

Warning

Whether you use medicinal herbs is your decision. If you choose to use them, be sure you take them with knowledge and understanding of what they are. Know the supplier, and be sure you know the possible dangers. Consider that self-medication with medicinal herbs may prevent you from receiving better help from more effective medications that have withstood critical scientific investigations.

Checklist for Safer Use of Medicinal Herbs

The most important caution regarding all medicinal herbs deals with the amount you take. Despite many popular articles in magazines and newspapers and reports on television, large doses of some of these substances can be hazardous to your health. Don't believe sensational advertisements and take large doses or megadoses. The belief "if a little does good, a lot will do much more" has no place in rational thinking regarding products to protect your health. Stay within safe-dose ranges!

1. Learn all you can about medicinal herbs *before* you take them. Information sources include this book, books from your public library, your doctor or your pharmacist.

2. Don't take medicinal herbs prescribed for someone else, even if your symptoms are the same. At the same time, keep prescription items to yourself. They may be harmful to someone else.

3. Tell your doctor or health-care professional about any symptoms you experience that you suspect may be caused by anything you take.

4. Take medicinal herbs in good light after you have identified the contents of the container. If you wear glasses, put them on to check and recheck labels.

5. Don't keep medicine by your bedside. You may unknowingly repeat a dose when you are half-asleep or confused.

6. Know the names of all the substances you take.

7. Read labels on medications you take. If the information is incomplete, ask your pharmacist for more details.

8. If the substance is in liquid form, shake it before you take it.

9. Store medicinal herbs in cool places away from sunlight and moisture. Bathroom medicine cabinets are usually unacceptable because they are too warm and humid.

10. If a herb requires refrigeration, don't freeze!

11. Obtain a standard measuring spoon from your pharmacy for liquid substances and a graduated dropper to use for liquid preparations for infants and children.

12. Follow manufacturer's or doctor's suggestions regarding diet instructions. Some products work best on a full stomach. Others work best on an empty stomach. Some products work best when you follow a special diet. For example, a low-salt diet enhances effectiveness of any product expected to lower blood pressure.

13. Avoid any substance you know you are allergic to.

14. If you become pregnant while taking a medicinal herb, tell your physician and discontinue taking it until you have discussed it with him or her. Try to remember the exact dose and the length of time you have taken the substance.

15. Tell any healthcare provider about medicinal herbs and other substances you take, even if you bought them without a prescription. During an illness or prior to surgery, this information is crucial. Even mention antacids, laxatives, tonics and over-the-counter preparations. Many people believe these products are completely safe and forget to tell doctors, nurses or pharmacists that they are using them.

16. Regard all medicinal herbs as potentially harmful to children. Store them safely away from their reach.

17. Alcohol, marijuana, cocaine, other mood-altering drugs and tobacco can cause life-threatening interactions when mixed with some medicinal herbs. They can also prevent treatment from being effective or delay your return to good health. Common sense dictates you avoid them, particularly during an illness.

Medicinal Herbs

The following section attempts to provide you with enough knowledge to avoid toxicity if you choose to self-prescribe medicinal herbs. If you collect and use herbal medications, you must be an expert botanist or herbologist. If you buy them, you have the right to know everything about possible side effects, adverse reactions, toxicity and other dangers in using materials that are not subjected to rigid control procedures.

Medicinal herbs have been effectively used in Eastern medicine for thousands of years; however, only a small percentage have undergone rigorous scientific study.

The most important warnings:

꙳ Don't use medicinal herbs for infants or children without guidance from an expert and your doctor's approval.

꙳ Don't use medicinal herbs at all unless you know enough to use them safely.

꙳ If you choose to use medicinal herbs, tell your doctor which ones you use and in what amounts when he or she asks if you take other medications. As you will see in the following charts, these substances could affect various medicines or courses of treatment your doctor may prescribe.

꙳ Be cautious with the use of medicinal herbs during pregnancy or lactation—check with a knowledgeable health professional before taking.

꙳ Lastly, it is most important to note that traditionally most medicinal herbs have been used in combination to treat the "whole" person rather than the single-symptom/single-herb approach more common to Western medicine.

Aconite (Blue Rocket, Fu-Tzu, Monkshood)

Basic Information

Biological name (genus and species):
Aconitum napellus

Parts used for medicinal purposes:
• Leaves
• Roots

Chemicals this herb contains:
• Aconine
• Aconitine
• Benzoylamine
• Neopelline
• Picraconitine

Known Effects

• Small amounts stimulate central nervous system and peripheral nerves.
• Large amounts depress central nervous system and peripheral nerves—dangerous.
• Normalizes heartbeat irregularities.
• A dose as low as 5ml (about 1 teaspoon) of the root can be lethal.
• Anti-inflammatory.

Miscellaneous information:

Used for centuries as an arrow poison.

Possible Additional Effects

• May decrease fever
• May soothe sore throats and laryngitis
• May reduce pain of rheumatoid arthritis and gout
• May help treat croup and bronchitis

Warnings and Precautions

Don't take if you:
• Are pregnant, think you may be pregnant or plan pregnancy in the near future
• Have any chronic disease of the gastrointestinal tract, such as stomach or duodenal ulcers, reflux esophagitis, ulcerative colitis, spastic colitis, diverticulosis or diverticulitis

Consult your doctor if you:
• Take this herb for any medical problem that doesn't improve in 2 weeks (There may be safer, more effective treatments.)
• Take any medicinal drugs or herbs including aspirin, laxatives, cold and cough remedies, antacids, vitamins, minerals, amino acids, supplements, other prescription or nonprescription drugs

Pregnancy:
Don't use.

Breastfeeding:
Don't use.

Infants and children:
Treating infants or children under 2 with any herbal preparation is hazardous.

Others:
Dangers outweigh any possible benefits. Don't use.

Storage:
• Store in cool, dry area away from direct light, but don't freeze.
• Store safely out of reach of children.
• Don't store in bathroom medicine cabinet. Heat and moisture may change the action of the herb.

Safe dosage:
Consult your doctor for the appropriate dose for your condition.

Toxicity
Rated dangerous, particularly in children, persons over 55 and those who take larger than appropriate quantities for extended periods of time

For symptoms of toxicity: See *Adverse Reactions, Side Effects or Overdose Symptoms* section below.

Adverse Reactions, Side Effects or Overdose Symptoms

Signs and symptoms	What to do
Burning or numbness of tongue and lips	Discontinue. Call doctor immediately.
Difficulty swallowing	Discontinue. Call doctor immediately.
Irritability	Discontinue. Call doctor when convenient.
Nausea or vomiting	Discontinue. Call doctor immediately.
Restlessness	Discontinue. Call doctor when convenient.
Speech difficulties	Discontinue. Call doctor immediately.
Vision doubled or blurred	Discontinue. Call doctor immediately.

Agave

Basic Information

Biological name (genus and species):
Agave lecheguilla

Parts used for medicinal purposes:
- Leaves
- Roots
- Sap

Chemicals this herb contains:
- Diosgenin
- Photosensitizing pigment (see Glossary)
- Steroidal chemicals (see Glossary)
- Vitamin C

Known Effects
- Causes disintegration of red blood cells
- Irritates skin
- Irritates lining of gastrointestinal tract
- Small amounts depress central nervous system
- Damages cells (dissolves membranes of red blood cells and changes tissue permeability)

Miscellaneous information:
- Agave is used to make mescal, an alcoholic beverage.
- Fibers are used for rope.
- Sap is used as a syrup.
- Roots and leaves contain active chemicals.

➜

Possible Additional Effects

- Roots and leaves used to relieve toothache
- May provide nutrition
- Potential hormone replacement
- May produce immunosuppressive effects on body
- May cause abortion or miscarriage
- May treat dysentery
- May relieve pain of sprains

Warnings and Precautions

Don't take if you:
- Are pregnant, think you may be pregnant or plan pregnancy in the near future
- Have symptoms of a disease caused by a hormone deficiency
- Have any chronic disease of the gastrointestinal tract, such as stomach or duodenal ulcers, reflux esophagitis, ulcerative colitis, spastic colitis, diverticulosis or diverticulitis

Consult your doctor if you:
- Have stomach problems
- Take cortisone, ACTH, testosterone or androgenic steroids

Pregnancy:
Don't use unless prescribed by your doctor.

Breastfeeding:
Don't use unless prescribed by your doctor.

Infants and children:
Treating infants or children under 2 with any herbal preparation is hazardous.

Others:
No problems expected if you are beyond childhood, under 45, not pregnant, basically healthy, take it for only a short time and do not exceed manufacturer's recommended dose.

Storage:
- Store in cool, dry area away from direct light, but don't freeze.
- Store safely out of reach of children.
- Don't store in bathroom medicine cabinet. Heat and moisture may change the action of the herb.

Safe dosage:
Consult your doctor for the appropriate dose for your condition.

Toxicity

Comparative-toxicity rating is not available from standard references.

For symptoms of toxicity: See *Adverse Reactions, Side Effects or Overdose Symptoms* section below.

Adverse Reactions, Side Effects or Overdose Symptoms

Signs and symptoms	What to do
Abortion (remote possibility if taken in large amounts)	Seek emergency treatment.
Diarrhea	Discontinue. Call doctor immediately.
Increased sensitivity to sunlight	Discontinue. Call doctor when convenient.
Jaundice (yellow skin and eyes)	Discontinue. Call doctor immediately.
Nausea or vomiting	Discontinue. Call doctor immediately.
Skin itching and rash	Discontinue. Call doctor when convenient.
Unusual bleeding	Discontinue. Call doctor immediately.

Alder, Black (Alder Buckthorn)

Basic Information

Biological name (genus and species):
Alnus glutinosa, Rhamnus frangula, Frangula

Parts used for medicinal purposes:
Various parts of the entire plant, frequently differing by country and culture

Chemicals this herb contains:
• Anthraquinone glycosides
• Emodin
• Rhamnose

Known Effects

• Irritates gastrointestinal tract
• Causes vomiting

Miscellaneous information:
• Alder is used in veterinary medicine for its cathartic properties.
• Emetic action (causing vomiting) is less when plant is dried for 1 year or more.

Possible Additional Effects

May temporarily relieve constipation

Warnings and Precautions

Don't take if you:
• Are pregnant, think you may be pregnant or plan pregnancy in the near future
• Have any chronic disease of the gastrointestinal tract, such as stomach or duodenal ulcers, reflux esophagitis, ulcerative colitis, spastic colitis, diverticulosis or diverticulitis

Consult your doctor if you:
• Take this herb for any medical problem that doesn't improve in 2 weeks (There may be safer, more effective treatments.)
• Take any medicinal drugs or herbs including aspirin, laxatives, cold and cough remedies, antacids, vitamins, minerals, amino acids, supplements, other prescription or nonprescription drugs

Pregnancy:
Don't use unless prescribed by your doctor.

Breastfeeding:
Don't use unless prescribed by your doctor.

Infants and children:
Treating infants or children under 2 with any herbal preparation is hazardous.

Others:
No problems expected if you are beyond childhood, under 45, not pregnant, basically healthy, take it for only a short time and do not exceed manufacturer's recommended dose.

Storage:
• Store in cool, dry area away from direct light, but don't freeze.
• Store safely out of reach of children.
• Don't store in bathroom medicine cabinet. Heat and moisture may change the action of the herb.

Safe dosage:
Consult your doctor for the appropriate dose for your condition.

➡

Toxicity

Rated slightly dangerous, particularly in children, persons over 55 and those who take larger than appropriate quantities for extended periods of time

For symptoms of toxicity: See *Adverse Reactions, Side Effects or Overdose Symptoms* section below.

 Adverse Reactions, Side Effects or Overdose Symptoms

Signs and symptoms	What to do
Abdominal cramps (severe)	Discontinue. Call doctor immediately.
Abdominal pain	Discontinue. Call doctor when convenient.
Nausea or vomiting	Discontinue. Call doctor immediately.

Alfalfa

 Basic Information

Biological name (genus and species): *Medicago sativa*

Parts used for medicinal purposes:
• Leaves
• Petals/flower
• Sprouts

Chemicals this herb contains:
• Proteins
• Saponins (see Glossary)
• Vitamins A, B, D, K

 Known Effects

• Provides useful proteins and vitamins for dietary use
• Stimulates menstruation
• Stimulates milk production in lactating women
• Has antifungal properties

Miscellaneous information:
Alfalfa is usually compressed into capsules or brewed as tea.

 Possible Additional Effects

• May treat arthritis
• May treat unusual bleeding
• May lower cholesterol
• May relieve constipation
• May treat morning sickness

 Warnings and Precautions

Don't take if you:
• Take anticoagulants such as warfarin sodium (coumadin) or heparin
• Have lupus erythematosus

Consult your doctor if you:
Have any bleeding disorder.

Pregnancy:
Pregnant women should experience no problems taking usual amounts as part of a balanced diet. Other products extracted from this herb have not been proved to cause problems.

Breastfeeding:
Breastfed infants of lactating mothers should experience no problems when mother takes usual amounts as part of a balanced diet. Other products extracted from this herb have not been proved to cause problems.

Infants and children:
Treating infants or children under 2 with any herbal preparation is hazardous.

Others:
- No problems expected if you are beyond childhood, under 45, basically healthy, take it for only a short time and do not exceed manufacturer's recommended dose.
- Alfalfa sprouts eaten in large amounts may cause a form of anemia.

Storage:
- Store in cool, dry area away from direct light, but don't freeze.
- Store safely out of reach of children.
- Don't store in bathroom medicine cabinet. Heat and moisture may change the action of the herb.

Safe dosage:
Consult your doctor for the appropriate dose for your condition.

Toxicity

Generally regarded as safe when taken in appropriate quantities for short periods of time

For symptoms of toxicity: See *Adverse Reactions, Side Effects or Overdose Symptoms* section below.

Adverse Reactions, Side Effects or Overdose Symptoms

Signs and symptoms	What to do
Abdominal cramps	Discontinue. Call doctor immediately.
Diarrhea	Discontinue. Call doctor when convenient.

Allspice (Cove Pepper, Jamaican Pepper)

Basic Information

Biological name (genus and species):
Pimenta dioica

Parts used for medicinal purposes:
Berries/fruits

Chemicals this herb contains:
- Acid-fixed oil
- Eugenol
- Resin (see Glossary)
- Tannic acid
- Volatile oils (see Glossary)

Known Effects

- Irritates mucous membranes, including lining of gastrointestinal tract
- Aids in expelling gas from intestines to relieve colic or griping

Miscellaneous information:
- Active chemicals are in berries
- Provides flavor in toothpaste and other products
- Used as an aromatic spice in foods

➔

Possible Additional Effects

May relieve diarrhea

Warnings and Precautions

Don't take if you:

- Are pregnant, think you may be pregnant or plan pregnancy in the near future
- Have any chronic disease of the gastrointestinal tract, such as stomach or duodenal ulcers, reflux esophagitis, ulcerative colitis, spastic colitis, diverticulosis or diverticulitis

Consult your doctor if you:

- Take this herb for any medical problem that doesn't improve in 2 weeks (There may be safer, more effective treatments.)
- Take any medicinal drugs or herbs including aspirin, laxatives, cold and cough remedies, antacids, vitamins, minerals, amino acids, supplements, other prescription or nonprescription drugs

Pregnancy:

Don't use unless prescribed by your doctor.

Breastfeeding:

Don't use unless prescribed by your doctor.

Infants and children:

Treating infants or children under 2 with any herbal preparation is hazardous.

Others:

No problems expected if you are beyond childhood, under 45, not pregnant, basically healthy, take it for only a short time and do not exceed manufacturer's recommended dose.

Storage:

- Store in cool, dry area away from direct light, but don't freeze.
- Store safely out of reach of children.
- Don't store in bathroom medicine cabinet. Heat and moisture may change the action of the herb.

Safe dosage:

Consult your doctor for the appropriate dose for your condition.

Toxicity

Rated relatively safe when taken in appropriate quantities for short periods of time

For symptoms of toxicity: See *Adverse Reactions, Side Effects or Overdose Symptoms* section below.

Adverse Reactions, Side Effects or Overdose Symptoms

Signs and symptoms	What to do
Excess of 5 ml (about 1 teaspoon) of eugenol (a volatile oil found in allspice) may cause convulsions, nausea, vomiting.	Discontinue. Call doctor immediately.

Aloe

 ## Basic Information

Aloe is also called *Mediterranean aloe*, *Barbados aloe*, *Curacao aloe* and *aloe vera*.

Biological name (genus and species): *Aloe vera, A. barbadensis, A. officinalis*

Parts used for medicinal purposes: Leaves

Chemicals this herb contains:
• Aloectin B
• Anthraquinones
• Polysaccharides
• Resins (see Glossary)
• Tannins (see Glossary)

 ## Known Effects

• Milky secretion (not dried preparations) from leaves helps reduce inflammation and hasten recovery in first- and second-degree burns.
• Acts as cathartic, but whether this is beneficial or dangerous depends on many factors.
• Treats X-ray or radiation burns.
• Interferes with absorption of iron and other minerals when taken internally.
• Has antibacterial and antiviral activity.
• General wound healing.
• Heals skin ulcers.

Miscellaneous information:
• Not useful for clearing intestinal tract before surgery because only cleanses small intestine
• Used as an ingredient in many over-the-counter laxatives
• Used as an ingredient in some cosmetics

 ## Possible Additional Effects

• May kill *Pseudomonas aeruginosa*, a bacterium, when applied to skin, but probably does not promote healing
• May treat amenorrhea (lack of menstrual periods) when taken internally
• May relieve headache when applied to head

 ## Warnings and Precautions

Don't take if you:
• Have gastric ulcers
• Have small-bowel problems, such as regional enteritis
• Have ulcerative colitis
• Have diverticulosis or diverticulitis
• Have proctitis or hemorrhoids

Consult your doctor if you:
• Have any digestive disorder
• Intend to take it internally

Pregnancy:
Don't use unless prescribed by your doctor.

Breastfeeding:
Don't use unless prescribed by your doctor.

Infants and children:
Treating infants or children under 2 with any herbal preparation is hazardous.

Others:
Healing properties of aloe taken internally are still tentative and need more study.

➜

Storage:
- Store in cool, dry area away from direct light, but don't freeze.
- Store safely out of reach of children.
- Don't store in bathroom medicine cabinet. Heat and moisture may change the action of the herb.

Safe dosage:
Consult your doctor for the appropriate dose for your condition.

 Toxicity

Generally regarded as safe when taken in appropriate quantities for short periods of time

For symptoms of toxicity: See *Adverse Reactions, Side Effects or Overdose Symptoms* section below.

 Adverse Reactions, Side Effects or Overdose Symptoms

Signs and symptoms	What to do
Abdominal cramps	Discontinue. Call doctor when convenient.
Bloody diarrhea, shock (with high doses)	Seek emergency treatment.
Bowel irritation	Discontinue. Call doctor when convenient.
Diarrhea	Discontinue. Call doctor immediately.
Minor skin irritation	Cleanse skin with clear water. Do not apply externally again.
Nausea or vomiting	Discontinue. Call doctor immediately.
Red urine	Discontinue. Call doctor when convenient.
Increased urinary frequency, backache pain on urination with long continued use	Discontinue. Call doctor immediately.

Alum Root

 Basic Information

Biological name (genus and species):
Heuchera

Parts used for medicinal purposes:
Roots

Chemicals this herb contains:
Tannins (see Glossary)

 Known Effects

- Shrinks tissues
- Prevents secretion of fluids

Miscellaneous information:
- Used externally and internally by some tribes of North American Indians for many disorders
- Used as a douche

Possible Additional Effects

- May treat heart disease
- May prevent infection in injured skin

 ## Warnings and Precautions

Don't take if you:
- Have liver or kidney disease
- Are pregnant, think you may be pregnant or plan pregnancy in the near future
- Have any chronic disease of the gastrointestinal tract, such as stomach or duodenal ulcers, reflux esophagitis, ulcerative colitis, spastic colitis, diverticulosis or diverticulitis

Consult your doctor if you:
- Take this herb for any medical problem that doesn't improve in 2 weeks (There may be safer, more effective treatments.)
- Take any medicinal drugs or herbs including aspirin, laxatives, cold and cough remedies, antacids, vitamins, minerals, amino acids, supplements, other prescription or nonprescription drugs

Pregnancy:
Don't use unless prescribed by your doctor.

Breastfeeding:
Don't use unless prescribed by your doctor.

Infants and children:
Treating infants or children under 2 with any herbal preparation is hazardous.

Others:
Toxic effects greatly outweigh any possible benefits. Don't take this herb internally!

Storage:
- Store in cool, dry area away from direct light, but don't freeze.
- Store safely out of reach of children.
- Don't store in bathroom medicine cabinet. Heat and moisture may change the action of the herb.

Safe dosage:
Consult your doctor for the appropriate dose for your condition.

 ## Toxicity

Comparative-toxicity rating is not available from standard references. However, it is believed toxic effects greatly outweigh any possible benefits.

For symptoms of toxicity: See *Adverse Reactions, Side Effects or Overdose Symptoms* section below.

 ## Adverse Reactions, Side Effects or Overdose Symptoms

Signs and symptoms	What to do
Burning indigestion	Discontinue. Call doctor when convenient.
Edema (swelling of hands and feet)	Discontinue. Call doctor when convenient.
Jaundice (yellow skin and eyes)	Discontinue. Call doctor immediately.
Nausea or vomiting	Discontinue. Call doctor immediately.

American Dogwood (American Boxwood, Dogwood)

Basic Information

Biological name (genus and species):
Cornus florida

Parts used for medicinal purposes:
Bark

Chemicals this herb contains:
• Betulic acid
• Cornin

Known Effects

• Irritates gastrointestinal tract and acts as a cathartic
• Causes uterine contractions

Possible Additional Effects

• May reduce fever
• May kill bacteria in boils, carbuncles, infected skin rashes, insect bites
• May treat malaria

Warnings and Precautions

Don't take if you:
Are pregnant. It may cause miscarriage.

Consult your doctor if you:
Take this herb for any medical problem that doesn't improve in 2 weeks. (There may be safer, more effective treatments.)

Pregnancy:
Dangers outweigh any possible benefits. Don't use.

Breastfeeding:
Dangers outweigh any possible benefits. Don't use.

Infants and children:
Treating infants or children under 2 with any herbal preparation is hazardous.

Storage:
• Store in cool, dry area away from direct light, but don't freeze.
• Store safely out of reach of children.
• Don't store in bathroom medicine cabinet. Heat and moisture may change the action of the herb.

Safe dosage:
Consult your doctor for the appropriate dose for your condition.

Toxicity

Rated relatively safe when taken in appropriate quantities for short periods of time

For symptoms of toxicity: See *Adverse Reactions, Side Effects or Overdose Symptoms* section below.

Adverse Reactions, Side Effects or Overdose Symptoms

Signs and symptoms	What to do
Abortion	Seek emergency treatment.
Dermatitis	Discontinue. Call doctor when convenient.

Angelica (European Angelica, Garden Angelica)

Basic Information

Biological name (genus and species):
Angelica archangelica

Parts used for medicinal purposes:
Entire plant

Chemicals this herb contains:
- Angelic acid
- Resin (see Glossary)
- Volatile oils (see Glossary)

Known Effects

*Volatile oil gives angelica the
following effects:*

- Decreases thickness and increases
  fluidity of mucus in lungs and
  bronchial tubes
- Increases perspiration

Possible Additional Effects

- Seeds and roots used to reduce odor
  and volume of intestinal gases
- May bring on menstruation
- May ease intestinal colic
  and flatulence

Warnings and Precautions

Don't take if you:
- Are pregnant, think you may be
  pregnant or plan pregnancy in the
  near future
- Have any chronic disease of the
  gastrointestinal tract, such as
  stomach or duodenal ulcers, reflux
  esophagitis, ulcerative colitis, spastic
  colitis, diverticulosis or diverticulitis

Consult your doctor if you:
- Take this herb for any medical
  problem that doesn't improve in
  2 weeks (There may be safer, more
  effective treatments.)
- Take any medicinal drugs or
  herbs including aspirin, laxatives,
  cold and cough remedies, antacids,
  vitamins, minerals, amino acids,
  supplements, other prescription
  or nonprescription drugs

Pregnancy:
Dangers outweigh any possible
benefits. Don't use.

Breastfeeding:
Dangers outweigh any possible
benefits. Don't use.

Infants and children:
Treating infants or children under
2 with any herbal preparation
is hazardous.

Others:
No problems expected if you are
beyond childhood, under 45, not
pregnant, basically healthy, take it for
only a short time and do not exceed
manufacturer's recommended dose.

Storage:
- Store in cool, dry area away from
  direct light, but don't freeze.
- Store safely out of reach of children.
- Don't store in bathroom medicine
  cabinet. Heat and moisture may
  change the action of the herb.

Safe dosage:
Consult your doctor for the
appropriate dose for your condition.

→

Toxicity

Rated relatively safe when taken in appropriate quantities for short periods of time

Adverse Reactions, Side Effects or Overdose Symptoms

None are expected.

Anise

Basic Information

Biological name (genus and species): *Pimpinella anisum*

Parts used for medicinal purposes: Seeds

Chemicals this herb contains:
- Anethole
- Creosol
- Dianethole
- Essential oils (see Glossary)
- Flavonoids (see Glossary)
- Proteins
- Sterols
- Terpenes (see Glossary)

Known Effects

- Helps expel gas from intestinal tract
- Helps body dispose of excess fluid by increasing amount of urine produced
- Reduces cough

Miscellaneous information:
- Anise is also used in perfumes, soaps, beverages, baked goods, liqueur and as a flavoring.
- It is available as a tincture or tea.

Possible Additional Effects

- May relieve indigestion
- May decrease colic
- May kill body lice when applied externally
- May treat bronchitis

Warnings and Precautions

Don't take if you:
- Are pregnant, think you may be pregnant or plan pregnancy in the near future
- Have any chronic disease of the gastrointestinal tract, such as stomach or duodenal ulcers, reflux esophagitis, ulcerative colitis, spastic colitis, diverticulosis or diverticulitis

Consult your doctor if you:
- Take this herb for any medical problem that doesn't improve in 2 weeks (There may be safer, more effective treatments.)
- Take any medicinal drugs or herbs including aspirin, laxatives, cold and cough remedies, antacids, vitamins, minerals, amino acids, supplements, other prescription or nonprescription drugs

Pregnancy:
Dangers outweigh any possible benefits. Don't use.

Breastfeeding:
Dangers outweigh any possible benefits. Don't use.

Infants and children:
Treating infants or children under 2 with any herbal preparation is hazardous.

Storage:
- Store in cool, dry area away from direct light, but don't freeze.
- Store safely out of reach of children.
- Don't store in bathroom medicine cabinet. Heat and moisture may change the action of the herb.

Safe dosage:
Consult your doctor for the appropriate dose for your condition.

 Toxicity

- Rated relatively safe when taken in appropriate quantities for short periods of time

- Japan: Poisonous Japeneses anise *(Illicium anisatum)*—do not mistake the two

For symptoms of toxicity: See *Adverse Reactions, Side Effects or Overdose Symptoms* section below.

 Adverse Reactions, Side Effects or Overdose Symptoms

Signs and symptoms	What to do
Oil may cause	
Diarrhea	Discontinue. Call doctor immediately.
Difficulty breathing	Seek emergency treatment.
Nausea or vomiting	Discontinue. Call doctor immediately.
Seizures	Seek emergency treatment.
Skin irritation, when applied to skin	Discontinue. Call doctor when convenient.

Asafetida (Devil's Dung)

 Basic Information

Biological name (genus and species): *Ferula assafoetida, F. foetida*

Parts used for medicinal purposes: Roots

Chemicals this herb contains:
- Gum (see Glossary)
- Resin (see Glossary)
- Volatile oils (see Glossary)

 Known Effects

Irritates lining of gastrointestinal tract and produces laxative effect

Miscellaneous information:
- Introduced by Arab physicians to European medical practitioners
- Has garlic-like odor and bitter taste, which may result in good placebo effect because it is so disagreeable
- Used in sack around the neck by some people to repel evil

→

- Used as a condiment
- Provides flavor as an ingredient in Worcestershire sauce

 ## Possible Additional Effects

- May decrease thickness and increase fluidity of mucus in lungs and bronchial tubes
- May treat colic (see Glossary)
- May treat nerve disorders

 ## Warnings and Precautions

Don't take if you:
- Are pregnant, think you may be pregnant or plan pregnancy in the near future
- Have any chronic disease of the gastrointestinal tract, such as stomach or duodenal ulcers, reflux esophagitis, ulcerative colitis, spastic colitis, diverticulosis or diverticulitis

Consult your doctor if you:
- Take this herb for any medical problem that doesn't improve in 2 weeks (There may be safer, more effective treatments.)
- Take any medicinal drugs or herbs including aspirin, laxatives, cold and cough remedies, antacids, vitamins, minerals, amino acids, supplements, other prescription or nonprescription drugs

Pregnancy:
Dangers outweigh any possible benefits. Don't use.

Breastfeeding:
Dangers outweigh any possible benefits. Don't use.

Infants and children:
Treating infants or children under 2 with any herbal preparation is hazardous.

Others:
No problems expected if you are beyond childhood, under 45, not pregnant, basically healthy, take it for only a short time and do not exceed manufacturer's recommended dose.

Storage:
- Store in cool, dry area away from direct light, but don't freeze.
- Store safely out of reach of children.
- Don't store in bathroom medicine cabinet. Heat and moisture may change the action of the herb.

Safe dosage:
Consult your doctor for the appropriate dose for your condition.

 ## Toxicity

Rated relatively safe when taken in appropriate quantities for short periods of time

For symptoms of toxicity: See *Adverse Reactions, Side Effects or Overdose Symptoms* section below.

 ## Adverse Reactions, Side Effects or Overdose Symptoms

Signs and symptoms	What to do
Diarrhea	Discontinue. Call doctor immediately.

Astragalus (Huang-Qi, Milk Vetch)

Basic Information

Biological name (genus and species):
Astragalus membranaceous

Parts used for medicinal purposes:
Root

Chemicals this herb contains:
- Asparagine
- Astragalosides
- Calcyosin
- Formononetin
- Kumatakenin
- Sterols

Known Effects

- Stimulates and protects the immune system
- Produces spontaneous sweating

Miscellaneous information:
Available as tea, fluid extract, capsules and dried root.

Possible Additional Effects

- May reduce fatigue/weakness
- Potential cold and flu treatment
- May increase stamina
- Potential treatment for immune-deficiency problems (AIDS, cancer)
- May reduce symptoms of chronic fatigue syndrome
- May improve appetite
- May alleviate diarrhea

Warnings and Precautions

Don't take if you:
- Are pregnant, think you may be pregnant or plan pregnancy in the near future
- Are currently feverish

Consult your doctor if you:
- Take this herb for any medical problem that doesn't improve in 2 weeks (There may be safer, more effective treatments.)
- Take any medicinal drugs or herbs including aspirin, laxatives, cold and cough remedies, antacids, vitamins, minerals, amino acids, supplements, other prescription or nonprescription drugs

Pregnancy:
Use only on the advice of your physician.

Breastfeeding:
Use only on the advice of your physician.

Infants and children:
Treating infants or children under 2 with any herbal preparation is hazardous.

Others:
None.

Storage:
- Store in cool, dry area away from direct light, but don't freeze.
- Store safely out of reach of children.
- Don't store in bathroom medicine cabinet. Heat and moisture may change the action of the herb.

Safe dosage:
Consult your doctor for the appropriate dose for your condition.

Toxicity

Comparative-toxicity rating is not available from standard references.

Adverse Reactions, Side Effects or Overdose Symptoms

None are expected.

Barberry (European Barberry)

Basic Information

Biological name (genus and species):
Berberis vulgaris

Parts used for medicinal purposes:
• Berries/fruits
• Rootbark

Chemicals this herb contains:
• Berbamine
• Berberine
• Berberrubine
• Columbamine
• Hydrastine
• Jatrorrhizine
• Oxyacanthine
• Palmatine

Known Effects

• Dilates blood vessels
• Decreases heart rate
• Stimulates intestinal movement, helps relieve constipation
• Reduces bronchial constriction

Miscellaneous information:
• Fruit is made into jelly.
• Roots are used to dye wool.

Possible Additional Effects

• May reduce diarrhea
• May reduce dyspepsia, indigestion, heartburn
• May treat skin infections
• May reduce symptoms of hepatitis, liver disease, jaundice
• May treat hangover

Warnings and Precautions

Don't take if you:
Are pregnant, think you may be pregnant or plan pregnancy in the near future.

Consult your doctor if you:
• Take this herb for any medical problem that doesn't improve in 2 weeks (There may be safer, more effective treatments.)
• Take any medicinal drugs or herbs including aspirin, laxatives, cold and cough remedies, antacids, vitamins, minerals, amino acids, supplements, other prescription or nonprescription drugs

Pregnancy:
Dangers outweigh any possible benefits. Don't use.

Breastfeeding:
Dangers outweigh any possible benefits. Don't use.

Infants and children:
Treating infants or children under 2 with any herbal preparation is hazardous.

Others:
No problems expected if you are beyond childhood, under 45, not pregnant, basically healthy, take it for only a short time and do not exceed manufacturer's recommended dose.

Storage:
• Store in cool, dry area away from direct light, but don't freeze.
• Store safely out of reach of children.
• Don't store in bathroom medicine cabinet. Heat and moisture may change the action of the herb.

Safe dosage:
Consult your doctor for the appropriate dose for your condition.

Toxicity

Rated slightly dangerous, particularly in children, persons over 55 and those who take larger than appropriate quantities for extended periods of time

For symptoms of toxicity: See *Adverse Reactions, Side Effects or Overdose Symptoms* section below.

Adverse Reactions, Side Effects or Overdose Symptoms

Signs and symptoms	What to do
Change in heart rate	Discontinue use. Call doctor immediately.
Convulsions	Discontinue use. Call doctor immediately.
Nausea, vomiting	Discontinue use. Call doctor immediately.
Upset stomach, diarrhea	Discontinue use. Call doctor when convenient.

Barley

Basic Information

Biological name (genus and species):
Hordeum distichon

Parts used for medicinal purposes:
Various parts of the entire plant, frequently differing by country and culture

Chemicals this herb contains:
• Ash
• Cellulose
• Hordenine
• Invert sugar (see Glossary)
• Lignin
• Malt
• Nitrogen
• Pectin
• Pentosan
• Protein
• Starch
• Sucrose

Known Effects

Provides nutrition to body

Miscellaneous information:
Barley is a grain and primarily contains nutrients.

Possible Additional Effects

Used as a "restorative" following stomach and intestinal irritation

Warnings and Precautions

Don't take if you:
Are allergic or sensitive to barley or gluten.

Consult your doctor if you:
• Take this herb for any medical problem that doesn't improve in

➔

2 weeks (There may be safer, more effective treatments.)
• Take any medicinal drugs or herbs including aspirin, laxatives, cold and cough remedies, antacids, vitamins, minerals, amino acids, supplements, other prescription or nonprescription drugs

Pregnancy:
Don't use unless prescribed by your doctor.

Breastfeeding:
Don't use unless prescribed by your doctor.

Infants and children:
Treating infants or children under 2 with any herbal preparation is hazardous.

Others:
Barley infested with fungus can cause poisoning in animals.

Storage:
• Store in cool, dry area away from direct light, but don't freeze.
• Store safely out of reach of children.
• Don't store in bathroom medicine cabinet. Heat and moisture may change the action of the herb.

Safe dosage:
Consult your doctor for the appropriate dose for your condition.

 Toxicity

Comparative-toxicity rating is not available from standard references.

 Adverse Reactions, Side Effects or Overdose Symptoms

None are expected.

Bayberry (Wax Myrtle)

 Basic Information

Biological name (genus and species):
Myrica cerifera

Parts used for medicinal purposes:
• Bark
• Berries/fruits
• Leaves

Chemicals this herb contains:
• Albumin
• Berberine
• Essential oil (see Glossary)
• Flavonoids (see Glossary)
• Gallic acid
• Gum (see Glossary)
• Myricinic acid, related to saponin (see Glossary)
• Myricitrin
• Palmitin
• Resin (see Glossary)
• Starch
• Sucrose
• Tannic acid
• Triterpenes

 Known Effects

• Reduces nasal congestion
• Reduces fever
• Interferes with absorption of iron and other minerals when taken internally

Miscellaneous information:
- Injections of bark extract have caused cancer in laboratory animals.
- Bayberry is frequently used as a basic ingredient in cosmetics, pharmaceuticals and candles.

Possible Additional Effects

Internal use:
- May cause vomiting
- May treat the common cold
- May treat diarrhea
- May treat jaundice

External use:
- May heal ulcers
- May treat gum problems
- May reduce varicose veins
- May increase circulation

Warnings and Precautions

Don't take if you:
- Are pregnant, think you may be pregnant or plan pregnancy in the near future
- Have a history of cancer (bayberry not recommended due to high tannin content)

Consult your doctor if you:
- Take this herb for any medical problem that doesn't improve in 2 weeks (There may be safer, more effective treatments.)
- Take any medicinal drugs or herbs including aspirin, laxatives, cold and cough remedies, antacids, vitamins, minerals, amino acids, supplements, other prescription or nonprescription drugs

Pregnancy:
Don't use unless prescribed by your doctor.

Breastfeeding:
Don't use unless prescribed by your doctor.

Infants and children:
Treating infants or children under 2 with any herbal preparation is hazardous.

Others:
- No problems expected if you are beyond childhood, under 45, not pregnant, basically healthy, take it for only a short time and do not exceed manufacturer's recommended dose
- Can effect electrolyte balance by increasing sodium but decreasing potassium, which can lead to high blood pressure and edema

Storage:
- Store in cool, dry area away from direct light, but don't freeze.
- Store safely out of reach of children.
- Don't store in bathroom medicine cabinet. Heat and moisture may change the action of the herb.

Safe dosage:
Consult your doctor for the appropriate dose for your condition.

Toxicity

Rated relatively safe when taken in appropriate quantities for short periods of time

Adverse Reactions, Side Effects or Overdose Symptoms

None are expected.

Bearberry (Uva-Ursi)

 Basic Information

Biological name (genus and species):
Arctostaphylos uva-ursi

Parts used for medicinal purposes:
Leaves

Chemicals this herb contains:
• Arbutin
• Chlorine
• Ellagic acid
• Ericolin
• Gallic acid
• Hydroquinone
• Malic acid
• Myricetin
• Quercetin
• Tannins (see Glossary)
• Ursolic acid
• Volatile oils (see Glossary)

 Known Effects

• Shrinks urinary tissues
• Prevents secretion of fluids
• Relieves urinary pain
• Helps body dispose of excess fluid
  by increasing amount of urine
  produced
• Antibacterial
• Interferes with absorption of iron
  and other minerals when
  taken internally

Miscellaneous information:
• Bearberry turns urine green.
• It was used extensively for urinary
  tract infections before the
  development of more
  effective drugs.

 Possible Additional Effects

Boiled, bruised leaves:
• May be good for kidney infections
• Potential sedative
• May relieve nausea
• May decrease ringing in ears
• May treat breathing problems

 Warnings and Precautions

Don't take if you:
Are pregnant, think you may be
pregnant or plan pregnancy in the
near future.

Consult your doctor if you:
• Take this herb for any medical
  problem that doesn't improve in
  2 weeks (There may be safer, more
  effective treatments.)
• Take any medicinal drugs or
  herbs including aspirin, laxatives,
  cold and cough remedies, antacids,
  vitamins, minerals, amino acids,
  supplements, other prescription
  or nonprescription drugs

Pregnancy:
Don't use unless prescribed by
your doctor.

Breastfeeding:
Don't use unless prescribed by
your doctor.

Infants and children:
Treating infants or children under
2 with any herbal preparation
is hazardous.

Others:

No problems expected if you are beyond childhood, under 45, not pregnant, basically healthy, take it for only a short time and do not exceed manufacturer's recommended dose.

Storage:

- Store in cool, dry area away from direct light, but don't freeze.
- Store safely out of reach of children.
- Don't store in bathroom medicine cabinet. Heat and moisture may change the action of the herb.

Safe dosage:

Consult your doctor for the appropriate dose for your condition.

 Toxicity

Rated relatively safe when taken in appropriate quantities for short periods of time (no more than one week)

 Adverse Reactions, Side Effects or Overdose Symptoms

None are expected.

Bilberry

 Basic Information

Biological name (genus and species): *Vaccinium myrtillus*

Parts used for medicinal purposes: Whole plant, especially fruits

Chemicals this herb contains:

- Anthocyanins
- Flavonoids (see Glossary)
- Hydroquinone
- Loeanolic acid
- Neomyrtillin
- Sodium
- Tannins (see Glossary)
- Ursolic acid

 Known Effects

- Acts as a diuretic
- Treats urinary tract infections
- Antioxidant
- Reduces acute diarrhea (dried berries only)
- Astringent

 Possible Additional Effects

- Potential anti-inflammatory
- May treat vision problems, including cataracts, diabetic retinopathy
- May reduce inflammation of oral cavity
- May treat hemorrhoids

 Warnings and Precautions

Don't take if you:

Are pregnant, think you may be pregnant or plan pregnancy in the near future.

→

Consult your doctor if you:
- Take this herb for any medical problem that doesn't improve in 2 weeks (There may be safer, more effective treatments.)
- Take any medicinal drugs or herbs including aspirin, laxatives, cold and cough remedies, antacids, vitamins, minerals, amino acids, supplements, other prescription or nonprescription drugs

Pregnancy:
Use only on the advice of your physician.

Breastfeeding:
Use only on the advice of your physician.

Infants and children:
Treating infants or children under 2 with any herbal preparation is hazardous.

Storage:
- Store in cool, dry area away from direct light, but don't freeze.
- Store safely out of reach of children.
- Don't store in bathroom medicine cabinet. Heat and moisture may change the action of the herb.

Safe dosage:
Consult your doctor for the appropriate dose for your condition.

 Toxicity

Comparative-toxicity rating is not available from standard references.

 Adverse Reactions, Side Effects or Overdose Symptoms

None are expected.

Birch

 Basic Information

Biological name (genus and species):
Betula alba, B. lenta

Parts used for medicinal purposes:
- Bark
- Leaves

Chemicals this herb contains:
- Betulin
- Methyl salicylate (similar to aspirin)
- Resin (see Glossary)
- Tar (creosol, phenol, creosote, guaiacol)

 Known Effects

- Provides counterirritation (see Glossary) when applied to skin overlying an inflamed or irritated joint
- Decreases inflammation in tissues

Miscellaneous information:
- Leaves have an agreeable aromatic odor but bitter taste.
- When treating urinary tract infections, drink plenty of water.

Possible Additional Effects

- May treat rheumatism and congestive heart failure when steeped to extract its medicinal properties
- May treat skin disorders when applied topically
- May shrink tissues
- May treat arthritis
- May prevent secretion of fluids

Warnings and Precautions

Don't take if you:
Are pregnant, think you may be pregnant or plan pregnancy in the near future.

Consult your doctor if you:
- Take this herb for any medical problem that doesn't improve in 2 weeks (There may be safer, more effective treatments.)
- Take any medicinal drugs or herbs including aspirin, laxatives, cold and cough remedies, antacids, vitamins, minerals, amino acids, supplements, other prescription or nonprescription drugs

Pregnancy:
Don't use unless prescribed by your doctor.

Breastfeeding:
Don't use unless prescribed by your doctor.

Infants and children:
Treating infants or children under 2 with any herbal preparation is hazardous.

Others:
No problems expected if you are beyond childhood, under 45, not pregnant, basically healthy, take it for only a short time and do not exceed manufacturer's recommended dose.

Storage:
- Store in cool, dry area away from direct light, but don't freeze.
- Store safely out of reach of children.
- Don't store in bathroom medicine cabinet. Heat and moisture may change the action of the herb.

Safe dosage:
Consult your doctor for the appropriate dose for your condition.

Toxicity

Comparative-toxicity rating is not available from standard references.

Adverse Reactions, Side Effects or Overdose Symptoms

None are expected.

Birthroot (Bethroot)

Basic Information

Biological name (genus and species):
Trillium erectum, T. pendulum

Parts used for medicinal purposes:
Various parts of the entire plant,
frequently differing by country
and culture

Chemicals this herb contains:
- Resin (see Glossary)
- Saponins (see Glossary)
- Starch
- Tannins (see Glossary)
- Volatile oils (see Glossary)

Known Effects

- Irritates mucous membranes
- Treats gastrointestinal upsets

Miscellaneous information:
- The name *birthroot* resulted from
  pioneers using this herb to stop
  bleeding after childbirth.
- It is used as an aphrodisiac by
  Indians in the southeastern United
  States.
- It is also used as an astringent
  poultice (see Glossary).

Possible Additional Effects

May treat menstrual irregularity or
increased menstrual frequency

Warnings and Precautions

Don't take if you:
Are pregnant, think you may be
pregnant or plan pregnancy in the
near future.

Consult your doctor if you:
- Take this herb for any medical
  problem that doesn't improve in
  2 weeks (There may be safer, more
  effective treatments.)
- Take any medicinal drugs or
  herbs including aspirin, laxatives,
  cold and cough remedies, antacids,
  vitamins, minerals, amino acids,
  supplements, other prescription
  or nonprescription drugs

Pregnancy:
Don't use unless prescribed by
your doctor.

Breastfeeding:
Don't use unless prescribed by
your doctor.

Infants and children:
Treating infants or children under
2 with any herbal preparation
is hazardous.

Others:
No problems expected if you are
beyond childhood, under 45, not
pregnant, basically healthy, take it for
only a short time and do not exceed
manufacturer's recommended dose.

Storage:
- Store in cool, dry area away from
  direct light, but don't freeze.
- Store safely out of reach of children.

- Don't store in bathroom medicine cabinet. Heat and moisture may change the action of the herb.

Safe dosage:
Consult your doctor for the appropriate dose for your condition.

 Toxicity

Comparative-toxicity rating is not available from standard references.

 Adverse Reactions, Side Effects or Overdose Symptoms

None are expected.

Bistort (Snakeweed)

 Basic Information

Biological name (genus and species):
Polygonum bistorta

Parts used for medicinal purposes:
Various parts of the entire plant, frequently differing by country and culture

Chemicals this herb contains:
Tannins (see Glossary)

 Known Effects

Roots are used for astringent gargle.

 Possible Additional Effects

Roots may cause vomiting.

 Warnings and Precautions

Don't take if you:
- Are pregnant, think you may be pregnant or plan pregnancy in the near future
- Have any chronic disease of the gastrointestinal tract, such as stomach or duodenal ulcers, reflux esophagitis, ulcerative colitis, spastic colitis, diverticulosis or diverticulitis

Consult your doctor if you:
- Take this herb for any medical problem that doesn't improve in 2 weeks (There may be safer, more effective treatments.)
- Take any medicinal drugs or herbs including aspirin, laxatives, cold and cough remedies, antacids, vitamins, minerals, amino acids, supplements, other prescription or nonprescription drugs

Pregnancy:
Dangers outweigh any possible benefits. Don't use.

➜

Breastfeeding:
Dangers outweigh any possible
benefits. Don't use.

Infants and children:
Treating infants or children under
2 with any herbal preparation
is hazardous.

Others:
No problems expected if you are
beyond childhood, under 45, not
pregnant, basically healthy, take it for
only a short time and do not exceed
manufacturer's recommended dose.

Storage:
• Store in cool, dry area away from
  direct light, but don't freeze.
• Store safely out of reach of children.
• Don't store in bathroom medicine
  cabinet. Heat and moisture may
  change the action of the herb.

Safe dosage:
Consult your doctor for the
appropriate dose for your condition.

Toxicity

Comparative-toxicity rating is not
available from standard references.

For symptoms of toxicity: See
*Adverse Reactions, Side Effects or
Overdose Symptoms* section below.

Adverse Reactions, Side Effects or Overdose Symptoms

Signs and symptoms	What to do
Bleeding from stomach characterized by vomiting bright red blood or material that looks like coffee grounds	Discontinue. Call doctor immediately.
Kidney damage characterized by blood in urine, decreased urine flow, swelling of hands and feet	Seek emergency treatment.
Nausea or vomiting	Discontinue. Call doctor immediately.

Bitter Lettuce (Prickly Lettuce)

Basic Information

Biological name (genus and species):
Lactuca virosa, L. scariola

Parts used for medicinal purposes:
Latex, which exudes from stem of
flower stalks

Chemicals this herb contains:
• Caoutchouc
• Hyoscyamine
• Lactucerol
• Lactucic acid
• Lactucin
• Mannite
• Nitrates
• Volatile oils (see Glossary)

Known Effects

Depresses central nervous system

Possible Additional Effects

- Potential sedative to relieve anxiety or nervous disorders
- May treat coughs
- May treat chest pain due to coronary artery disease (angina)
- May cause a "high" when smoked

Warnings and Precautions

Don't take if you:
Are pregnant, think you may be pregnant or plan pregnancy in the near future.

Consult your doctor if you:
- Take this herb for any medical problem that doesn't improve in 2 weeks (There may be safer, more effective treatments.)
- Take any medicinal drugs or herbs including aspirin, laxatives, cold and cough remedies, antacids, vitamins, minerals, amino acids, supplements, other prescription or nonprescription drugs

Pregnancy:
Dangers outweigh any possible benefits. Don't use.

Breastfeeding:
Dangers outweigh any possible benefits. Don't use.

Infants and children:
Treating infants or children under 2 with any herbal preparation is hazardous.

Others:
Use only under medical supervision.

Storage:
- Store in cool, dry area away from direct light, but don't freeze.
- Store safely out of reach of children.
- Don't store in bathroom medicine cabinet. Heat and moisture may change the action of the herb.

Safe dosage:
Consult your doctor for the appropriate dose for your condition.

Toxicity

Rated relatively safe when taken in appropriate quantities for short periods of time

For symptoms of toxicity: See *Adverse Reactions, Side Effects or Overdose Symptoms* section below.

Adverse Reactions, Side Effects or Overdose Symptoms

Signs and symptoms	What to do
Breathing difficulties	Seek emergency treatment.

Bitter Root (Rheumatism Weed, Spreading Dogbane, Wild Ipecac)

 ## Basic Information

Biological name (genus and species):
Apocynum androsaemifolium

Parts used for medicinal purposes:
- Bark
- Petals/flower
- Rhizomes
- Roots

Chemicals this herb contains:
- Apocynein
- Apocynin
- Cymarin
- Saponins (see Glossary)

 ## Known Effects

- Slows heartbeat
- Helps body dispose of excess fluid by increasing amount of urine produced
- Causes vomiting

Miscellaneous information:
- Bitter root has a marked effect on the heart. Prescribed FDA-approved digitalis preparations are far superior in treating heart disorders such as congestive heart failure and heartbeat irregularities.
- Many plants of varying potency and toxicity are called by this name. Be sure you know what you buy and take.
- You will need increased potassium if you take this herb. Take potassium supplements or eat more food high in potassium, such as apricots, citrus fruits and bananas.

 ## Possible Additional Effects

- May help treat congestive heart failure
- May help treat palpitations
- May help treat gallstones
- May "correct" bile flow
- May restore normal tone to tissues or stimulate appetite when roots and rhizomes are used to make a medicinal preparation

 ## Warnings and Precautions

Don't take if you:
- Are pregnant, think you may be pregnant or plan pregnancy in the near future
- Have any chronic disease of the gastrointestinal tract, such as stomach or duodenal ulcers, reflux esophagitis, ulcerative colitis, spastic colitis, diverticulosis or diverticulitis

Consult your doctor if you:
- Take this herb for any medical problem that doesn't improve in 2 weeks (There may be safer, more effective treatments.)
- Take any medicinal drugs or herbs including aspirin, laxatives, cold and cough remedies, antacids, vitamins, minerals, amino acids, supplements, other prescription or nonprescription drugs

Pregnancy:
Don't use unless prescribed by your doctor.

Breastfeeding:
Don't use unless prescribed by your doctor.

Infants and children:
Treating infants or children under 2 with any herbal preparation is hazardous.

Others:
Use only under medical supervision.

Storage:
- Store in cool, dry area away from direct light, but don't freeze.
- Store safely out of reach of children.
- Don't store in bathroom medicine cabinet. Heat and moisture may change the action of the herb.

Safe dosage:
Consult your doctor for the appropriate dose for your condition.

 Toxicity

Rated slightly dangerous, particularly in children, persons over 55 and those who take larger than appropriate quantities for extended periods of time

For symptoms of toxicity: See *Adverse Reactions, Side Effects or Overdose Symptoms* section below.

 Adverse Reactions, Side Effects or Overdose Symptoms

Signs and symptoms	What to do
Gastritis	Discontinue. Call doctor when convenient.
Heartbeat irregularities	Seek emergency treatment.
Precipitous blood-pressure drop: symptoms include faintness, cold sweat, paleness, rapid pulse	Seek emergency treatment.
Vomiting	Discontinue. Call doctor immediately.

Bittersweet (Bitter Nightshade, European Bittersweet)

 Basic Information

Biological name (genus and species):
Solanum dulcamara

Parts used for medicinal purposes:
- Leaves
- Roots

Chemicals this herb contains:
- Dulcamarin
- Saponins (see Glossary)
- Solanidine
- Solanine

 Known Effects

Depresses central nervous system

Miscellaneous information:
Bittersweet is a potentially dangerous herb. Toxic amounts depress the nervous system and cause drowsiness. Berries are poisonous.

➔

Possible Additional Effects

- May treat eczema (see Glossary)
- May reduce pain
- Potential aphrodisiac

Warnings and Precautions

Don't take if you:

- Are pregnant, think you may be pregnant or plan pregnancy in the near future
- Have any chronic disease of the gastrointestinal tract, such as stomach or duodenal ulcers, reflux esophagitis, ulcerative colitis, spastic colitis, diverticulosis or diverticulitis

Consult your doctor if you:

- Take this herb for any medical problem that doesn't improve in 2 weeks (There may be safer, more effective treatments.)
- Take any medicinal drugs or herbs including aspirin, laxatives, cold and cough remedies, antacids, vitamins, minerals, amino acids, supplements, other prescription or nonprescription drugs

Pregnancy:

Dangers outweigh any possible benefits. Don't use.

Breastfeeding:

Dangers outweigh any possible benefits. Don't use.

Infants and children:

Treating infants or children under 2 with any herbal preparation is hazardous.

Others:

Dangers outweigh any possible benefits. Don't use.

Storage:

- Store in cool, dry area away from direct light, but don't freeze.
- Store safely out of reach of children.
- Don't store in bathroom medicine cabinet. Heat and moisture may change the action of the herb.

Safe dosage:

Consult your doctor for the appropriate dose for your condition.

Toxicity

Rated slightly dangerous, particularly in children, persons over 55 and those who take larger than appropriate quantities for extended periods of time

For symptoms of toxicity: See *Adverse Reactions, Side Effects or Overdose Symptoms* section below.

Adverse Reactions, Side Effects or Overdose Symptoms

Signs and symptoms	What to do
Toxins are mostly in unripe fruit, which cause the following symptoms:	
Burning throat	Discontinue. Call doctor when convenient.
Coma	Seek emergency treatment.
Dilated pupils	Discontinue. Call doctor immediately.
Dizziness	Discontinue. Call doctor immediately.
Headache	Discontinue. Call doctor when convenient.
Muscle weakness	Discontinue. Call doctor immediately.
Nausea, vomiting	Discontinue. Call doctor immediately.
Slow pulse	Seek emergency treatment.

Black Walnut

Basic Information

Biological name (genus and species): *Juglans nigra*

Parts used for medicinal purposes:
- Husks
- Inner bark
- Leaves
- Nuts

Chemicals this herb contains:
- Ellagic acid
- Juglone
- Mucin

Known Effects

- Reduces constipation
- Reduces intestinal parasites

Miscellaneous information:
- Nut husks yield brown dye for hair and clothing.
- Black walnut is available as tincture, extract, dried bark or leaves and fruit rind.

Possible Additional Effects

- May treat fungal infections of skin
- May treat poison ivy and warts
- May treat herpes and cold sores
- May treat athlete's foot and jock itch
- May relieve toxic blood conditions
- May help treat acne
- May help treat mouth canker sores

Warnings and Precautions

Don't take if you:
- Are pregnant, think you may be pregnant or plan pregnancy in the near future
- Have any chronic disease of the gastrointestinal tract, such as stomach or duodenal ulcers, reflux esophagitis, ulcerative colitis, spastic colitis, diverticulosis or diverticulitis

Consult your doctor if you:
- Take this herb for any medical problem that doesn't improve in 2 weeks (There may be safer, more effective treatments.)
- Take any medicinal drugs or herbs including aspirin, laxatives, cold and cough remedies, antacids, vitamins, minerals, amino acids, supplements, other prescription or nonprescription drugs

Pregnancy:
Don't use unless prescribed by your doctor.

Breastfeeding:
Don't use unless prescribed by your doctor.

Infants and children:
Treating infants or children under 2 with any herbal preparation is hazardous.

Others:
No problems expected if you are beyond childhood, under 45, not pregnant, basically healthy, take it for only a short time and do not exceed manufacturer's recommended dose.

➔

Storage:
- Store in cool, dry area away from direct light, but don't freeze.
- Store safely out of reach of children.
- Don't store in bathroom medicine cabinet. Heat and moisture may change the action of the herb.

Safe dosage:
Consult your doctor for the appropriate dose for your condition.

 Toxicity

Comparative-toxicity rating is not available from standard references.

For symptoms of toxicity: See *Adverse Reactions, Side Effects or Overdose Symptoms* section below.

 Adverse Reactions, Side Effects or Overdose Symptoms

Signs and symptoms	What to do
Mild laxative effect	Discontinue. Call doctor when convenient.
Nausea	Discontinue. Call doctor immediately.
Upper abdominal pain	Discontinue. Call doctor when convenient.

Bladderwrack

 Basic Information

Biological name (genus and species):
Fuycus vesiculosus

Parts used for medicinal purposes:
Various parts of the entire plant, frequently differing by country and culture

Chemicals this herb contains:
- Alginic acid
- Bromine iodine
- Fucodin
- Laminarin

 Known Effects

Absorbs water in intestines to form bulk

 Possible Additional Effects

- May treat obesity
- May increase thyroid activity
- May kill intestinal parasites

 Warnings and Precautions

Don't take if you:
Are pregnant, think you may be pregnant or plan pregnancy in the near future.

Consult your doctor if you:
- Take this herb for any medical problem that doesn't improve in 2 weeks (There may be safer, more effective treatments.)
- Take any medicinal drugs or herbs including aspirin, laxatives, cold and cough remedies, antacids,

vitamins, minerals, amino acids, supplements, other prescription or nonprescription drugs

Pregnancy:
Don't use unless prescribed by your doctor.

Breastfeeding:
Don't use unless prescribed by your doctor.

Infants and children:
Treating infants or children under 2 with any herbal preparation is hazardous.

Others:
No problems expected if you are beyond childhood, under 45, not pregnant, basically healthy, take it for only a short time and do not exceed manufacturer's recommended dose.

Storage:
• Store in cool, dry area away from direct light, but don't freeze.

• Store safely out of reach of children.
• Don't store in bathroom medicine cabinet. Heat and moisture may change the action of the herb.

Safe dosage:
Consult your doctor for the appropriate dose for your condition.

 Toxicity

Comparative-toxicity rating is not available from standard references.

 Adverse Reactions, Side Effects or Overdose Symptoms

None are expected.

Blessed Thistle

 Basic Information

Biological name (genus and species):
Cnicus benedictus

Parts used for medicinal purposes:
Various parts of the entire plant, frequently differing by country and culture

Chemicals this herb contains:
• Cincin
• Volatile oils (see Glossary)

 Known Effects

• Stimulates milk production in lactating women
• Antibacterial
• Anti-inflammatory
• Coagulant

Miscellaneous information:
• Applied to skin overlying a joint to cause an irritant to relieve another irritant
• Effects have not been studied to any great extent
• Careful handling necessary to avoid toxic effects on skin

→

Possible Additional Effects

- May help reduce fever
- May reduce headache
- May regulate menses
- May induce vomiting
- May treat cuts, bruises and wounds when applied externally

Warnings and Precautions

Don't take if you:

- Are pregnant, think you may be pregnant or plan pregnancy in the near future
- Have any chronic disease of the gastrointestinal tract, such as stomach or duodenal ulcers, reflux esophagitis, ulcerative colitis, spastic colitis, diverticulosis or diverticulitis

Consult your doctor if you:

- Take this herb for any medical problem that doesn't improve in 2 weeks (There may be safer, more effective treatments.)
- Take any medicinal drugs or herbs including aspirin, laxatives, cold and cough remedies, antacids, vitamins, minerals, amino acids, supplements, other prescription or nonprescription drugs

Pregnancy:
Don't use unless prescribed by your doctor.

Breastfeeding:
Don't use unless prescribed by your doctor.

Infants and children:
Treating infants or children under 2 with any herbal preparation is hazardous.

Others:
No problems expected if you are beyond childhood, under 45, not pregnant, basically healthy, take it for only a short time and do not exceed manufacturer's recommended dose.

Storage:

- Store in cool, dry area away from direct light, but don't freeze.
- Store safely out of reach of children.
- Don't store in bathroom medicine cabinet. Heat and moisture may change the action of the herb.

Safe dosage:
Consult your doctor for the appropriate dose for your condition.

Toxicity

Comparative-toxicity rating is not available from standard references.

For symptoms of toxicity: See *Adverse Reactions, Side Effects or Overdose Symptoms* section below.

Adverse Reactions, Side Effects or Overdose Symptoms

Signs and symptoms	What to do
Vomiting	Discontinue. Call doctor immediately.

Blueberry

 Basic Information

Biological name (genus and species):
Vaccinium (many species exist)

Parts used for medicinal purposes:
• Leaves
• Stems

Chemicals this herb contains:
• Fatty acids (see Glossary)
• Hydroquinone
• Loeanolic acid
• Neomyrtillin
• Tannins (see Glossary)
• Ursolic acid

 Known Effects

• Decreases blood sugar
• Interferes with absorption of iron and other minerals when taken internally
• Treats diarrhea

 Possible Additional Effects

• May treat ulcers
• May treat gastroenteritis
• May help body dispose of excess fluid by increasing amount of urine produced
• May treat and prevent scurvy

 Warnings and Precautions

Don't take if you:
Are pregnant, think you may be pregnant or plan pregnancy in the near future.

Consult your doctor if you:
• Take this herb for any medical problem that doesn't improve in 2 weeks (There may be safer, more effective treatments.)
• Take any medicinal drugs or herbs including aspirin, laxatives, cold and cough remedies, antacids, vitamins, minerals, amino acids, supplements, other prescription or nonprescription drugs

Pregnancy:
Don't use unless prescribed by your doctor.

Breastfeeding:
Don't use unless prescribed by your doctor.

Infants and children:
Treating infants or children under 2 with any herbal preparation is hazardous.

Others:
No problems expected if you are beyond childhood, under 45, not pregnant, basically healthy, take it for only a short time and do not exceed manufacturer's recommended dose.

Storage:
• Store in cool, dry area away from direct light, but don't freeze.
• Store safely out of reach of children.
• Don't store in bathroom medicine cabinet. Heat and moisture may change the action of the herb.

Safe dosage:
Consult your doctor for the appropriate dose for your condition.

Toxicity

Comparative-toxicity rating is not available from standard references.

 Adverse Reactions, Side Effects or Overdose Symptoms

None are expected.

Boneset (Ague Weed, Richweed, White Snakeroot)

 Basic Information

Biological name (genus and species):
Eupatorium perfoliatum, E. rugosum

Parts used for medicinal purposes:
• Leaves
• Petals/flower

Chemicals this herb contains:
• Eupatorin
• Resin (see Glossary)
• Sugar
• Tremetone
• Volatile oils (see Glossary)
• Wax (see Glossary)

 Known Effects

• Can produce "milk sickness" in humans, an acute disease characterized by trembling, vomiting and severe abdominal pain caused by eating dairy products or beef from cattle poisoned by eating boneset
• Causes vomiting

Miscellaneous information:
Tremetone can accumulate slowly in animal bodies and cause toxic symptoms. It may do the same in humans.

 Possible Additional Effects

• May decrease blood sugar
• May treat malaria
• May treat fever
• May treat flu, colds and coughs
• Potential anti-inflammatory
• May treat arthritis

 Warnings and Precautions

Don't take if you:
• Are pregnant, think you may be pregnant or plan pregnancy in the near future
• Have any chronic disease of the gastrointestinal tract, such as stomach or duodenal ulcers, reflux esophagitis, ulcerative colitis, spastic colitis, diverticulosis or diverticulitis

Consult your doctor if you:
• Take this herb for any medical problem that doesn't improve in 2 weeks (There may be safer, more effective treatments.)
• Take any medicinal drugs or herbs including aspirin, laxatives, cold and cough remedies, antacids, vitamins, minerals, amino acids, supplements, other prescription or nonprescription drugs

Pregnancy:
Dangers outweigh any possible benefits. Don't use.

Breastfeeding:
Dangers outweigh any possible benefits. Don't use.

Infants and children:
Treating infants or children under 2 with any herbal preparation is hazardous.

Others:
Dangers outweigh any possible benefits. Don't use.

Storage:
• Store in cool, dry area away from direct light, but don't freeze.
• Store safely out of reach of children.
• Don't store in bathroom medicine cabinet. Heat and moisture may change the action of the herb.

Safe dosage:
Consult your doctor for the appropriate dose for your condition.

 Toxicity

Comparative-toxicity rating is not available from standard references.

For symptoms of toxicity: See *Adverse Reactions, Side Effects or Overdose Symptoms* section below.

 Adverse Reactions, Side Effects or Overdose Symptoms

Signs and symptoms	What to do
Breathing difficulties	Seek emergency treatment.
Coma	Seek emergency treatment.
Diarrhea	Discontinue. Call doctor immediately.
Drooling	Discontinue. Call doctor when convenient.
Muscle trembling	Discontinue. Call doctor immediately.
Nausea or vomiting	Discontinue. Call doctor immediately.
Stiffness	Discontinue. Call doctor when convenient.
Weakness	Discontinue. Call doctor when convenient.

Buchu (Honey Buchu, Short-Leaf Mountain Buchu)

 Basic Information

Biological name (genus and species):
Barosma betulina

Parts used for medicinal purposes:
Leaves

Chemicals this herb contains:
• Camphor
• Diosmine
• Hesperidin
• Isomenthone
• Mucilage (see Glossary)
• Resin (see Glossary)
• Volatile oils (see Glossary)

Known Effects

- Helps body dispose of excess fluid by increasing amount of urine produced
- Works as a urinary antiseptic
- Helps expel gas from intestinal tract

Miscellaneous information:
Buchu has a peppermint-like odor.

Possible Additional Effects

- May treat bladder irritation
- May treat urethral irritation
- May treat bloating associated with premenstrual syndrome (PMS)
- Potential diuretic

Warnings and Precautions

Don't take if you:
- Are pregnant, think you may be pregnant or plan pregnancy in the near future
- Have any chronic disease of the gastrointestinal tract, such as stomach or duodenal ulcers, reflux esophagitis, ulcerative colitis, spastic colitis, diverticulosis or diverticulitis

Consult your doctor if you:
- Take this herb for any medical problem that doesn't improve in 2 weeks (There may be safer, more effective treatments.)
- Take any medicinal drugs or herbs including aspirin, laxatives, cold and cough remedies, antacids, vitamins, minerals, amino acids, supplements, other prescription or nonprescription drugs

Pregnancy:
Dangers outweigh any possible benefits. Don't use.

Breastfeeding:
Dangers outweigh any possible benefits. Don't use.

Infants and children:
Treating infants or children under 2 with any herbal preparation is hazardous.

Others:
No problems expected if you are beyond childhood, under 45, not pregnant, basically healthy, take it for only a short time and do not exceed manufacturer's recommended dose.

Storage:
- Store in cool, dry area away from direct light, but don't freeze.
- Store safely out of reach of children.
- Don't store in bathroom medicine cabinet. Heat and moisture may change the action of the herb.

Safe dosage:
Consult your doctor for the appropriate dose for your condition.

Toxicity

Rated relatively safe when taken in appropriate quantities for short periods of time

For symptoms of toxicity: See *Adverse Reactions, Side Effects or Overdose Symptoms* section below.

Adverse Reactions, Side Effects or Overdose Symptoms

Signs and symptoms	What to do
Diarrhea	Discontinue. Call doctor when convenient.
Nausea or vomiting	Discontinue. Call doctor immediately.

Buckthorn

Basic Information

Biological name (genus and species):
Rhamnus cathartica

Parts used for medicinal purposes:
• Bark
• Berries/fruits

Chemicals this herb contains:
• Anthraquinone
• Emodin

Known Effects

• Irritates gastrointestinal tract and may cause watery, explosive bowel movements
• Used to treat constipation short term

Miscellaneous information:
• Several dyes are made from the juice of the berries.
• Children can have toxic symptoms after eating as few as 20 berries.
• The syrup of buckthorn is made from berries.

Possible Additional Effects

No additional effects are known.

Warnings and Precautions

Don't take if you:
• Are pregnant, think you may be pregnant or plan pregnancy in the near future
• Have any chronic disease of the gastrointestinal tract, such as stomach or duodenal ulcers, reflux esophagitis, ulcerative colitis, spastic colitis, diverticulosis or diverticulitis

Consult your doctor if you:
• Take this herb for any medical problem that doesn't improve in 2 weeks (There may be safer, more effective treatments.)
• Take any medicinal drugs or herbs including aspirin, laxatives, cold and cough remedies, antacids, vitamins, minerals, amino acids, supplements, other prescription or nonprescription drugs

Pregnancy:
Dangers outweigh any possible benefits. Don't use.

Breastfeeding:
Dangers outweigh any possible benefits. Don't use.

Infants and children:
Treating infants or children under 2 with any herbal preparation is hazardous.

Others:
• No problems expected if you are beyond childhood, under 45, not pregnant, basically healthy, take it for only a short time and do not exceed manufacturer's recommended dose.
• Do not use in combination with other laxatives.

Storage:
• Store in cool, dry area away from direct light, but don't freeze.
• Store safely out of reach of children.
• Don't store in bathroom medicine cabinet. Heat and moisture may change the action of the herb.

Safe dosage:
Consult your doctor for the appropriate dose for your condition.

→

Toxicity

Comparative-toxicity rating is not available from standard references.

For symptoms of toxicity: See *Adverse Reactions, Side Effects or Overdose Symptoms* section below.

 Adverse Reactions, Side Effects or Overdose Symptoms

Signs and symptoms	What to do
Diarrhea, severe and watery	Discontinue. Call doctor immediately.
Diarrhea, violent	Seek emergency treatment if uncontrollable.
Kidney damage (with large amounts over long period of time) characterized by blood in urine, decreased urine flow, swelling of hands and feet	Seek emergency treatment.
Nausea or vomiting	Discontinue. Call doctor immediately.
Stomach cramps	Discontinue. Call doctor immediately.

Burdock (Edible Burdock, Great Burdock, Lappa)

 Basic Information

Biological name (genus and species): *Arctium lappa*

Parts used for medicinal purposes:
- Roots
- Seeds

Chemicals this herb contains:
- Arctiin
- Inulin
- Tannins (see Glossary)
- Vitamins B and E
- Volatile oils (see Glossary)

 Known Effects

Stimulates the immune system

 Possible Additional Effects

- May treat skin disorders
- May treat gout
- May relieve urinary tract infections
- May treat fungal and bacterial infections
- May treat arthritis and rheumatism

 Warnings and Precautions

Don't take if you:
Are pregnant, think you may be pregnant or plan pregnancy in the near future.

Consult your doctor if you:
- Take this herb for any medical problem that doesn't improve in 2 weeks (There may be safer, more effective treatments.)
- Take any medicinal drugs or herbs including aspirin, laxatives, cold and cough remedies, antacids, vitamins, minerals, amino acids, supplements, other prescription or nonprescription drugs

Pregnancy:
Dangers outweigh any possible benefits. Don't use.

Breastfeeding:
Dangers outweigh any possible benefits. Don't use.

Infants and children:
Treating infants or children under 2 with any herbal preparation is hazardous.

Storage:
- Store in cool, dry area away from direct light, but don't freeze.
- Store safely out of reach of children.
- Don't store in bathroom medicine cabinet. Heat and moisture may change the action of the herb.

Safe dosage:
Consult your doctor for the appropriate dose for your condition.

Toxicity

Rated relatively safe when taken in appropriate quantities for short periods of time

For symptoms of toxicity: See *Adverse Reactions, Side Effects or Overdose Symptoms* section below.

Adverse Reactions, Side Effects or Overdose Symptoms

Signs and symptoms	What to do
Dilated pupils	Discontinue. Call doctor immediately.
Dry mouth	Discontinue. Call doctor when convenient.
Hallucinations	Seek emergency treatment.
Stomach discomfort	Discontinue. Call doctor immediately.

Calamus Root

Basic Information

Calamus root is also called *sweet root, acore, rat root, sweet flag, sweet myrtle, sweet cane, sweet sedge, flagroot* and *calamus*.

Biological name (genus and species):
Acorus calamus

Parts used for medicinal purposes:
Roots

Chemicals this herb contains:
- Asarone
- Beta-asarone
- Camphene
- Caryophyllene
- Eugenol
- Pinene
- Volatile oils (see Glossary)

Known Effects
- Aids in expelling gas from the intestinal tract

➜

- Depresses central nervous system
- Causes hallucinations

Miscellaneous information:
- Calamus root is used primarily in India for many illnesses.
- Essential oil extracted from the root causes cancer in rats. The FDA has banned all varieties of this plant for human use.

Possible Additional Effects

- May treat asthma
- May treat coughs
- May treat dyspepsia
- May treat convulsions
- May treat epilepsy
- May treat hysteria
- May treat insanity
- May treat intestinal parasites
- Potential aphrodisiac
- May reduce fever

Warnings and Precautions

Don't take if you:
Possible risks outweigh any benefits. Don't take.

Consult your doctor if you:
Take this herb.

Pregnancy:
Don't use.

Breastfeeding:
Don't use unless prescribed by your doctor.

Infants and children:
Treating infants or children under 2 with any herbal preparation is hazardous.

Storage:
- Store in cool, dry area away from direct light, but don't freeze.
- Store safely out of reach of children.
- Don't store in bathroom medicine cabinet. Heat and moisture may change the action of the herb.

Safe dosage:
Consult your doctor for the appropriate dose for your condition.

Toxicity

Rated dangerous, particularly in children, persons over 55 and those who take larger than appropriate quantities for extended periods of time

For symptoms of toxicity: See *Adverse Reactions, Side Effects or Overdose Symptoms* section below.

Adverse Reactions, Side Effects or Overdose Symptoms

Signs and symptoms	What to do
Drowsiness	Discontinue. Call doctor when convenient.
Hallucinations	Seek emergency treatment.

Calendula (Pot Marigold)

Basic Information

Biological name (genus and species):
Calendula officinalis

Parts used for medicinal purposes:
• Florets
• Flower
• Petals

Chemicals this herb contains:
• Calenduline
• Chlorogenic acid
• Flavonoids (see Glossary)
• Triterpenes
• Volatile oils (see Glossary)

Known Effects

• Promotes wound healing by reducing inflammation and promoting new tissue growth
• Aids in the treatment of psoriasis, acne and eczema
• Antifungal properties to treat skin rashes including diaper rash and athlete's foot
• Anti-inflammatory

Miscellaneous information:

Available as lotions, ointments, oils, tinctures and fresh or dried leaves/florets.

Possible Additional Effects

• May be good for gastritis, colitis and peptic ulcers
• May alleviate menstrual pain
• May treat gallbladder problems
• May treat canker sores

Warnings and Precautions

Don't take if you:

Are pregnant, think you may be pregnant or plan pregnancy in the near future.

Consult your doctor if you:

• Take this herb for any medical problem that doesn't improve in 2 weeks (There may be safer, more effective treatments.)
• Take any medicinal drugs or herbs including aspirin, laxatives, cold and cough remedies, antacids, vitamins, minerals, amino acids, supplements, other prescription or nonprescription drugs
• Have a severe burn or deep wound

Pregnancy:

Don't use unless prescribed by your doctor.

Breastfeeding:

Don't use unless prescribed by your doctor.

Infants and children:

Treating infants or children under 2 with any herbal preparation is hazardous.

Storage:

• Store in cool, dry area away from direct light, but don't freeze.
• Store safely out of reach of children.
• Don't store in bathroom medicine cabinet. Heat and moisture may change the action of the herb.

Safe dosage:

Consult your doctor for the appropriate dose for your condition.

➜

Toxicity

Comparative-toxicity rating is not available from standard references.

Adverse Reactions, Side Effects or Overdose Symptoms

None are expected.

California Poppy

Basic Information

Biological name (genus and species):
Eschscholzia californica

Parts used for medicinal purposes:
Entire plant, except roots

Chemicals this herb contains:
• Coptisine
• Sanguinarine

Known Effects

• Feeble narcotic action
• Increases perspiration
• Depresses central nervous system

Miscellaneous information:
California poppy does not contain any narcotic derivatives, such as morphine or codeine. The poppy plant that has narcotic properties is different from this one.

Possible Additional Effects

Used by drug abusers for sedative or mind-altering effects

Warnings and Precautions

Don't take if you:
Are pregnant, think you may be pregnant or plan pregnancy in the near future.

Consult your doctor if you:
• Take this herb for any medical problem that doesn't improve in 2 weeks (There may be safer, more effective treatments.)
• Take any medicinal drugs or herbs including aspirin, laxatives, cold and cough remedies, antacids, vitamins, minerals, amino acids, supplements, other prescription or nonprescription drugs

Pregnancy:
Don't use unless prescribed by your doctor.

Breastfeeding:
Don't use unless prescribed by your doctor.

Infants and children:
Treating infants or children under 2 with any herbal preparation is hazardous.

Others:

No problems expected if you are beyond childhood, under 45, not pregnant, basically healthy, take it for only a short time and do not exceed manufacturer's recommended dose.

Storage:

- Store in cool, dry area away from direct light, but don't freeze.
- Store safely out of reach of children.
- Don't store in bathroom medicine cabinet. Heat and moisture may change the action of the herb.

Safe dosage:

Consult your doctor for the appropriate dose for your condition.

 Toxicity

Rated slightly dangerous, particularly in children, persons over 55 and those who take larger than appropriate quantities for extended periods of time

For symptoms of toxicity: See *Adverse Reactions, Side Effects or Overdose Symptoms* section below.

 Adverse Reactions, Side Effects or Overdose Symptoms

Signs and symptoms	What to do
Change in heart rate	Discontinue. Call doctor immediately.
Drowsiness	Discontinue. Call doctor immediately.

Caraway

 Basic Information

Biological name (genus and species): *Carum carvi*

Parts used for medicinal purposes:
- Leaves
- Seeds

Chemicals this herb contains:
- Calcium oxalate
- Carveol
- Carvone, a volatile oil (see Glossary)
- Dihydrocarvone
- Fatty acids (see Glossary)
- Proteins

 Known Effects

- Aromatic (see Glossary)
- Helps expel gas from intestinal tract

Miscellaneous information:
- Caraway is used as a flavoring agent in baking.
- The oil is used in making ice cream.
- No effects are expected on the body, either good or bad, when this herb is used in very small amounts to enhance the flavor of food.

➔

Possible Additional Effects

- May reduce flatulence in infants
- May treat abdominal cramping
- May treat nausea
- May treat scabies

Warnings and Precautions

Don't take if you:

- Are pregnant, think you may be pregnant or plan pregnancy in the near future
- Have any chronic disease of the gastrointestinal tract, such as stomach or duodenal ulcers, reflux esophagitis, ulcerative colitis, spastic colitis, diverticulosis or diverticulitis

Consult your doctor if you:

- Take this herb for any medical problem that doesn't improve in 2 weeks (There may be safer, more effective treatments.)
- Take any medicinal drugs or herbs including aspirin, laxatives, cold and cough remedies, antacids, vitamins, minerals, amino acids, supplements, other prescription or nonprescription drugs

Pregnancy:

Don't use unless prescribed by your doctor.

Breastfeeding:

Don't use unless prescribed by your doctor.

Infants and children:

Treating infants or children under 2 with any herbal preparation is hazardous.

Others:

No problems expected if you are beyond childhood, under 45, not pregnant, basically healthy, take it for only a short time and do not exceed manufacturer's recommended dose.

Storage:

- Store in cool, dry area away from direct light, but don't freeze.
- Store safely out of reach of children.
- Don't store in bathroom medicine cabinet. Heat and moisture may change the action of the herb.

Safe dosage:

Consult your doctor for the appropriate dose for your condition.

Toxicity

Comparative-toxicity rating is not available from standard references.

For symptoms of toxicity: See *Adverse Reactions, Side Effects or Overdose Symptoms* section below.

Adverse Reactions, Side Effects or Overdose Symptoms

Signs and symptoms	What to do
In very large amounts only:	
Central-nervous-system depression	Seek emergency treatment.
Nausea or vomiting	Discontinue. Call doctor immediately.

Cardamom Seed

Basic Information

Biological name (genus and species):
Ellettaria cardamonum

Parts used for medicinal purposes:
Seeds

Chemicals this herb contains:
- Fixed oil (see Glossary)
- Gum (see Glossary)
- Limonene
- Starch
- Terpene alcohol (see Glossary)
- Terpinene
- Volatile oils (see Glossary)
- Yellow coloring

Known Effects

- Helps expel gas from intestinal tract
- Causes explosive watery diarrhea

Miscellaneous information:
Provides flavor in foods.

Possible Additional Effects

- May treat bronchitis
- May treat urinary incontinence

Warnings and Precautions

Don't take if you:
- Are pregnant, think you may be pregnant or plan pregnancy in the near future
- Have any chronic disease of the gastrointestinal tract, such as stomach or duodenal ulcers, reflux esophagitis, ulcerative colitis, spastic colitis, diverticulosis or diverticulitis

Consult your doctor if you:
- Take this herb for any medical problem that doesn't improve in 2 weeks (There may be safer, more effective treatments.)
- Take any medicinal drugs or herbs including aspirin, laxatives, cold and cough remedies, antacids, vitamins, minerals, amino acids, supplements, other prescription or nonprescription drugs

Pregnancy:
Don't use unless prescribed by your doctor.

Breastfeeding:
Don't use unless prescribed by your doctor.

Infants and children:
Treating infants or children under 2 with any herbal preparation is hazardous.

Others:
No problems expected if you are beyond childhood, under 45, not pregnant, basically healthy, take it for only a short time and do not exceed manufacturer's recommended dose.

Storage:
- Store in cool, dry area away from direct light, but don't freeze.
- Store safely out of reach of children.
- Don't store in bathroom medicine cabinet. Heat and moisture may change the action of the herb.

Safe dosage:
Consult your doctor for the appropriate dose for your condition.

→

Toxicity

Comparative-toxicity rating is not available from standard references.

For symptoms of toxicity: See *Adverse Reactions, Side Effects or Overdose Symptoms* section below.

Adverse Reactions, Side Effects or Overdose Symptoms

Signs and symptoms	What to do
Diarrhea	Discontinue. Call doctor immediately.
Nausea or vomiting	Discontinue. Call doctor immediately.

Cascara Sagrada (Cascara Buckthorn)

Basic Information

Biological name (genus and species): *Rhamnus purshiana*

Parts used for medicinal purposes: Bark

Chemicals this herb contains:
- Anthraquinone
- Cascarosides
- Volatile oils (see Glossary)

Known Effects

- Used as a mild laxative
- Stimulant

Miscellaneous information:
- Not recommended for prolonged use
- Standard medicinal product listed in the United States Pharmacopeia
- Available as extract or fluid extract dried into capsule form

Possible Additional Effects

May treat intermittent constipation

Warnings and Precautions

Don't take if you:
- Are pregnant, think you may be pregnant or plan pregnancy in the near future
- Have any chronic disease of the gastrointestinal tract, such as stomach or duodenal ulcers, reflux esophagitis, ulcerative colitis, spastic colitis, diverticulosis or diverticulitis

Consult your doctor if you:
- Take this herb for any medical problem that doesn't improve in 2 weeks (There may be safer, more effective treatments.)
- Take any medicinal drugs or herbs including aspirin, laxatives, cold and cough remedies, antacids, vitamins, minerals, amino acids, supplements, other prescription or nonprescription drugs

Pregnancy:
Don't use.

Breastfeeding:
Don't use.

Infants and children:
Treating infants or children under 2 with any herbal preparation is hazardous.

Others:
No problems expected if you are beyond childhood, under 45, not pregnant, basically healthy, take it for only a short time and do not exceed manufacturer's recommended dose.

Storage:
• Store in cool, dry area away from direct light, but don't freeze.
• Store safely out of reach of children.
• Don't store in bathroom medicine cabinet. Heat and moisture may change the action of the herb.

Safe dosage:
Consult your doctor for the appropriate dose for your condition.

 Toxicity

• Cascara sagrada is rated slightly dangerous, particularly in children,

persons over 55 and those who take larger than appropriate quantities for extended periods of time.
• It is for short-term use only. Long-term use can lead to lazy-bowel syndrome.

For symptoms of toxicity: See *Adverse Reactions, Side Effects or Overdose Symptoms* section below.

 Adverse Reactions, Side Effects or Overdose Symptoms

Signs and symptoms	What to do
With excessive dosage:	
Diarrhea, violent and watery	Discontinue. Call doctor immediately.
Nausea or vomiting	Discontinue. Call doctor immediately.
Stomach cramps	Discontinue. Call doctor immediately.

Catalpa

 Basic Information

Biological name (genus and species):
Catalpa bignonioides

Parts used for medicinal purposes:
Various parts of the entire plant, frequently differing by country and culture

Chemicals this herb contains:
• Catalpin
• Catalposide

 Known Effects

Irritates gastrointestinal tract

 Possible Additional Effects

May treat asthma

→

Warnings and Precautions

Don't take if you:

- Are pregnant, think you may be pregnant or plan pregnancy in the near future
- Have any chronic disease of the gastrointestinal tract, such as stomach or duodenal ulcers, reflux esophagitis, ulcerative colitis, spastic colitis, diverticulosis or diverticulitis

Consult your doctor if you:

- Take this herb for any medical problem that doesn't improve in 2 weeks (There may be safer, more effective treatments.)
- Take any medicinal drugs or herbs including aspirin, laxatives, cold and cough remedies, antacids, vitamins, minerals, amino acids, supplements, other prescription or nonprescription drugs

Pregnancy:

Dangers outweigh any possible benefits. Don't use.

Breastfeeding:

Dangers outweigh any possible benefits. Don't use.

Infants and children:

Treating infants or children under 2 with any herbal preparation is hazardous.

Others:

Dangers outweigh any possible benefits. Don't use.

Storage:

- Store in cool, dry area away from direct light, but don't freeze.
- Store safely out of reach of children.
- Don't store in bathroom medicine cabinet. Heat and moisture may change the action of the herb.

Safe dosage:

Consult your doctor for the appropriate dose for your condition.

 Toxicity

Comparative-toxicity rating is not available from standard references.

For symptoms of toxicity: See *Adverse Reactions, Side Effects or Overdose Symptoms* section below.

 Adverse Reactions, Side Effects or Overdose Symptoms

Signs and symptoms	What to do
Cold, clammy skin	Discontinue. Call doctor when convenient.
Diarrhea	Discontinue. Call doctor immediately.
Nausea or vomiting	Discontinue. Call doctor immediately.
Precipitous blood-pressure drop: symptoms include faintness, cold sweat, paleness, rapid pulse	Seek emergency treatment.
Rapid, weak pulse	Seek emergency treatment.

Catechu, Black

 Basic Information

Biological name (genus and species):
Acacia catechu

Parts used for medicinal purposes:
Various parts of the entire plant,
frequently differing by country
and culture

Chemical this herb contains:
Tannins (see Glossary)

 Known Effects

- Shrinks tissues
- Prevents secretion of fluids
- Interferes with absorption of iron
  and other minerals when
  taken internally

 Possible
Additional Effects

- May decrease unusual bleeding
- May treat chronic diarrhea
- Used as gargle for sore throat

 Warnings and
Precautions

Don't take if you:
- Are pregnant, think you may be
  pregnant or plan pregnancy in the
  near future
- Have any chronic disease of the
  gastrointestinal tract, such as
  stomach or duodenal ulcers, reflux
  esophagitis, ulcerative colitis, spastic
  colitis, diverticulosis or diverticulitis

Consult your doctor if you:
- Take this herb for any medical
  problem that doesn't improve in
  2 weeks (There may be safer, more
  effective treatments.)
- Take any medicinal drugs or
  herbs including aspirin, laxatives,
  cold and cough remedies, antacids,
  vitamins, minerals, amino acids,
  supplements, other prescription
  or nonprescription drugs

Pregnancy:
Dangers outweigh any possible
benefits. Don't use.

Breastfeeding:
Dangers outweigh any possible
benefits. Don't use.

Infants and children:
Treating infants or children under
2 with any herbal preparation
is hazardous.

Others:
No problems expected if you are
beyond childhood, under 45, not
pregnant, basically healthy, take it for
only a short time and do not exceed
manufacturer's recommended dose.

Storage:
- Store in cool, dry area away from
  direct light, but don't freeze.
- Store safely out of reach of children.
- Don't store in bathroom medicine
  cabinet. Heat and moisture may
  change the action of the herb.

Safe dosage:
Consult your doctor for the
appropriate dose for your condition.

Toxicity

Comparative-toxicity rating is not available from standard references.

For symptoms of toxicity: See *Adverse Reactions, Side Effects or Overdose Symptoms* section below.

Adverse Reactions, Side Effects or Overdose Symptoms

Signs and symptoms	What to do
Diarrhea	Discontinue. Call doctor immediately.
Kidney damage characterized by blood in urine, decreased urine flow, swelling of hands and feet	Seek emergency treatment.
Vomiting	Discontinue. Call doctor immediately.

Catha (Khat Plant)

Basic Information

Biological name (genus and species): *Catha edulis*

Parts used for medicinal purposes: Leaves

Chemicals this herb contains:
• Cathidine
• Cathine (a form of ephedrine)
• Cathinone
• Celastrin
• Choline
• Katine
• Tannins (see Glossary)

Known Effects
• Stimulates brain and spinal cord through synapses
• Interferes with absorption of iron and other minerals when taken internally

Miscellaneous information:
Can be habit forming—addicts become talkative then depressed and apathetic.

Possible Additional Effects
• May treat fatigue when leaves are chewed or steeped to make tea
• May suppress appetite

Warnings and Precautions

Don't take if you:
• Are pregnant, think you may be pregnant or plan pregnancy in the near future
• Have heart trouble
• Have high blood pressure

Consult your doctor if you:
• Take this herb for any medical problem that doesn't improve in 2 weeks (There may be safer, more effective treatments.)

- Take any medicinal drugs or herbs including aspirin, laxatives, cold and cough remedies, antacids, vitamins, minerals, amino acids, supplements, other prescription or nonprescription drugs

Pregnancy:
Dangers outweigh any possible benefits. Don't use.

Breastfeeding:
Dangers outweigh any possible benefits. Don't use.

Infants and children:
Treating infants or children under 2 with any herbal preparation is hazardous.

Storage:
- Store in cool, dry area away from direct light, but don't freeze.
- Store safely out of reach of children.
- Don't store in bathroom medicine cabinet. Heat and moisture may change the action of the herb.

Safe dosage:
Consult your doctor for the appropriate dose for your condition.

Toxicity

Rated slightly dangerous, particularly in children, persons over 55 and those who take larger than appropriate quantities for extended periods of time

For symptoms of toxicity: See *Adverse Reactions, Side Effects or Overdose Symptoms* section below.

Adverse Reactions, Side Effects or Overdose Symptoms

Signs and symptoms	What to do
Large amounts:	
Breathing difficulties	Seek emergency treatment.
Depression	Discontinue. Call doctor when convenient.
Euphoria	Discontinue. Call doctor when convenient.
Increased blood pressure	Discontinue. Call doctor immediately.
Increased heart rate	Seek emergency treatment.
Paralysis	Seek emergency treatment.
Stomach irritation, with bleeding	Discontinue. Call doctor immediately.

Catnip (Catmint, Catnep)

Basic Information

Biological name (genus and species):
Nepeta cataria

Parts used for medicinal purposes:
Leaves

Chemicals this herb contains:
- Acetic acid
- Buteric acid
- Citral
- Dipentene
- Lifronella
- Limonene
- Nepetalic acid
- Tannins (see Glossary)
- Terpenes (see Glossary)
- Valeric acid
- Volatile oils (see Glossary)

→

Known Effects

- Affects central nervous system
- Relieves spasm in skeletal or smooth muscle
- Relieves indigestion

Miscellaneous information:
Catnip is not a psychedelic or euphoria-producing drug, despite several reports to the contrary.

Possible Additional Effects

- May increase sweating to reduce fevers when leaves are steeped
- May treat colic (see Glossary) when leaves used as snuff
- May treat insomnia
- May treat colds and flu
- May relieve bronchial congestion

Warnings and Precautions

Don't take if you:
Are pregnant, think you may be pregnant or plan pregnancy in the near future.

Consult your doctor if you:
- Take this herb for any medical problem that doesn't improve in 2 weeks (There may be safer, more effective treatments.)
- Take any medicinal drugs or herbs including aspirin, laxatives, cold and cough remedies, antacids, vitamins, minerals, amino acids, supplements, other prescription or nonprescription drugs

Pregnancy:
Don't use unless prescribed by your doctor.

Breastfeeding:
Don't use unless prescribed by your doctor.

Infants and children:
Treating infants or children under 2 with any herbal preparation is hazardous.

Others:
No problems expected if you are beyond childhood, under 45, not pregnant, basically healthy, take it for only a short time and do not exceed manufacturer's recommended dose.

Storage:
- Store in cool, dry area away from direct light, but don't freeze.
- Store safely out of reach of children.
- Don't store in bathroom medicine cabinet. Heat and moisture may change the action of the herb.

Safe dosage:
Consult your doctor for the appropriate dose for your condition.

Toxicity

Generally regarded as safe when taken in appropriate quantities for short periods of time

For symptoms of toxicity: See *Adverse Reactions, Side Effects or Overdose Symptoms* section below.

Adverse Reactions, Side Effects or Overdose Symptoms

Signs and symptoms	What to do
Upset stomach	Discontinue. Call doctor immediately.

Cat's Claw (Una de Gato)

 Basic Information

Biological name (genus and species):
Uncaria tomentosa

Parts used for medicinal purposes:
- Root
- Bark

Chemicals this herb contains:
- Glycosides (see Glossary)
- Oxindole alkaloids
- Polyphenols
- Proanthocyanidins
- Quinovic acid
- Triterpenes

 Known Effects

- Anti-inflammatory
- Stimulates the immune system (antiviral)

Miscellaneous information:
Commonly available in capsules, teas and liquid extracts.

 Possible Additional Effects

- May reduce symptoms of gastritis
- May help treat asthma
- May have antioxidant properties
- May provide relief from nausea and side effects of chemotherapy
- Being tested in conjunction with AZT to treat AIDS patients
- May promote healing of gastric ulcers
- May increase blood circulation
- May reduce bowel inflammation
- May promote normal bowel function
- Potential anticarcinogenic

 Warnings and Precautions

Don't take if you:
- Are pregnant, think you may be pregnant or plan pregnancy in the near future
- Are a tissue- or organ-transplant patient, because this herb tends to cause the immune system to reject foreign cells

Consult your doctor if you:
- Take this herb for any medical problem that doesn't improve in 2 weeks (There may be safer, more effective treatments.)
- Take any medicinal drugs or herbs including aspirin, laxatives, cold and cough remedies, antacids, vitamins, minerals, amino acids, supplements, other prescription or nonprescription drugs

Pregnancy:
Don't use.

Breastfeeding:
Don't use unless prescribed by your doctor.

Infants and children:
Treating infants or children under 2 with any herbal preparation is hazardous.

Storage:
- Store in cool, dry area away from direct light, but don't freeze.
- Store safely out of reach of children.
- Don't store in bathroom medicine cabinet. Heat and moisture may change the action of the herb.

Safe dosage:
Consult your doctor for the appropriate dose for your condition.

→

Toxicity

Comparative-toxicity rating is not available from standard references.

For symptoms of toxicity: See *Adverse Reactions, Side Effects or Overdose Symptoms* section below.

Adverse Reactions, Side Effects or Overdose Symptoms

Signs and symptoms	What to do
Diarrhea	Lower dose and monitor for 1 to 2 weeks. May occur for 1 to 2 weeks but should then resolve. Call doctor when convenient.

Cayenne (Capsicum)

Basic Information

Cayenne is also known as *red-hot pepper, hot pepper, capsaicin, chili pepper, Africa pepper, American pepper, red pepper* and *Spanish pepper*.

Biological name (genus and species): *Capsicum frutescens, Capsicum annuum*

Parts used for medicinal purposes: Berries/fruits

Chemicals this herb contains:
- Apsaicine
- Capsacutin
- Capsaicin
- Capsanthine
- Capsico
- Folic acid
- Vitamins A, B and C

Known Effects

- Provides counterirritation (see Glossary) when applied to skin overlying an inflamed or irritated joint

- Stimulant
- Antioxidant
- Reduces pain of diabetic neuropathy
- Treats cluster headache

Miscellaneous information:
- Available in powder form
- Available as oil capsules
- Available as fresh food
- Used in small amounts as a condiment
- No effects are expected on the body, either good or bad, when herb is used in very small amounts to enhance the flavor of food

Possible Additional Effects

- May promote healing of oral lesions associated with chemotherapy, as well as canker sores
- May settle "upset stomach" and help relieve gas and indigestion
- Is used as external rub or poultice to relieve pain
- May reduce pain of arthritis
- May promote blood flow
- May influence healing of duodenal ulcers

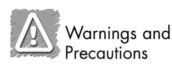 Warnings and Precautions

Don't take if you:
- Are pregnant, think you may be pregnant or plan pregnancy in the near future
- Have any chronic disease of the gastrointestinal tract, such as stomach or duodenal ulcers, reflux esophagitis, ulcerative colitis, spastic colitis, diverticulosis or diverticulitis
- Have a bleeding problem

Consult your doctor if you:
- Take this herb for any medical problem that doesn't improve in 2 weeks (There may be safer, more effective treatments.)
- Take any medicinal drugs or herbs including aspirin, laxatives, cold and cough remedies, antacids, vitamins, minerals, amino acids, supplements, other prescription or nonprescription drugs

Pregnancy:
Problems in pregnant women taking small or usual amounts have not been proved, but the chance of problems does exist. Don't use unless prescribed by your doctor.

Breastfeeding:
Problems in breastfed infants of lactating mothers taking small or usual amounts have not been proved, but the chance of problems does exist. Don't use unless prescribed by your doctor.

Infants and children:
Treating infants or children under 2 with any herbal preparation is hazardous.

Others:
Inhalation of cayenne can cause allergic alveolitis.

Storage:
- Store in cool, dry area away from direct light, but don't freeze.
- Store safely out of reach of children.
- Don't store in bathroom medicine cabinet. Heat and moisture may change the action of the herb.

Safe dosage:
Consult your doctor for the appropriate dose for your condition.

 Toxicity

- Cayenne is rated relatively safe when taken in appropriate quantities for short periods of time.
- Excessive intake may cause gastroenteritis, hepatic or renal damage.

For symptoms of toxicity: See *Adverse Reactions, Side Effects or Overdose Symptoms* section below.

 Adverse Reactions, Side Effects or Overdose Symptoms

Signs and symptoms	What to do
Diarrhea, regular or bloody	Discontinue. Call doctor immediately.
Nausea or vomiting	Discontinue. Call doctor immediately.
Vomiting blood	Seek emergency treatment.

Celery Fruit (Celery)

 Basic Information

Biological name (genus and species):
Apium graveolens

Parts used for medicinal purposes:
• Juice
• Roots
• Seeds

Chemicals this herb contains:
• D-limonene
• Nitrates
• Resin (see Glossary)
• Sedanoic anhydrides
• Sedanolide
• Volatile oils (see Glossary)

 Known Effects

• Relieves spasm in skeletal or smooth muscle
• Causes uterine contractions, whether pregnant or not
• Reduces blood pressure, when in juice form
• Reduces gas in gastrointestinal tract

Miscellaneous information:
• No effects are expected on the body, either good or bad, when this herb is used in very small amounts to enhance the flavor of food or when eaten as a common food.
• Workers in celery fields may develop skin rashes.

 Possible Additional Effects

• Potential antioxidant (seeds)
• Potential sedative
• May treat dysmenorrhea (menstrual cramps)
• May treat arthritis
• Potential aphrodisiac (roots)

 Warnings and Precautions

Don't take if you:
Are in your third trimester of a pregnancy.

Consult your doctor if you:
• Take this herb for any medical problem that doesn't improve in 2 weeks (There may be safer, more effective treatments.)
• Take any medicinal drugs or herbs including aspirin, laxatives, cold and cough remedies, antacids, vitamins, minerals, amino acids, supplements, other prescription or nonprescription drugs

Pregnancy:
Pregnant women should experience no problems taking usual amounts as part of a balanced diet. Don't drink large quantities of celery juice.

Breastfeeding:
Breastfed infants of lactating mothers should experience no problems when mother takes usual amounts as part of a balanced diet. Other products extracted from this herb have not been proved to cause problems.

Infants and children:
Treating infants or children under 2 with any herbal preparation is hazardous.

Others:
No problems expected if you are beyond childhood, under 45, basically healthy, take it for only a short time and do not exceed manufacturer's recommended dose.

Storage:
- Store in cool, dry area away from direct light, but don't freeze.
- Store safely out of reach of children.
- Don't store in bathroom medicine cabinet. Heat and moisture may change the action of the herb.

Safe dosage:
Consult your doctor for the appropriate dose for your condition.

Toxicity

Rated relatively safe when taken in appropriate quantities for short periods of time

For symptoms of toxicity: See *Adverse Reactions, Side Effects or Overdose Symptoms* section below.

Adverse Reactions, Side Effects or Overdose Symptoms

Signs and symptoms	What to do
Deep sedation (with large amounts)	Seek emergency treatment.
Premature labor	Seek emergency treatment.

Centaury (Minor Centaury)

Basic Information

Biological name (genus and species):
Centaurium erythraea,
C. umbellatum

Parts used for medicinal purposes:
Petals/flower

Chemicals this herb contains:
- Amarogentin
- Erytaurin
- Erythrocentaurin
- Gentiopicrin
- Gentisin

Known Effects
- Reduces indigestion
- May stimulate appetite

Possible Additional Effects

No additional effects are known.

Warnings and Precautions

Don't take if you:
- Are pregnant, think you may be pregnant or plan pregnancy in the near future
- Have any chronic disease of the gastrointestinal tract, such as stomach or duodenal ulcers, reflux esophagitis, ulcerative colitis, spastic colitis, diverticulosis or diverticulitis

Consult your doctor if you:
- Take this herb for any medical problem that doesn't improve in 2 weeks (There may be safer, more effective treatments.)

➜

• Take any medicinal drugs or herbs including aspirin, laxatives, cold and cough remedies, antacids, vitamins, minerals, amino acids, supplements, other prescription or nonprescription drugs

Pregnancy:
Don't use unless prescribed by your doctor.

Breastfeeding:
Don't use unless prescribed by your doctor.

Infants and children:
Treating infants or children under 2 with any herbal preparation is hazardous.

Others:
No problems expected if you are beyond childhood, under 45, not pregnant, basically healthy, take it for only a short time and do not exceed manufacturer's recommended dose.

Storage:
• Store in cool, dry area away from direct light, but don't freeze.
• Store safely out of reach of children.

• Don't store in bathroom medicine cabinet. Heat and moisture may change the action of the herb.

Safe dosage:
Consult your doctor for the appropriate dose for your condition.

Toxicity

Comparative-toxicity rating is not available from standard references.

For symptoms of toxicity: See *Adverse Reactions, Side Effects or Overdose Symptoms* section below.

Adverse Reactions, Side Effects or Overdose Symptoms

Signs and symptoms	What to do
Only with very large amounts or accidental overdose:	
Nausea or vomiting	Discontinue. Call doctor immediately.

Chamomile

Basic Information

Biological name (genus and species):
Anthemis nobilis, A. flores

Parts used for medicinal purposes:
Various parts of the entire plant, frequently differing by country or culture

Chemicals this herb contains:
• Antheme
• Anthemic acid
• Anthesterol
• Apigenin
• Chamazulene
• Resin (see Glossary)
• Tannic acid
• Tiglic acid
• Volatile oils (see Glossary)

Known Effects

- Decreases spasm of smooth or skeletal muscle
- Alleviates menstrual cramps
- Anti-inflammatory
- Mild sedative
- Interferes with absorption of iron and other minerals when taken internally
- Kills bacteria on skin
- Reduces stomach cramps, gas, indigestion

Miscellaneous information:

- Flowers are used to make extract and herbal tea.
- Chamomile is available as tea, tincture, oil, dried or fresh flowers.

Possible Additional Effects

Internal use:

- Potential insomnia treatment
- Potential diarrhea treatment
- May treat bronchial infections
- Used as a gargle for gingivitis and sore throat
- May soothe sunburn, cuts and scrapes, sore or inflamed eyes

External use:

- Used as a poultice (see Glossary)
- May help medicate skin abscesses
- Potential hemorrhoid treatment

Warnings and Precautions

Don't take if you:

- Are pregnant, think you may be pregnant or plan pregnancy in the near future
- Have any chronic disease of the gastrointestinal tract, such as stomach or duodenal ulcers, reflux esophagitis, ulcerative colitis, spastic colitis, diverticulosis or diverticulitis

Consult your doctor if you:

- Take this herb for any medical problem that doesn't improve in 2 weeks (There may be safer, more effective treatments.)
- Take any medicinal drugs or herbs including aspirin, laxatives, cold and cough remedies, antacids, vitamins, minerals, amino acids, supplements, other prescription or nonprescription drugs

Pregnancy:

Dangers outweigh any benefits. Don't use.

Breastfeeding:

Dangers outweigh any benefits. Don't use.

Infants and children:

Treating infants or children under 2 with any herbal preparation is hazardous.

Storage:

- Store in cool, dry area away from direct light, but don't freeze.
- Store safely out of reach of children.
- Don't store in bathroom medicine cabinet. Heat and moisture may change the action of the herb.

Safe dosage:

Consult your doctor for the appropriate dose for your condition.

Toxicity

Comparative-toxicity rating is not available from standard references.

For symptoms of toxicity: See *Adverse Reactions, Side Effects or Overdose Symptoms* section below.

→

Adverse Reactions, Side Effects or Overdose Symptoms

Signs and symptoms	What to do
Allergic reactions in individuals who are sensitive to ragweed pollens (rare)	Discontinue. Call doctor immediately.
Life-threatening anaphylaxis may follow injections—symptoms include immediate severe itching, paleness, low blood pressure, loss of consciousness, coma	Yell for help. Don't leave victim. Begin CPR (cardio-pulmonary resuscitation), mouth-to-mouth breathing and external cardiac massage. Have someone dial "0" (operator) or 911 (emergency). Don't stop CPR until help arrives.
Skin irritation	Discontinue. Call doctor when convenient.
Vomiting	Discontinue. Call doctor immediately.

Chickweed

Basic Information

Biological name (genus and species):
Stellaria media

Parts used for medicinal purposes:
Various parts of the entire plant, frequently differing by country or culture

Chemicals this herb contains:
• Ascorbic acid (vitamin C)
• Potash salts
• Rutin

Known Effects

Internal use:
• Protects scraped tissues
• Vitamin-C supplement
• Relieves constipation

External use:
• Ointment for rashes and sores
• Soothes cuts and wounds

Miscellaneous information:
• Due to high vitamin-C content, chickweed can treat scurvy.
• It is available as dried bulk, oil, ointment and tincture.

Possible Additional Effects

Internal use:
- May treat fatigue
- May treat bronchitis by reducing thickness of mucus in lungs
- May increase urine production

External use:
- May treat insect bites
- May treat eczema and itchy scalp conditions

 ## Warnings and Precautions

Don't take if you:
Are pregnant, think you may be pregnant or plan pregnancy in the near future.

Consult your doctor if you:
- Take this herb for any medical problem that doesn't improve in 2 weeks (There may be safer, more effective treatments.)
- Take any medicinal drugs or herbs including aspirin, laxatives, cold and cough remedies, antacids, vitamins, minerals, amino acids, supplements, other prescription or nonprescription drugs

Pregnancy:
Don't use unless prescribed by your doctor.

Breastfeeding:
Don't use unless prescribed by your doctor.

Infants and children:
Treating infants or children under 2 with any herbal preparation is hazardous.

Others:
No problems expected if you are beyond childhood, under 45, not pregnant, basically healthy, take it for only a short time and do not exceed manufacturer's recommended dose.

Storage:
- Store in cool, dry area away from direct light, but don't freeze.
- Store safely out of reach of children.
- Don't store in bathroom medicine cabinet. Heat and moisture may change the action of the herb.

Safe dosage:
Consult your doctor for the appropriate dose for your condition.

 ## Toxicity

Rated relatively safe when taken in appropriate quantities for short periods of time

For symptoms of toxicity: See *Adverse Reactions, Side Effects or Overdose Symptoms* section below.

 ## Adverse Reactions, Side Effects or Overdose Symptoms

Signs and symptoms	What to do
Temporary paralysis (large amounts only)	Seek emergency treatment.

Chicory

Basic Information

Biological name (genus and species):
Cichorium intybus

Parts used for medicinal purposes:
Roots

Chemicals this herb contains:
- Ascorbic acid (vitamin C)
- Inulin
- Vitamin A

Known Effects

- Laxative
- Mild diuretic

Possible Additional Effects

- Potential dyspepsia treatment
- Potential jaundice treatment
- May treat rheumatism and gout
- May treat skin irritations as a compress

Warnings and Precautions

Don't take if you:
Are pregnant, think you may be pregnant or plan pregnancy in the near future.

Consult your doctor if you:
- Take this herb for any medical problem that doesn't improve in 2 weeks (There may be safer, more effective treatments.)
- Take any medicinal drugs or herbs including aspirin, laxatives, cold and cough remedies, antacids, vitamins, minerals, amino acids, supplements, other prescription or nonprescription drugs

Pregnancy:
Don't use unless prescribed by your doctor.

Breastfeeding:
Don't use unless prescribed by your doctor.

Infants and children:
Treating infants or children under 2 with any herbal preparation is hazardous.

Storage:
- Store in cool, dry area away from direct light, but don't freeze.
- Store safely out of reach of children.
- Don't store in bathroom medicine cabinet. Heat and moisture may change the action of the herb.

Safe dosage:
Consult your doctor for the appropriate dose for your condition.

Toxicity

Comparative-toxicity rating is not available from standard references.

For symptoms of toxicity: See *Adverse Reactions, Side Effects or Overdose Symptoms* section below.

Adverse Reactions, Side Effects or Overdose Symptoms

Signs and symptoms	What to do
Rapid heart rate	Seek medical care.
Red, swollen or irritated skin	Discontinue. Call doctor when convenient. Use gloves when handling.

Chinese Rhubarb (Canton Rhubarb)

Basic Information

Biological name (genus and species):
Rheum officinalis, R. palmatum

Parts used for medicinal purposes:
- Dried rhizomes
- Roots

Chemicals this herb contains:
- Aloe-emodin
- Anthraquinone
- Chrysophanol
- Emodin
- Tannins (see Glossary)

Known Effects

- Irritates mucous membranes of intestinal tract
- Strong laxative

Miscellaneous information:
This is not the garden variety of rhubarb.

Possible Additional Effects

No additional effects are known.

Warnings and Precautions

Don't take if you:
- Are pregnant, think you may be pregnant or plan pregnancy in the near future
- Have any chronic disease of the gastrointestinal tract, such as stomach or duodenal ulcers, reflux esophagitis, ulcerative colitis, spastic colitis, diverticulosis or diverticulitis

Consult your doctor if you:
- Take this herb for any medical problem that doesn't improve in 2 weeks (There may be safer, more effective treatments.)
- Take any medicinal drugs or herbs including aspirin, laxatives, cold and cough remedies, antacids, vitamins, minerals, amino acids, supplements, other prescription or nonprescription drugs

Pregnancy:
Avoid overeating this herb.

Breastfeeding:
Avoid overeating this herb.

Infants and children:
Treating infants or children under 2 with any herbal preparation is hazardous.

Others:
- No problems expected if you are beyond childhood, under 45, not pregnant, basically healthy, take it for only a short time and do not exceed manufacturer's recommended dose.
- Frequent use is not recommended. Less potent laxative herbs are available.

Storage:
- Store in cool, dry area away from direct light, but don't freeze.
- Store safely out of reach of children.
- Don't store in bathroom medicine cabinet. Heat and moisture may change the action of the herb.

Safe dosage:
Consult your doctor for the appropriate dose for your condition.

→

Toxicity

Rated relatively safe when taken in appropriate quantities for short periods of time

For symptoms of toxicity: See *Adverse Reactions, Side Effects or Overdose Symptoms* section below.

Adverse Reactions, Side Effects or Overdose Symptoms

Signs and symptoms	What to do
Cramping, abdominal pain	Discontinue. Call doctor immediately.
Diarrhea (explosive, watery)	Discontinue. Call doctor immediately.

Cinnamon (Camphor)

Basic Information

Biological name (genus and species):
Cinnamomum camphora

Parts used for medicinal purposes:
• Bark
• Leaves
• Roots

Chemicals this herb contains:
• Camphor oil
• Cineole
• Cinnamic aldehyde
• Fatty acids
• Gum (see Glossary)
• Limonene
• Mannitol
• Safrole
• Tannins (see Glossary)
• Oils

Known Effects

• Helps expel gas from intestinal tract
• Mouthwash
• Relieves diarrhea

Miscellaneous information:
• Used to make celluloid, explosives and other chemicals
• Available as powder, pill and tincture

Possible Additional Effects

• Safrole is possible carcinogen
• May soothe indigestion
• May prevent ulcers
• May fight tooth decay
• Potential nausea relief
• May lessen menstrual cramps
• May help treat asthma
• May help treat loss of appetite

Warnings and Precautions

Don't take if you:
• Are pregnant, think you may be pregnant or plan pregnancy in the near future
• Have any chronic disease of the gastrointestinal tract, such as stomach or duodenal ulcers, reflux esophagitis, ulcerative colitis, spastic colitis, diverticulosis or diverticulitis

Consult your doctor if you:

- Take this herb for any medical problem that doesn't improve in 2 weeks (There may be safer, more effective treatments.)
- Take any medicinal drugs or herbs including aspirin, laxatives, cold and cough remedies, antacids, vitamins, minerals, amino acids, supplements, other prescription or nonprescription drugs

Pregnancy:

Don't use.

Breastfeeding:

Don't use.

Infants and children:

Treating infants or children under 2 with any herbal preparation is hazardous.

Others:

No problems expected if you are beyond childhood, under 45, not pregnant, basically healthy, take it for only a short time and do not exceed manufacturer's recommended dose.

Storage:

- Store in cool, dry area away from direct light, but don't freeze.
- Store safely out of reach of children.
- Don't store in bathroom medicine cabinet. Heat and moisture may change the action of the herb.

Safe dosage:

Consult your doctor for the appropriate dose for your condition.

Toxicity

Rated dangerous, particularly in children, persons over 55 and those who take larger than appropriate quantities for extended periods of time

For symptoms of toxicity: See *Adverse Reactions, Side Effects or Overdose Symptoms* section below.

Adverse Reactions, Side Effects or Overdose Symptoms

Signs and symptoms	What to do
Convulsions	Seek emergency treatment.
Dizziness	Discontinue. Call doctor immediately.
Hallucinations	Seek emergency treatment.
Large overdose (0.5ml/kg body weight) can cause coma or kidney damage	Seek emergency treatment.
Nausea	Discontinue. Call doctor immediately.
Skin contact with oil can cause redness and burning sensation	Discontinue. Call doctor when convenient.
Vomiting	Discontinue. Call doctor immediately.

Coconut

Basic Information

Biological name (genus and species):
Cocus nucifera

Parts used for medicinal purposes:
Oil from seeds

Chemicals this herb contains:
• Fixed oil (see Glossary)
• Tannins (see Glossary)
• Trilaurin
• Trimyristin
• Triolein
• Tripalmatic acid
• Tripalmatin
• Tristearin

Known Effects

• Prevents secretion of fluids
• Interferes with absorption of iron
  and other minerals when
  taken internally

Miscellaneous information:
• Coconut is used in making soaps,
  scalp applications, hand creams and
  some foodstuffs.
• Coconut-oil–based soaps are useful
  for marine purposes because they
  are not easily separated by saltwater
  or salty solutions.

Possible Additional Effects

No additional effetcs are known.

Warnings and Precautions

Don't take if you:
Have any chronic disease of the
gastrointestinal tract, such as stomach
or duodenal ulcers, reflux esophagitis,
ulcerative colitis, spastic colitis, diverticulosis or diverticulitis.

Consult your doctor if you:
• Take this herb for any medical
  problem that doesn't improve in
  2 weeks (There may be safer, more
  effective treatments.)
• Take any medicinal drugs or
  herbs including aspirin, laxatives,
  cold and cough remedies, antacids,
  vitamins, minerals, amino acids,
  supplements, other prescription
  or nonprescription drugs

Pregnancy:
Pregnant women should experience
no problems taking usual amounts as
part of a balanced diet. Other products
extracted from this herb have not been
proved to cause problems.

Breastfeeding:
Breastfed infants of lactating mothers
should experience no problems when
mother takes usual amounts as part of
a balanced diet. Other products
extracted from this herb have not been
proved to cause problems.

Infants and children:
Treating infants or children under
2 with any herbal preparation
is hazardous.

Others:

No problems expected if you are beyond childhood, under 45, basically healthy, take it for only a short time and do not exceed manufacturer's recommended dose.

Storage:

- Store in cool, dry area away from direct light, but don't freeze.
- Store safely out of reach of children.
- Don't store in bathroom medicine cabinet. Heat and moisture may change the action of the herb.

Safe dosage:

Consult your doctor for the appropriate dose for your condition.

Toxicity

Comparative-toxicity rating is not available from standard references.

For symptoms of toxicity: See *Adverse Reactions, Side Effects or Overdose Symptoms* section below.

Adverse Reactions, Side Effects or Overdose Symptoms

Signs and symptoms	What to do
Diarrhea	Discontinue. Call doctor immediately.

Cohosh, Black (Black Snakeroot, Rattle Root, Squaw Root)

Basic Information

Biological name (genus and species):
Cimicifuga racemosa

Parts used for medicinal purposes:
- Rhizomes
- Roots

Chemicals this herb contains:
- Glycosides (see Glossary)
- Isoferulic acid
- Isoflavones
- Tannins (see Glossary)
- Volatile oils (see Glossary)

Known Effects

- Treats hot flashes and symptoms of menopause
- Treats PMS
- Treats dysmenorrhea

Possible Additional Effects

- May treat diarrhea
- Used as an antidote for rattlesnake poison
- May lower blood pressure

Warnings and Precautions

Don't take if you:

- Are pregnant, think you may be pregnant or plan pregnancy in the near future
- Have any chronic disease of the gastrointestinal tract, such as stomach or duodenal ulcers, reflux esophagitis, ulcerative colitis, spastic colitis, diverticulosis or diverticulitis

→

Consult your doctor if you:
- Take this herb for any medical problem that doesn't improve in 2 weeks (There may be safer, more effective treatments.)
- Take any medicinal drugs or herbs including aspirin, laxatives, cold and cough remedies, antacids, vitamins, minerals, amino acids, supplements, other prescription or nonprescription drugs

Pregnancy:
Don't use unless prescribed by your doctor.

Breastfeeding:
Don't use unless prescribed by your doctor.

Infants and children:
Treating infants or children under 2 with any herbal preparation is hazardous.

Others:
Limit use to 6 months.

Storage:
- Store in cool, dry area away from direct light, but don't freeze.
- Store safely out of reach of children.

- Don't store in bathroom medicine cabinet. Heat and moisture may change the action of the herb.

Safe dosage:
Consult your doctor for the appropriate dose for your condition.

 Toxicity

Rated slightly dangerous, particularly in children, persons over 55 and those who take larger than appropriate quantities for extended periods of time

For symptoms of toxicity: See *Adverse Reactions, Side Effects or Overdose Symptoms* section below.

 Adverse Reactions, Side Effects or Overdose Symptoms

Signs and symptoms	What to do
Gastroenteritis, characterized by stomach pain, nausea, diarrhea	Discontinue. Call doctor immediately.
Nausea or vomiting	Discontinue. Call doctor immediately.

Cohosh, Blue (Papoose Root, Squaw Root)

 Basic Information

Biological name (genus and species):
Caulophyllum thalictroides

Parts used for medicinal purposes:
Roots

Chemicals this herb contains:
- Coulosaponin

- Leontin, a saponin (see Glossary)
- Methylcystine

 Known Effects

- Stimulates contraction of smooth muscle (blood vessels and small muscles surrounding certain arteries and muscle fibers in the uterus)
- Raises blood pressure

Possible Additional Effects

- May treat menstrual problems
- May stimulate uterine contractions during labor

Warnings and Precautions

Don't take if you:

- Are pregnant, think you may be pregnant or plan pregnancy in the near future
- Have any chronic disease of the gastrointestinal tract, such as stomach or duodenal ulcers, reflux esophagitis, ulcerative colitis, spastic colitis, diverticulosis or diverticulitis

Consult your doctor if you:

- Take this herb for any medical problem that doesn't improve in 2 weeks (There may be safer, more effective treatments.)
- Take any medicinal drugs or herbs including aspirin, laxatives, cold and cough remedies, antacids, vitamins, minerals, amino acids, supplements, other prescription or nonprescription drugs

Pregnancy:

Dangers outweigh any possible benefits. Don't use.

Breastfeeding:

Dangers outweigh any possible benefits. Don't use.

Infants and children:

Treating infants or children under 2 with any herbal preparation is hazardous.

Others:

Don't self-medicate for any purpose. Cohosh may cause toxic symptoms.

Storage:

- Store in cool, dry area away from direct light, but don't freeze.
- Store safely out of reach of children.
- Don't store in bathroom medicine cabinet. Heat and moisture may change the action of the herb.

Safe dosage:

Consult your doctor for the appropriate dose for your condition.

Toxicity

Rated slightly dangerous, particularly in children, persons over 55 and those who take larger than appropriate quantities for extended periods of time

For symptoms of toxicity: See *Adverse Reactions, Side Effects or Overdose Symptoms* section below.

Adverse Reactions, Side Effects or Overdose Symptoms

Signs and symptoms	What to do
Chest pain	Seek emergency treatment.
Convulsions	Seek emergency treatment.
Dilated pupils	Discontinue. Call doctor immediately.
Headache	Discontinue. Call doctor immediately.
Nausea or vomiting	Discontinue. Call doctor immediately.
Stomach irritation, with possible bleeding	Discontinue. Call doctor immediately.
Thirst	Discontinue. Call doctor when convenient.
Weakness	Discontinue. Call doctor immediately.

Cohosh, White

Basic Information

Biological name (genus and species):
Actaea alba, A. arguta

Parts used for medicinal purposes:
Various parts of the entire plant,
frequently differing by country
and culture

Chemicals this herb contains:
- Glycosides (see Glossary)
- Protoanemonin
- Volatile oils (see Glossary)

Known Effects

Irritates mucous membranes

Possible Additional Effects

- Potential mild sedative to relieve anxiety
- May help bring on menstruation

Warnings and Precautions

Don't take if you:
- Are pregnant, think you may be pregnant or plan pregnancy in the near future
- Have any chronic disease of the gastrointestinal tract, such as stomach or duodenal ulcers, reflux esophagitis, ulcerative colitis, spastic colitis, diverticulosis or diverticulitis

Consult your doctor if you:
- Take this herb for any medical problem that doesn't improve in 2 weeks (There may be safer, more effective treatments.)

- Take any medicinal drugs or herbs including aspirin, laxatives, cold and cough remedies, antacids, vitamins, minerals, amino acids, supplements, other prescription or nonprescription drugs

Pregnancy:
Dangers outweigh any possible benefits. Don't use.

Breastfeeding:
Dangers outweigh any possible benefits. Don't use.

Infants and children:
Treating infants or children under 2 with any herbal preparation is hazardous.

Others:
This product will not help you and may cause toxic symptoms.

Storage:
- Store in cool, dry area away from direct light, but don't freeze.
- Store safely out of reach of children.
- Don't store in bathroom medicine cabinet. Heat and moisture may change the action of the herb.

Safe dosage:
Consult your doctor for the appropriate dose for your condition.

Toxicity

Comparative-toxicity rating is not available from standard references.

For symptoms of toxicity: See *Adverse Reactions, Side Effects or Overdose Symptoms* section below.

Adverse Reactions,
Side Effects or
Overdose Symptoms

Signs and symptoms	What to do
Diarrhea (sometimes bloody)	Discontinue. Call doctor immediately.
Hallucinations	Seek emergency treatment.
Nausea or vomiting	Discontinue. Call doctor immediately.
Skin rashes or eye irritation, if used on skin or in eye	Discontinue. Call doctor immediately.

Coltsfoot (Coughwort, Horse-Hoof)

 Basic Information

Biological name (genus and species):
Tussilago farfara

Parts used for medicinal purposes:
- Berries/fruits
- Leaves

Chemicals this herb contains:
- Caoutchouc
- Pectin
- Resin (see Glossary)
- Tannins (see Glossary)
- Volatile oils (see Glossary)

 Known Effects

No proven medicinal effects are known.

Miscellaneous information:
- Has been found to have carcinogenic properties
- Available as tincture, capsule, bulk

 Possible
Additional Effects

Internal use:
May treat persistent cough—bronchitis, allergic, whooping

External use:
May soothe various skin disorders

 Warnings and
Precautions

Don't take if you:
Are pregnant, think you may be pregnant or plan pregnancy in the near future.

Consult your doctor if you:
- Take this herb for any medical problem that doesn't improve in 2 weeks (There may be safer, more effective treatments.)
- Take any medicinal drugs or herbs including aspirin, laxatives,

➡

cold and cough remedies, antacids, vitamins, minerals, amino acids, supplements, other prescription or nonprescription drugs

Pregnancy:
Don't use unless prescribed by your doctor.

Breastfeeding:
Don't use unless prescribed by your doctor.

Infants and children:
Treating infants or children under 2 with any herbal preparation is hazardous.

Others:
No problems expected if you are beyond childhood, under 45, not pregnant, basically healthy, take it for only a short time and do not exceed manufacturer's recommended dose.

Storage:
• Store in cool, dry area away from direct light, but don't freeze.
• Store safely out of reach of children.
• Don't store in bathroom medicine cabinet. Heat and moisture may change the action of the herb.

Safe dosage:
Consult your doctor for the appropriate dose for your condition.

Toxicity

Coltsfoot is rated relatively safe when taken in small quantities for short periods of time; however, cumulative effects may produce malignant growths.

For symptoms of toxicity: See *Adverse Reactions, Side Effects or Overdose Symptoms* section below.

Adverse Reactions, Side Effects or Overdose Symptoms

Signs and symptoms	What to do
Abdominal pain	Discontinue. Call doctor immediately.
Fever	Discontinue. Call doctor immediately.
Jaundice (yellow skin and eyes)	Discontinue. Call doctor immediately.
Nausea or vomiting	Discontinue. Call doctor immediately.

Comfrey (Knitbone)

Basic Information

Biological name (genus and species):
Symphytum officinale

Parts used for medicinal purposes:
• Leaves
• Roots

Chemicals this herb contains:
• Allantoin
• Consolidine
• Mucilage (see Glossary)
• Phosphorus
• Potassium
• Pyrrolizidine
• Starch
• Symphytocynglossine
• Tannins (see Glossary)
• Vitamins A and C

Known Effects

- Reduces inflammation associated with injury
- Promotes healing of cuts, insect bites

Miscellaneous information:

- Taken internally, comfrey may cause liver damage.
- It may be toxic when applied to skin as well.

Possible Additional Effects

- Used in poultices (see Glossary) to heal wounds and ulcers
- May protect scraped tissues
- May treat sunburns
- May treat psoriasis and skin rashes
- Potential dermatitis treatment
- May help body dispose of excess fluid by increasing the amount of urine produced

Warnings and Precautions

Don't take if you:

Are pregnant, think you may be pregnant or plan pregnancy in the near future, because you need to restrict the potassium in your diet.

Consult your doctor if you:

- Take this herb for any medical problem that doesn't improve in 2 weeks (There may be safer, more effective treatments.)
- Take any medicinal drugs or herbs including aspirin, laxatives, cold and cough remedies, antacids, vitamins, minerals, amino acids, supplements, other prescription or nonprescription drugs

Pregnancy:

Do not use.

Breastfeeding:

Problems in breastfed infants of lactating mothers taking small or usual amounts have not been proved, but the chance of problems does exist. Don't use unless prescribed by your doctor.

Infants and children:

Treating infants or children under 2 with any herbal preparation is hazardous.

Others:

Do not take internally.

Storage:

- Store in cool, dry area away from direct light, but don't freeze.
- Store safely out of reach of children.
- Don't store in bathroom medicine cabinet. Heat and moisture may change the action of the herb.

Safe dosage:

Consult your doctor for the appropriate dose for your condition.

Toxicity

Comfrey is toxic if taken internally.

For symptoms of toxicity: See *Adverse Reactions, Side Effects or Overdose Symptoms* section below.

Adverse Reactions, Side Effects or Overdose Symptoms

Signs and symptoms	What to do
Coma	Seek emergency treatment.
Drowsiness	Discontinue. Call doctor immediately.
Lethargy	Discontinue. Call doctor immediately.
Rash	Call doctor when convenient.

Cottonwood (Balm of Gilead)

 ## Basic Information

Biological name (genus and species):
Populus deltoides, P. candicans

Parts used for medicinal purposes:
Roots

Chemicals this herb contains:
Salicin

 ## Known Effects

• Anti-inflammatory
• Reduces pain
• Reduces fever

Miscellaneous information:
Used extensively by Native Americans
for many disorders.

 ## Possible Additional Effects

• May relieve toothache
• May treat arthritis
• May treat heart diseases
• May treat any illness accompanied by
  fever, pain or inflammation

 ## Warnings and Precautions

Don't take if you:
Are pregnant, think you may be
pregnant or plan pregnancy in the
near future.

Consult your doctor if you:
• Take this herb for any medical
  problem that doesn't improve in
  2 weeks (There may be safer, more
  effective treatments.)
• Take any medicinal drugs or
  herbs including aspirin, laxatives,
  cold and cough remedies, antacids,
  vitamins, minerals, amino acids,
  supplements, other prescription
  or nonprescription drugs

Pregnancy:
Don't use unless prescribed by
your doctor.

Breastfeeding:
Don't use unless prescribed by
your doctor.

Infants and children:
Treating infants or children under
2 with any herbal preparation
is hazardous.

Others:
No problems expected if you are
beyond childhood, under 45, not
pregnant, basically healthy, take it for
only a short time and do not exceed
manufacturer's recommended dose.

Storage:
• Store in cool, dry area away from
  direct light, but don't freeze.
• Store safely out of reach of children.
• Don't store in bathroom medicine
  cabinet. Heat and moisture may
  change the action of the herb.

Safe dosage:
Consult your doctor for the
appropriate dose for your condition.

 ## Toxicity

Comparative-toxicity rating is not
available from standard references.

For symptoms of toxicity: See
*Adverse Reactions, Side Effects or
Overdose Symptoms* section below.

Adverse Reactions, Side Effects or Overdose Symptoms

Signs and symptoms	What to do
Coma	Seek emergency treatment.
Confusion	Discontinue. Call doctor immediately.
Convulsions	Seek emergency treatment.

Couch Grass (Dog Grass, Triticum)

Basic Information

Biological name (genus and species):
Agropyrum repens

Parts used for medicinal purposes:
Roots

Chemicals this herb contains:
- Dextrose
- Gum (see Glossary)
- Inosite
- Lactic acid
- Levulose
- Mannite
- Silica
- Vannilin

Known Effects

- Helps body dispose of excess fluid by increasing amount of urine produced
- If contaminated with ergot, causes constriction of blood vessels and muscular spasm of uterus

Miscellaneous information:
Couch grass is frequently contaminated with a poisonous fungus containing ergot. Discard any grass that has a black coating.

Possible Additional Effects

- May protect scraped tissues
- Potential nutrient
- May treat bladder infections
- May treat arthritis

Warnings and Precautions

Don't take if you:
- Are pregnant, think you may be pregnant or plan pregnancy in the near future
- Have any chronic disease of the gastrointestinal tract, such as stomach or duodenal ulcers, reflux esophagitis, ulcerative colitis, spastic colitis, diverticulosis or diverticulitis

Consult your doctor if you:

• Take this herb for any medical problem that doesn't improve in 2 weeks (There may be safer, more effective treatments.)

• Take any medicinal drugs or herbs including aspirin, laxatives, cold and cough remedies, antacids, vitamins, minerals, amino acids, supplements, other prescription or nonprescription drugs

Pregnancy:

Dangers outweigh any possible benefits. Don't use.

Breastfeeding:

Dangers outweigh any possible benefits. Don't use.

Infants and children:

Treating infants or children under 2 with any herbal preparation is hazardous.

Others:

No problems expected if you are beyond childhood, under 45, not pregnant, basically healthy, take it for only a short time and do not exceed manufacturer's recommended dose.

Storage:

• Store in cool, dry area away from direct light, but don't freeze.

• Store safely out of reach of children.

• Don't store in bathroom medicine cabinet. Heat and moisture may change the action of the herb.

Safe dosage:

Consult your doctor for the appropriate dose for your condition.

 Toxicity

Comparative-toxicity rating is not available from standard references.

For symptoms of toxicity: See *Adverse Reactions, Side Effects or Overdose Symptoms* section below.

 Adverse Reactions, Side Effects or Overdose Symptoms

Signs and symptoms	What to do
Only if contaminated with ergot:	
Coma	Seek emergency treatment.
Diarrhea	Discontinue. Call doctor when convenient.
Rapid, weak pulse	Seek emergency treatment.
Tingling, itching	Discontinue. Call doctor when convenient.
Unquenchable thirst	Discontinue. Call doctor immediately.
Vomiting	Discontinue. Call doctor immediately.

Cow Parsnip (Hogweed, Keck)

Basic Information

Biological name (genus and species):
Heracleum lanatum

Parts used for medicinal purposes:
- Fruit
- Leaves
- Roots
- Seeds

Chemicals this herb contains:
Volatile oils (see Glossary)

Known Effects

- Decreases thickness and increases fluidity of mucus in lungs and bronchial tubes
- Depresses central nervous system
- Decreases spasm of smooth muscle or skeletal muscle

Miscellaneous information:
Young plants may look like hemlock, which is poisonous.

Possible Additional Effects

Fruits and leaves are potential sedatives.

Warnings and Precautions

Don't take if you:
Are pregnant, think you may be pregnant or plan pregnancy in the near future.

Consult your doctor if you:
- Take this herb for any medical problem that doesn't improve in 2 weeks (There may be safer, more effective treatments.)
- Take any medicinal drugs or herbs including aspirin, laxatives, cold and cough remedies, antacids, vitamins, minerals, amino acids, supplements, other prescription or nonprescription drugs

Pregnancy:
Dangers outweigh any possible benefits. Don't use.

Breastfeeding:
Dangers outweigh any possible benefits. Don't use.

Infants and children:
Treating infants or children under 2 with any herbal preparation is hazardous.

Others:
No problems expected if you are beyond childhood, under 45, not pregnant, basically healthy, take it for only a short time and do not exceed manufacturer's recommended dose.

Storage:
- Store in cool, dry area away from direct light, but don't freeze.
- Store safely out of reach of children.
- Don't store in bathroom medicine cabinet. Heat and moisture may change the action of the herb.

Safe dosage:
Consult your doctor for the appropriate dose for your condition.

Toxicity

Comparative-toxicity rating is not available from standard references.

 Adverse Reactions, Side Effects or Overdose Symptoms

None are expected.

Cranesbill (Crowfoot)

 Basic Information

Biological name (genus and species):
Geranium maculatum

Parts used for medicinal purposes:
- Leaves
- Roots

Chemicals this herb contains:
- Coloring materials
- Gallic acid
- Gum (see Glossary)
- Pectin
- Starch
- Sugar
- Tannins (see Glossary)

 Known Effects

- Produces puckering
- Shrinks tissues
- Prevents secretion of fluids
- Interferes with absorption of iron and other minerals when taken internally

Miscellaneous information:
- Used as a mouthwash and a gargle for sore throat
- Used in traps to kill Japanese beetles (They die when they eat cranesbill leaves.)
- Used as a poultice (see Glossary)
- Occasionally used as a means of applying medications

 Possible Additional Effects

- May increase blood clotting
- Potential astringent
- May decrease nosebleeds
- May treat bleeding from stomach, mouth, intestines
- May treat diarrhea

 Warnings and Precautions

Don't take if you:
- Are pregnant, think you may be pregnant or plan pregnancy in the near future
- Have any chronic disease of the gastrointestinal tract, such as stomach or duodenal ulcers, reflux esophagitis, ulcerative colitis, spastic colitis, diverticulosis or diverticulitis

Consult your doctor if you:
- Take this herb for any medical problem that doesn't improve in 2 weeks (There may be safer, more effective treatments.)
- Take any medicinal drugs or herbs including aspirin, laxatives, cold and cough remedies, antacids, vitamins, minerals, amino acids, supplements, other prescription or nonprescription drugs

Pregnancy:
Don't use unless prescribed by
your doctor.

Breastfeeding:
Don't use unless prescribed by
your doctor.

Infants and children:
Treating infants or children under
2 with any herbal preparation
is hazardous.

Others:
No problems expected if you are
beyond childhood, under 45, not
pregnant, basically healthy, take it for
only a short time and do not exceed
manufacturer's recommended dose.

Storage:
• Store in cool, dry area away from
  direct light, but don't freeze.
• Store safely out of reach of children.
• Don't store in bathroom medicine
  cabinet. Heat and moisture may
  change the action of the herb.

Safe dosage:
Consult your doctor for the
appropriate dose for your condition.

Toxicity

Comparative-toxicity rating is not
available from standard references.

For symptoms of toxicity: See
*Adverse Reactions, Side Effects or
Overdose Symptom* section below.

Adverse Reactions, Side Effects or Overdose Symptoms

Signs and symptoms	What to do
Diarrhea	Discontinue. Call doctor immediately.
Kidney damage characterized by blood in urine, decreased urine flow, swelling of hands and feet	Seek emergency treatment.
Nausea or vomiting	Discontinue. Call doctor immediately.

Cubeb (Java Pepper, Tailed Pepper)

Basic Information

Biological name (genus and species):
Piper cubeba

Parts used for medicinal purposes:
Berries/fruits

Chemicals this herb contains:
• Cubebic acid
• Cubebin
• Fixed oil (see Glossary)
• Gum (see Glossary)
• Resin (see Glossary)
• Sesquiterpene alcohol
• Terpenes (see Glossary)
• Volatile oils (see Glossary)

Known Effects

Cubebic acid irritates the ureter,
bladder and urethra.

Miscellaneous information:
Active chemicals are in fully grown,
unripe fruit.

➔

Possible
Additional Effects

- May help body dispose of excess fluid by increasing amount of urine produced
- Potential urinary antiseptic
- May decrease thickness and increase fluidity of mucus in lungs and bronchial tubes
- May help expel gas from intestinal tract

 Warnings and
Precautions

Don't take if you:

- Are pregnant, think you may be pregnant or plan pregnancy in the near future
- Have any chronic disease of the gastrointestinal tract, such as stomach or duodenal ulcers, reflux esophagitis, ulcerative colitis, spastic colitis, diverticulosis or diverticulitis

Consult your doctor if you:

- Take this herb for any medical problem that doesn't improve in 2 weeks (There may be safer, more effective treatments.)
- Have chronic intestinal disease; cubeb may make it worse

Pregnancy:
Don't use unless prescribed by your doctor.

Breastfeeding:
Don't use unless prescribed by your doctor.

Infants and children:
Treating infants or children under 2 with any herbal preparation is hazardous.

Others:
No problems expected if you are beyond childhood, under 45, not pregnant, basically healthy, take it for only a short time and do not exceed manufacturer's recommended dose.

Storage:

- Store in cool, dry area away from direct light, but don't freeze.
- Store safely out of reach of children.
- Don't store in bathroom medicine cabinet. Heat and moisture may change the action of the herb.

Safe dosage:
Consult your doctor for the appropriate dose for your condition.

 Toxicity

Comparative-toxicity rating is not available from standard references.

For symptoms of toxicity: See *Adverse Reactions, Side Effects or Overdose Symptoms* section below.

 Adverse Reactions,
Side Effects or
Overdose Symptoms

Signs and symptoms	What to do
Nausea or vomiting	Discontinue. Call doctor immediately.

Damiana

 Basic Information

Biological name (genus and species):
Turnera diffusa

Parts used for medicinal purposes:
Leaves

Chemicals this herb contains:
• Arbutin
• Chlorophyll
• Damianian
• Resin (see Glossary)
• Starch
• Sugar
• Tannins (see Glossary)
• Volatile oils (see Glossary)

 Known Effects

No proven medicinal effects are known.

Miscellaneous information:
• Tastes very bitter
• Used as food additive in baked goods and liqueurs

 Possible Additional Effects

• Used as an aphrodisiac
• May alleviate headaches
• May reduce depression, anxiety or listlessness
• May improve sexual potency
• Used as a mild laxative

 Warnings and Precautions

Don't take if you:
• Are pregnant, think you may be pregnant or plan pregnancy in the near future
• Have any chronic disease of the gastrointestinal tract, such as stomach or duodenal ulcers, reflux esophagitis, ulcerative colitis, spastic colitis, diverticulosis or diverticulitis
• Have kidney or urinary tract disease

Consult your doctor if you:
• Take this herb for any medical problem that doesn't improve in 2 weeks (There may be safer, more effective treatments.)
• Take any medicinal drugs or herbs including aspirin, laxatives, cold and cough remedies, antacids, vitamins, minerals, amino acids, supplements, other prescription or nonprescription drugs

Pregnancy:
Don't use.

Breastfeeding:
Don't use.

Infants and children:
Treating infants or children under 2 with any herbal preparation is hazardous.

Others:
No problems expected if you are beyond childhood, under 45, not pregnant, basically healthy, take it for only a short time and do not exceed manufacturer's recommended dose.

Storage:
• Store in cool, dry area away from direct light, but don't freeze.
• Store safely out of reach of children.
• Don't store in bathroom medicine cabinet. Heat and moisture may change the action of the herb.

Safe dosage:
Consult your doctor for the appropriate dose for your condition.

Toxicity

Rated relatively safe when taken in appropriate quantities for short periods of time

For symptoms of toxicity: See *Adverse Reactions, Side Effects or Overdose Symptoms* section below.

Adverse Reactions, Side Effects or Overdose Symptoms

Signs and symptoms	What to do
No documented cases reported. Theoretically:	
Change in urinary frequency	Discontinue. Call doctor when convenient.
Diarrhea	Discontinue. Call doctor immediately.
Headache	Discontinue. Call doctor immediately.
Insomnia	Discontinue. Call doctor immediately.
Nausea or vomiting	Discontinue. Call doctor immediately.

Dandelion

Basic Information

Biological name (genus and species): *Taraxacum officinale*

Parts used for medicinal purposes:
• Leaves
• Roots
• Young tops

Chemicals this herb contains:
• Bitters (see Glossary)
• Fats
• Gluten
• Gum (see Glossary)
• Inulin
• Iron
• Niacin
• Potash
• Proteins
• Resin (see Glossary)
• Taraxacerin
• Vitamins A, B, C and E

Known Effects

No proven medicinal effects are known.

Possible Additional Effects

• May treat dyspepsia
• May treat constipation
• May treat hepatitis
• May treat jaundice
• May treat rheumatism
• May treat anemia
• Potential diuretic
• May stimulate appetite

Warnings and Precautions

Don't take if you:
Are pregnant, think you may be pregnant or plan pregnancy in the near future.

Consult your doctor if you:

- Take this herb for any medical problem that doesn't improve in 2 weeks (There may be safer, more effective treatments.)
- Take any medicinal drugs or herbs including aspirin, laxatives, cold and cough remedies, antacids, vitamins, minerals, amino acids, supplements, other prescription or nonprescription drugs

Pregnancy:

Don't use unless prescribed by your doctor.

Breastfeeding:

Don't use unless prescribed by your doctor.

Infants and children:

Treating infants or children under 2 with any herbal preparation is hazardous.

Others:

No problems expected if you are beyond childhood, under 45, not pregnant, basically healthy, take it for only a short time and do not exceed manufacturer's recommended dose.

Storage:

- Store in cool, dry area away from direct light, but don't freeze.
- Store safely out of reach of children.
- Don't store in bathroom medicine cabinet. Heat and moisture may change the action of the herb.

Safe dosage:

Consult your doctor for the appropriate dose for your condition.

Toxicity

Dandelion is generally regarded as safe when taken in appropriate quantities for short periods of time.

For symptoms of toxicity: See *Adverse Reactions, Side Effects or Overdose Symptoms* section below.

Adverse Reactions, Side Effects or Overdose Symptoms

Signs and symptoms	What to do
Heartburn and diarrhea (rare)	Discontinue. Call doctor when convenient.

Dong Quai (Chinese Angelica, Dang Gui, Tank Kwei)

Basic Information

Biological name (genus and species):
Angelica sinensis

Parts used for medicinal purposes:

- Rhizomes
- Root

Chemicals this herb contains:

- Coumarins
- Vitamin B-12
- Volatile oils (see Glossary)

Known Effects

- Treats menstrual irregularity
- Reduces pain of menstrual cramps

➜

Miscellaneous information:
Available as teas, tablets and alcohol extracts.

Possible Additional Effects

- May lower blood pressure
- Potential muscle relaxant
- May reduce menopausal symptoms, including hot flashes
- May improve circulation
- May relax bowel
- Potential anti-inflammatory
- May inhibit platelet aggregation, thus protecting against heart disease

Warnings and Precautions

Don't take if you:
- Are pregnant, think you may be pregnant or plan pregnancy in the near future
- Take medication for high blood pressure
- If you are prone to heavy menstrual flow
- Plan to have surgery in 2 weeks or less, due to risk of increased bleeding time

Consult your doctor if you:
- Use this herb at all
- Take this herb for any medical problem that doesn't improve in 2 weeks (There may be safer, more effective treatments.)
- Take any medicinal drugs or herbs including aspirin, laxatives, cold and cough remedies, antacids, vitamins, minerals, amino acids, supplements, other prescription or nonprescription drugs

Pregnancy:
Don't use unless prescribed by your doctor.

Breastfeeding:
Don't use unless prescribed by your doctor.

Infants and children:
Treating infants or children under 2 with any herbal preparation is hazardous.

Others:
Use caution if taking with other blood-thinning medicines or herbs.

Storage:
- Store in cool, dry area away from direct light, but don't freeze.
- Store safely out of reach of children.
- Don't store in bathroom medicine cabinet. Heat and moisture may change the action of the herb.

Safe dosage:
4 to 7 grams (200mg), 3 times daily between meals.

Toxicity

Comparative-toxicity rating is not available from standard references.

For symptoms of toxicity: See *Adverse Reactions, Side Effects or Overdose Symptoms* section below.

Adverse Reactions, Side Effects or Overdose Symptoms

Signs and symptoms	What to do
Diarrhea	Discontinue. Call doctor immediately.
Irritability, restlessness	Discontinue. Call doctor when convenient.
Nausea	Discontinue. Call doctor immediately.

Echinacea (Purple Coneflower)

 Basic Information

Biological name (genus and species):
Echinacea angustifolia, E. pallida

Parts used for medicinal purposes:
Various parts of the entire plant,
frequently differing by country or
culture

Chemicals this herb contains:
- Alkaloids
- Echinacoside
- Flavonoids (see Glossary)
- Isobutyl amides
- Polyacetylenes
- Polysaccharides
- Volatile oils (see Glossary)

 Known Effects

Stimulates the immune system

Miscellaneous information:
Another herb, *Rudbeckia laciniata,* is
also called *coneflower* and has been
reported to be toxic. If you take any
coneflower, be sure it is *Echinacea
angustifolia.*

 Possible Additional Effects

- Potential natural antitoxin for
  internal and external infections
- May relieve symptoms of cold
  and flu
- May help heal wounds
- Possible antitumor activity
- May increase immune function after
  cancer treatment

 Warnings and Precautions

Don't take if you:
- Are pregnant, think you may be
  pregnant or plan pregnancy in the
  near future
- Have tuberculosis, multiple sclerosis
  or collagen disease
- Have been diagnosed with an
  autoimmune disease, such as
  pernicious anemia

Consult your doctor if you:
- Take this herb for any medical
  problem that doesn't improve in
  2 weeks (There may be safer, more
  effective treatments.)
- Take any medicinal drugs or
  herbs including aspirin, laxatives,
  cold and cough remedies, antacids,
  vitamins, minerals, amino acids,
  supplements, other prescription
  or nonprescription drugs
- Are a transplant patient

Pregnancy:
Don't use unless prescribed by
your doctor.

Breastfeeding:
Don't use unless prescribed by
your doctor.

Infants and children:
Treating infants or children under
2 with any herbal preparation
is hazardous.

Others:
No problems expected if you are
beyond childhood, under 45, not
pregnant, basically healthy, take it for
only a short time and do not exceed
manufacturer's recommended dose.

Storage:

- Store in cool, dry area away from direct light, but don't freeze.
- Store safely out of reach of children.
- Don't store in bathroom medicine cabinet. Heat and moisture may change the action of the herb.

Safe dosage:

- Consult your doctor for the appropriate dose for your condition.
- More effective if used intermittently at first symptoms of an illness and only for 6 weeks or less.

Toxicity

Comparative-toxicity rating is not available from standard references.

For symptoms of toxicity: See *Adverse Reactions, Side Effects or Overdose Symptoms* section below.

Adverse Reactions, Side Effects or Overdose Symptoms

Signs and symptoms	What to do
Dermatitis (in sensitive patients)	Discontinue. Call doctor when convenient.

Elderberry (Elder)

Basic Information

Biological name (genus and species): *Sambucus nigra*

Parts used for medicinal purposes:

- Bark
- Berries/fruits
- Inner bark
- Leaves

Chemicals this herb contains:

- Albumin
- Cyanide
- Hydrocyanic acid
- Resin (see Glossary)
- Rutin
- Sambucine
- Sambunigrin (found in stem; breaks down to cyanide)
- Tannic acid

- Tyrosine
- Viburnic acid
- Vitamin C
- Volatile oils (see Glossary)
- Wax (see Glossary)

Known Effects

- Irritates the gastrointestinal tract and acts as a laxative and purgative
- Causes vomiting (sometimes)

Miscellaneous information:

Stems contain cyanide and can be extremely toxic.

Possible Additional Effects

- May help treat headache
- May help treat arthritis
- May help treat gout

- May help treat the common cold
- May help treat fevers
- May help treat sore throat
- May ease discomfort of menstrual cramps
- May promote healing of bruises and sprains when used as a poultice (see Glossary)
- May help treat skin irritations

Warnings and Precautions

Don't take if you:

- Are pregnant, think you may be pregnant or plan pregnancy in the near future
- Have any chronic disease of the gastrointestinal tract, such as stomach or duodenal ulcers, reflux esophagitis, ulcerative colitis, spastic colitis, diverticulosis or diverticulitis

Consult your doctor if you:

- Take this herb for any medical problem that doesn't improve in 2 weeks (There may be safer, more effective treatments.)
- Take any medicinal drugs or herbs including aspirin, laxatives, cold and cough remedies, antacids, vitamins, minerals, amino acids, supplements, other prescription or nonprescription drugs

Pregnancy:

Dangers outweigh any possible benefits. Don't use.

Breastfeeding:

Dangers outweigh any possible benefits. Don't use.

Infants and children:

Treating infants or children under 2 with any herbal preparation is hazardous.

Others:

- Ripe berries are probably nontoxic. They should be eaten only after cooking.
- Beware of stems. Enough cyanide from them could be fatal.

Storage:

- Store in cool, dry area away from direct light, but don't freeze.
- Store safely out of reach of children.
- Don't store in bathroom medicine cabinet. Heat and moisture may change the action of the herb.

Safe dosage:

Consult your doctor for the appropriate dose for your condition.

Toxicity

- Elderberry is rated slightly dangerous, particularly in children, persons over 55 and those who take larger than appropriate quantities for extended periods of time.
- Raw seeds are toxic.
- Roots, stems and leaves can cause cyanide poisoning.

For symptoms of toxicity: See *Adverse Reactions, Side Effects or Overdose Symptoms* section below.

Adverse Reactions, Side Effects or Overdose Symptoms

Signs and symptoms	What to do
Abdominal pain	Discontinue. Call doctor immediately.
Diarrhea	Discontinue. Call doctor immediately.
Nausea or vomiting	Discontinue. Call doctor immediately.

Evening Primrose

Basic Information

Biological name (genus and species):
Oenothera biennis

Parts used for medicinal purposes:
Oil from seeds

Chemicals this herb contains:
Gamma linolenic acid (GLA)

Known Effects

- Anti-inflammatory
- Reduces high blood pressure
- Treats atopic eczema

Possible Additional Effects

- Potential muscle relaxant
- May reduce effects of premenstrual syndrome (PMS)
- May lubricate hair, eyes, nails
- May treat all forms of eczema and other skin disorders
- Potential anticoagulant
- Potential astringent

Warnings and Precautions

Don't take if you:
- Are pregnant, think you may be pregnant or plan pregnancy in the near future
- Take medication for high blood pressure
- Are prone to heavy menstrual flow
- Are taking anticoagulant drugs (such as warfarin/coumadin)

Consult your doctor if you:
- Take this herb for any medical problem that doesn't improve in 2 weeks (There may be safer, more effective treatments.)
- Take any medicinal drugs or herbs including aspirin, laxatives, cold and cough remedies, antacids, vitamins, minerals, amino acids, supplements, other prescription or nonprescription drugs

Pregnancy:
Don't use unless prescribed by your doctor.

Breastfeeding:
Don't use unless prescribed by your doctor.

Infants and children:
Treating infants or children under 2 with any herbal preparation is hazardous.

Storage:
- Store in cool, dry area away from direct light, but don't freeze.
- Store safely out of reach of children.
- Don't store in bathroom medicine cabinet. Heat and moisture may change the action of the herb.

Safe dosage:
Consult your doctor for the appropriate dose for your condition.

Toxicity

Comparative-toxicity rating is not available from standard references.

For symptoms of toxicity: See *Adverse Reactions, Side Effects or Overdose Symptoms* section below.

Adverse Reactions,
Side Effects or
Overdose Symptoms

Signs and symptoms	What to do
Abdominal discomfort	Discontinue. Call doctor when convenient.
Headache	Discontinue. Call doctor when convenient.
Nausea	Discontinue. Call doctor when convenient.
Skin rash	Discontinue. Call doctor when convenient.

Eyebright

 Basic Information

Biological name (genus and species):
Euphrasia officinalis

Parts used for medicinal purposes:
Entire plant, except roots

Chemicals this herb contains:
- Bitters (see Glossary)
- Pantothenic acid
- Tannins (see Glossary)
- Vitamins A, B-12, C, E and D
- Volatile oils (see Glossary)

 Known Effects

Reduces inflammation

 Possible
Additional Effects

Internal use:
- May treat nasal congestion
- May treat cough
- May treat sinusitis
- May treat allergies

External use:
- Used as an eyewash to relieve discomfort caused from eyestrain or minor irritation
- May treat conjunctivitis

 Warnings and
Precautions

Don't take if you:
Are pregnant, think you may be pregnant or plan pregnancy in the near future.

Consult your doctor if you:
- Take this herb for any medical problem that doesn't improve in 2 weeks (There may be safer, more effective treatments.)
- Take any medicinal drugs or herbs including aspirin, laxatives, cold and cough remedies, antacids, vitamins, minerals, amino acids, supplements, other prescription or nonprescription drugs

→

Pregnancy:
Don't use unless prescribed by your doctor.

Breastfeeding:
Don't use unless prescribed by your doctor.

Infants and children:
Treating infants or children under 2 with any herbal preparation is hazardous.

Others:
No problems expected if you are beyond childhood, under 45, not pregnant, basically healthy, take it for only a short time and do not exceed manufacturer's recommended dose.

Storage:
- Store in cool, dry area away from direct light, but don't freeze.
- Store safely out of reach of children.
- Don't store in bathroom medicine cabinet. Heat and moisture may change the action of the herb.

Safe dosage:
Consult your doctor for the appropriate dose for your condition.

 Toxicity

Rated relatively safe when taken in appropriate quantities for short periods of time

For symptoms of toxicity: See *Adverse Reactions, Side Effects or Overdose Symptoms* section below.

 Adverse Reactions, Side Effects or Overdose Symptoms

Signs and symptoms	What to do
Nausea	Discontinue. Call doctor immediately.
Skin rash	Discontinue. Call doctor when convenient.

Fennel (Finocchio)

 Basic Information

Biological name (genus and species):
Foeniculum vulgare

Parts used for medicinal purposes:
- Berries/fruits
- Roots
- Stems

Chemicals this herb contains:
- Anethole
- Fixed oil (see Glossary)
- Volatile oils (see Glossary)

 Known Effects

- Helps expel gas from intestinal tract
- Stimulates respiration
- Increases stomach acidity
- Treats dyspepsia
- Helps treat common colds
- Treats coughs
- Treats colic

Miscellaneous information:
- Used as a flavoring
- Available in dry bulk, oil and tinctures

Possible Additional Effects

May treat diarrhea

Warnings and Precautions

Don't take if you:

- Are pregnant, think you may be pregnant or plan pregnancy in the near future
- Have any chronic disease of the gastrointestinal tract, such as stomach or duodenal ulcers, reflux esophagitis, ulcerative colitis, spastic colitis, diverticulosis or diverticulitis

Consult your doctor if you:

- Take this herb for any medical problem that doesn't improve in 2 weeks (There may be safer, more effective treatments.)
- Take any medicinal drugs or herbs including aspirin, laxatives, cold and cough remedies, antacids, vitamins, minerals, amino acids, supplements, other prescription or nonprescription drugs

Pregnancy:

Dangers outweigh any possible benefits. Don't use.

Breastfeeding:

Dangers outweigh any possible benefits. Don't use.

Infants and children:

Treating infants or children under 2 with any herbal preparation is hazardous.

Others:

No problems expected if you are beyond childhood, under 45, not pregnant, basically healthy, take it for only a short time and do not exceed manufacturer's recommended dose.

Storage:

- Store in cool, dry area away from direct light, but don't freeze.
- Store safely out of reach of children.
- Don't store in bathroom medicine cabinet. Heat and moisture may change the action of the herb.

Safe dosage:

Consult your doctor for the appropriate dose for your condition.

Toxicity

Generally regarded as safe when taken in appropriate quantities for short periods of time

For symptoms of toxicity: See
Adverse Reactions, Side Effects or Overdose Symptoms section below.

Adverse Reactions, Side Effects or Overdose Symptoms

Signs and symptoms	What to do
Oil extracted from fennel may cause	
Congestive heart failure	Seek emergency treatment.
Nausea or vomiting	Discontinue. Call doctor immediately.
Rash	Discontinue. Call doctor when convenient.
Seizures	Seek emergency treatment.

Fenugreek

 Basic Information

Biological name (genus and species):
Trigonella foenumgraecum

Parts used for medicinal purposes:
Seeds

Chemicals this herb contains:
- Choline
- Fixed oil (see Glossary)
- Iron
- Lecithin
- Mucilage (see Glossary)
- Phosphates (see Glossary)
- Protein
- Trigonelline
- Trimethylamine
- Volatile oils (see Glossary)

 Known Effects

- Increases stomach acidity
- Reduces sore throat

Miscellaneous information:
- Fenugreek has a disagreeable odor and bitter taste.
- It is prescribed frequently by veterinarians, particularly for horses.
- Fenugreek is available in bulk seeds, capsules and tinctures.

 Possible Additional Effects

- Potential bulk laxative (seeds)
- May protect scraped tissues
- May reduce arthritic pain
- May promote lactation

 Warnings and Precautions

Don't take if you:
Are pregnant, think you may be pregnant or plan pregnancy in the near future.

Consult your doctor if you:
- Take this herb for any medical problem that doesn't improve in 2 weeks (There may be safer, more effective treatments.)
- Take any medicinal drugs or herbs including aspirin, laxatives, cold and cough remedies, antacids, vitamins, minerals, amino acids, supplements, other prescription or nonprescription drugs

Pregnancy:
Don't use unless prescribed by your doctor.

Breastfeeding:
Don't use unless prescribed by your doctor.

Infants and children:
Treating infants or children under 2 with any herbal preparation is hazardous.

Storage:
- Store in cool, dry area away from direct light, but don't freeze.
- Store safely out of reach of children.
- Don't store in bathroom medicine cabinet. Heat and moisture may change the action of the herb.

Safe dosage:
Consult your doctor for the appropriate dose for your condition.

Toxicity

Rated relatively safe when taken in appropriate quantities for short periods of time

Adverse Reactions, Side Effects or Overdose Symptoms

None are expected.

Feverfew (Altamisa, Bachelor's Buttons)

Basic Information

Biological name (genus and species): *Tanacetum parthenium*

Parts used for medicinal purposes:
• Bark
• Dried flowers
• Leaves

Chemicals this herb contains:
• Parthenolide
• Pyrethrins
• Santamarin
• Volatile oils (see Glossary)

Known Effects

• Decreases thickness and increases fluidity of mucus in lungs and bronchial tubes
• Lessens severity and reduces frequency of migraine attacks
• Antispasmodic

Possible Additional Effects

Leaves:
• May treat menstrual disorders
• May treat common cold
• May treat indigestion and diarrhea
• May stimulate appetite

Dried flowers:
• May treat intestinal parasites (worms)
• Potential aid in expelling gas from intestinal tract
• May relieve arthritis
• Potential anti-inflammatory
• May reduce fever

Warnings and Precautions

Don't take if you:
• Are allergic to pyrethrins
• Are pregnant, think you may be pregnant or plan pregnancy in the near future

Consult your doctor if you:
• Take this herb for any medical problem that doesn't improve in 2 weeks (There may be safer, more effective treatments.)
• Take any medicinal drugs or herbs including aspirin, laxatives, cold and cough remedies, antacids, vitamins, minerals, amino acids, supplements, other prescription or nonprescription drugs

Pregnancy:
Don't use.

Breastfeeding:
Don't use.

Infants and children:
Treating infants or children under 2 with any herbal preparation is hazardous.

Others:
Chewing leaves may cause mouth sores.

Storage:
- Store in cool, dry area away from direct light, but don't freeze.
- Store safely out of reach of children.
- Don't store in bathroom medicine cabinet. Heat and moisture may change the action of the herb.

Safe dosage:
- Consult your doctor for the appropriate dose for your condition.
- Pause occasionally in your treatment to enhance long-term efficacy.

 Toxicity

Feverfew is generally regarded as safe when taken in very small quantities for short periods of time.

For symptoms of toxicity: See *Adverse Reactions, Side Effects or Overdose Symptoms* section below.

 Adverse Reactions, Side Effects or Overdose Symptoms

Signs and symptoms	What to do
Abdominal pain	Seek medical care.
Internal mouth sores	Seek medical care.
Life-threatening anaphylaxis may follow injections—symptoms include immediate severe itching, paleness, low blood pressure, loss of consciousness, coma	Yell for help. Don't leave victim. Begin CPR (cardiopulmonary resuscitation), mouth-to-mouth breathing and external cardiac massage. Have someone dial 0 (operator) or 911 (emergency). Don't stop CPR until help arrives.

Flax (Linseed)

 Basic Information

Biological name (genus and species):
Linum usitatissimum

Parts used for medicinal purposes:
- Oil
- Seeds

Chemicals this herb contains:
- Fixed oil (see Glossary)
- Glycosides (see Glossary)
- Gum (see Glossary)
- Linamarin
- Linoleic acid
- Linolenic acid
- Mucilage (see Glossary)
- Protein
- Tannins (see Glossary)
- Wax (see Glossary)

 Known Effects

- Treats skin disorders
- Forms bulk in intestinal tract
- Anti-inflammatory
- Laxative
- Contains essential fatty acids

Miscellaneous information:
- Purification has improved
- Increasingly being used in cereal, grain products
- Good for increasing fiber in your diet

Possible Additional Effects

- May ease symptoms of menopause
- May reduce cholesterol and triglyceride levels
- May soothe coughs
- Oil may soften or smooth skin
- Used for poultices (see Glossary) to apply to chest for colds and coughs
- May treat burns when applied externally
- May protect scraped tissues
- May reduce inflammation associated with arthritis
- May stimulate immune system

Warnings and Precautions

Don't take if you:
- Are pregnant, think you may be pregnant or plan pregnancy in the near future
- Are on anticoagulant therapy

Consult your doctor if you:
- Take this herb for any medical problem that doesn't improve in 2 weeks (There may be safer, more effective treatments.)
- Take any medicinal drugs or herbs including aspirin, laxatives, cold and cough remedies, antacids, vitamins, minerals, amino acids, supplements, other prescription or nonprescription drugs

Pregnancy:
Dangers outweigh any possible benefits. Don't use.

Breastfeeding:
Dangers outweigh any possible benefits. Don't use.

Infants and children:
Treating infants or children under 2 with any herbal preparation is hazardous.

Others:
No problems expected if you are beyond childhood, under 45, not pregnant, basically healthy, take it for only a short time and do not exceed manufacturer's recommended dose.

Storage:
- Store in cool, dry area away from direct light, but don't freeze.
- Store safely out of reach of children.
- Don't store in bathroom medicine cabinet. Heat and moisture may change the action of the herb.

Safe dosage:
Consult your doctor for the appropriate dose for your condition.

Toxicity

Comparative-toxicity rating is not available from standard references.

Adverse Reactions, Side Effects or Overdose Symptoms

None are expected.

Fritillaria (Bei Mu, Snake's Head)

Basic Information

Biological name (genus and species):
Fritillaria verticillata, F. meleagris

Parts used for medicinal purposes:
Roots

Chemicals this herb contains:
- Fritilline
- Fritimine
- Peimine
- Peiminine
- Verticilline
- Verticine

(Peimine and peiminine may resemble steroid hormones.)

Known Effects

No proven medicinal effects are known.

Possible Additional Effects

- May affect the electrical system of the heart (because of peimine and peiminine)
- May reduce fevers
- May decrease thickness and increase fluidity of mucus in lungs and bronchial tubes
- May increase flow of breast milk in lactating women
- May decrease blood pressure
- May increase blood sugar

Warnings and Precautions

Don't take if you:
- Are pregnant, think you may be pregnant or plan pregnancy in the near future
- Have heart disease

Consult your doctor if you:
- Take this herb for any medical problem that doesn't improve in 2 weeks (There may be safer, more effective treatments.)
- Take any medicinal drugs or herbs including aspirin, laxatives, cold and cough remedies, antacids, vitamins, minerals, amino acids, supplements, other prescription or nonprescription drugs

Pregnancy:
Dangers outweigh any possible benefits. Don't use.

Breastfeeding:
Dangers outweigh any possible benefits. Don't use.

Infants and children:
Treating infants or children under 2 with any herbal preparation is hazardous.

Others:
No problems expected if you are beyond childhood, under 45, not pregnant, basically healthy, take it for only a short time and do not exceed manufacturer's recommended dose.

Storage:
- Store in cool, dry area away from direct light, but don't freeze.

- Store safely out of reach of children.
- Don't store in bathroom medicine cabinet. Heat and moisture may change the action of the herb.

Safe dosage:
Consult your doctor for the appropriate dose for your condition.

Toxicity

Comparative-toxicity rating is not available from standard references.

For symptoms of toxicity: See *Adverse Reactions, Side Effects or Overdose Symptoms* section below.

Adverse Reactions, Side Effects or Overdose Symptoms

Signs and symptoms	What to do
Heart block characterized by slow heart rate (below 50)	Seek emergency treatment.
Heartbeat irregularity	Discontinue. Call doctor immediately.

Galanga Major & Minor
(Chinese Ginger, India Root)

Basic Information

Biological name (genus and species):
Alpinia galanga, A. officinarum

Parts used for medicinal purposes:
Various parts of the entire plant, frequently differing by country and culture

Chemicals this herb contains:
- Cineole
- Galangin
- Galangol
- Kaempferid
- Resin (see Glossary)
- Volatile oils (see Glossary)

Known Effects

Antibacterial effect acts against bacterial germs, such as streptococci, staphylococci and coliform bacteria.

Miscellaneous information:
- Related botanically and pharmacologically to ginger
- Used by ancient Greeks and Arabs

Possible Additional Effects

- May help expel gas from intestinal tract
- May treat impotence
- May reduce excess phlegm caused by allergies
- May treat painful teeth and gums
- May stimulate respiration

Warnings and Precautions

Don't take if you:
- Are pregnant, think you may be pregnant or plan pregnancy in the near future

➜

- Have any chronic disease of the gastrointestinal tract, such as stomach or duodenal ulcers, reflux esophagitis, ulcerative colitis, spastic colitis, diverticulosis or diverticulitis

Consult your doctor if you:
- Take this herb for any medical problem that doesn't improve in 2 weeks (There may be safer, more effective treatments.)
- Take any medicinal drugs or herbs including aspirin, laxatives, cold and cough remedies, antacids, vitamins, minerals, amino acids, supplements, other prescription or nonprescription drugs

Pregnancy:
Don't use unless prescribed by your doctor.

Breastfeeding:
Don't use unless prescribed by your doctor.

Infants and children:
Treating infants or children under 2 with any herbal preparation is hazardous.

Others:
No problems expected if you are beyond childhood, under 45, not pregnant, basically healthy, take it for only a short time and do not exceed manufacturer's recommended dose.

Storage:
- Store in cool, dry area away from direct light, but don't freeze.
- Store safely out of reach of children.
- Don't store in bathroom medicine cabinet. Heat and moisture may change the action of the herb.

Safe dosage:
Consult your doctor for the appropriate dose for your condition.

Toxicity

Comparative-toxicity rating is not available from standard references.

For symptoms of toxicity: See *Adverse Reactions, Side Effects or Overdose Symptoms* section below.

Adverse Reactions, Side Effects or Overdose Symptoms

Signs and symptoms	What to do
Diarrhea	Discontinue. Call doctor immediately.
Nausea or vomiting	Discontinue. Call doctor immediately.

Galega (European Goat Rue)

Basic Information

Biological name (genus and species):
Galega officinalis

Parts used for medicinal purposes:
Various parts of the entire plant, frequently differing by country and culture

Chemicals this herb contains:
- Bitters (see Glossary)
- Galegine
- Tannins (see Glossary)

Known Effects

- Reduces blood sugar
- Interferes with absorption of iron and other minerals when taken internally

Miscellaneous information:
Plant smells bad when it is bruised.

Possible Additional Effects

- May treat diabetes
- May increase flow of breast milk in lactating women

Warnings and Precautions

Don't take if you:
Are pregnant, think you may be pregnant or plan pregnancy in the near future.

Consult your doctor if you:
- Take this herb for any medical problem that doesn't improve in 2 weeks (There may be safer, more effective treatments.)
- Take any medicinal drugs or herbs including aspirin, laxatives, cold and cough remedies, antacids, vitamins, minerals, amino acids, supplements, other prescription or nonprescription drugs

Pregnancy:
Don't use unless prescribed by your doctor.

Breastfeeding:
Don't use unless prescribed by your doctor.

Infants and children:
Treating infants or children under 2 with any herbal preparation is hazardous.

Others:
No problems expected if you are beyond childhood, under 45, not pregnant, basically healthy, take it for only a short time and do not exceed manufacturer's recommended dose.

Storage:
- Store in cool, dry area away from direct light, but don't freeze.
- Store safely out of reach of children.
- Don't store in bathroom medicine cabinet. Heat and moisture may change the action of the herb.

Safe dosage:
Consult your doctor for the appropriate dose for your condition.

Toxicity

Comparative-toxicity rating is not available from standard references.

For symptoms of toxicity: See *Adverse Reactions, Side Effects or Overdose Symptoms* section below.

Adverse Reactions, Side Effects or Overdose Symptoms

Signs and symptoms	What to do
Headache	Discontinue. Call doctor when convenient.
Jitters	Discontinue. Call doctor when convenient.
Weakness	Discontinue. Call doctor immediately.

Gambier (Gambir, Pale Catechu)

Basic Information

Biological name (genus and species):
Uncaria gambir

Parts used for medicinal purposes:
• Leaves
• Twigs

Chemicals this herb contains:
• Catechin
• Catechu-tannic acid
• Tannins (see Glossary)

Known Effects

• Shrinks tissues
• Prevents secretion of fluids
• Interferes with absorption of iron and other minerals when taken internally

Possible Additional Effects

• May decrease unusual bleeding
• May treat chronic diarrhea
• May treat sore throats as a gargle

Warnings and Precautions

Don't take if you:
Have any chronic disease of the gastrointestinal tract, such as stomach or duodenal ulcers, reflux esophagitis, ulcerative colitis, spastic colitis, diverticulosis or diverticulitis.

Consult your doctor if you:
• Take this herb for any medical problem that doesn't improve in 2 weeks (There may be safer, more effective treatments.)
• Take any medicinal drugs or herbs including aspirin, laxatives, cold and cough remedies, antacids, vitamins, minerals, amino acids, supplements, other prescription or nonprescription drugs

Pregnancy:
Dangers outweigh any possible benefits. Don't use.

Breastfeeding:
Dangers outweigh any possible benefits. Don't use.

Infants and children:
Treating infants or children under 2 with any herbal preparation is hazardous.

Storage:
• Store in cool, dry area away from direct light, but don't freeze.
• Store safely out of reach of children.
• Don't store in bathroom medicine cabinet. Heat and moisture may change the action of the herb.

Safe dosage:
Consult your doctor for the appropriate dose for your condition.

Toxicity

Rated relatively safe when taken in appropriate quantities for short periods of time

For symptoms of toxicity: See *Adverse Reactions, Side Effects or Overdose Symptoms* section below.

Adverse Reactions, Side Effects or Overdose Symptoms

Signs and symptoms	What to do
Diarrhea	Discontinue. Call doctor immediately.
Kidney damage characterized by blood in urine, decreased urine flow, swelling of hands and feet	Seek emergency treatment.
Vomiting	Discontinue. Call doctor immediately.

Garlic

Basic Information

Biological name (genus and species):
Allium sativum

Parts used for medicinal purposes:
Bulb

Chemicals this herb contains:
- Allicin
- Allyl disulfides
- Iron
- Magnesium
- Manganese
- Phytoncides
- Potassium
- Selenium
- Sulfur
- Unsaturated aldehydes
- Vitamins A, B-1 and C
- Volatile oils (see Glossary)

Known Effects
- Protects against infection
- Relieves indigestion
- Decreases thickness and increases fluidity of mucus in lungs and bronchial tubes
- Helps body dispose of excess fluid by increasing amount of urine produced
- Promotes blood-pressure control
- Decreases cholesterol in hypercholesterolemic (see Glossary) males
- Antioxidant
- Antiviral and antibacterial
- Reduces platelet aggregation
- Anticoagulant

Miscellaneous information:
- Garlic is used as a condiment.
- Avoid using garlic as a medicinal herb in any amount for children!
- It is acceptable to use garlic as a flavoring in children's food.

Possible Additional Effects
- May treat cramping, abdominal pain in adults
- May inhibit certain forms of cancer
- May redden skin by increasing blood flow to it

→

- May treat sinusitis
- May improve circulation
- May treat burns when used externally as a moist pulp

Warnings and Precautions

Don't take if you:
Are being treated for any medical problem—consult your doctor first.

Consult your doctor if you:
- Take this herb for any medical problem that doesn't improve in 2 weeks (There may be safer, more effective treatments.)
- Take any medicinal drugs or herbs including aspirin, laxatives, cold and cough remedies, antacids, vitamins, minerals, amino acids, supplements, anticoagulants or other prescription or nonprescription drugs

Pregnancy:
Don't use unless prescribed by your doctor.

Breastfeeding:
Don't use unless prescribed by your doctor.

Infants and children:
Treating infants or children under 2 with any herbal preparation is hazardous.

Storage:
- Store in cool, dry area away from direct light, but don't freeze.
- Store safely out of reach of children.
- Don't store in bathroom medicine cabinet. Heat and moisture may

change the action of the herb.

Safe dosage:
- Limit intake to 5 cloves a day.
- 2-3 cloves of chopped fresh garlic daily are adequate to achieve therapeutic benefits.

Toxicity

Comparative-toxicity rating is not available from standard references.

For symptoms of toxicity: See *Adverse Reactions, Side Effects or Overdose Symptoms* section below.

Adverse Reactions, Side Effects or Overdose Symptoms

Signs and symptoms	What to do
Contact dermatitis	Wear gloves.
Gastrointestinal upset, nausea	Decrease dose.
Increased number of circulating white blood cells as determined by laboratory studies	Discontinue. Call doctor immediately.
Precipitous blood-pressure drop: symptoms include faintness, cold sweat, paleness, rapid pulse	Seek emergency treatment.
Skin eruptions	Discontinue. Call doctor when convenient.

Gentian (Yellow Gentian)

Basic Information

Biological name (genus and species):
Gentiana lutea

Parts used for medicinal purposes:
Roots

Chemicals this herb contains:
- Gentiamarin
- Gentiin
- Gentiopicrin
- Gentisin
- Sugar
- Xanthone pigment

Known Effects

- Irritates mucous membranes
- Kills plasmodium, which causes malaria

Miscellaneous information:
Used since ancient times in Greece.

Possible Additional Effects

- May increase contractions of stomach muscles
- May stimulate gastric secretions
- May stimulate appetite when used as a tonic
- May aid digestion

Warnings and Precautions

Don't take if you:
- Are pregnant, think you may be pregnant or plan pregnancy in the near future
- Have any chronic disease of the gastrointestinal tract, such as stomach or duodenal ulcers, reflux esophagitis, ulcerative colitis, spastic colitis, diverticulosis or diverticulitis

Consult your doctor if you:
- Take this herb for any medical problem that doesn't improve in 2 weeks (There may be safer, more effective treatments.)
- Take any medicinal drugs or herbs including aspirin, laxatives, cold and cough remedies, antacids, vitamins, minerals, amino acids, supplements, other prescription or nonprescription drugs

Pregnancy:
Don't use unless prescribed by your doctor.

Breastfeeding:
Don't use unless prescribed by your doctor.

Infants and children:
Treating infants or children under 2 with any herbal preparation is hazardous.

Others:
No problems expected if you are beyond childhood, under 45, not pregnant, basically healthy, take it for only a short time and do not exceed manufacturer's recommended dose.

Storage:
- Store in cool, dry area away from direct light, but don't freeze.
- Store safely out of reach of children.
- Don't store in bathroom medicine cabinet. Heat and moisture may change the action of the herb.

Safe dosage:
Consult your doctor for the appropriate dose for your condition.

Toxicity

Rated relatively safe when taken in appropriate quantities for short periods of time

For symptoms of toxicity: See *Adverse Reactions, Side Effects or Overdose Symptoms* section below.

Adverse Reactions, Side Effects or Overdose Symptoms

Signs and symptoms	What to do
Nausea or vomiting	Discontinue. Call doctor immediately.

German Chamomile (Hungarian Chamomile, Matricaria)

Basic Information

Biological name (genus and species): *Matricaria chamomilla*

Parts used for medicinal purposes: Petals/flower

Chemicals this herb contains:
• Alphabisabolol
• Azulene
• Fatty acid
• Furfural
• Paraffin hydrocarbons
• Sesquiterpene
• Sesquiterpene alcohol
• Tannins (see Glossary)

Known Effects

• Anti-inflammatory
• Weakens muscles
• Interferes with absorption of iron and other minerals when taken internally

Miscellaneous information:
• Ice cream, candy and liqueur manufacturers use small, nontoxic amounts for flavoring.
• It is also used as a tonic.

Possible Additional Effects

• Relieves spasms in skeletal or smooth muscle
• Potential sedative
• May help expel gas from intestinal tract

Warnings and Precautions

Don't take if you:
• Are pregnant, think you may be pregnant or plan pregnancy in the near future
• Have any chronic disease of the gastrointestinal tract, such as stomach or duodenal ulcers, reflux esophagitis, ulcerative colitis, spastic colitis, diverticulosis or diverticulitis

Consult your doctor if you:
• Take this herb for any medical problem that doesn't improve in 2 weeks (There may be safer, more effective treatments.)
• Take any medicinal drugs or herbs including aspirin, laxatives, cold and cough remedies, antacids, vitamins, minerals, amino acids,

supplements, other prescription or nonprescription drugs

Pregnancy:
Don't use unless prescribed by your doctor.

Breastfeeding:
Don't use unless prescribed by your doctor.

Infants and children:
Treating infants or children under 2 with any herbal preparation is hazardous.

Others:
No problems expected if you are beyond childhood, under 45, not pregnant, basically healthy, take it for only a short time and do not exceed manufacturer's recommended dose.

Storage:
- Store in cool, dry area away from direct light, but don't freeze.
- Store safely out of reach of children.
- Don't store in bathroom medicine cabinet. Heat and moisture may change the action of the herb.

Safe dosage:
Consult your doctor for the appropriate dose for your condition.

 Toxicity

Generally regarded as safe when taken in appropriate quantities for short periods of time

For symptoms of toxicity: See *Adverse Reactions, Side Effects or Overdose Symptoms* section below.

 Adverse Reactions, Side Effects or Overdose Symptoms

Signs and symptoms	What to do
Diarrhea	Discontinue. Call doctor immediately.
Excess sedation	Discontinue. Call doctor immediately.
Nausea or vomiting	Discontinue. Call doctor immediately.
Skin eruptions	Discontinue. Call doctor when convenient.

Ginger (Ginger Rhizome)

 Basic Information

Biological name (genus and species):
Zingiber officinale

Parts used for medicinal purposes:
Roots

Chemicals this herb contains:
- Bisabolene
- Borneal
- Camphene
- Choline
- Cineole
- Citral
- Sesquiterpene
- Volatile oils (see Glossary)
- Zingerone
- Zingiberene

 Known Effects

- Helps expel gas from intestinal tract
- Provides counterirritation (see Glossary) when applied to

➜

skin overlying an inflamed or irritated joint
• Treats nausea and vomiting
• Treats motion sickness

Miscellaneous information:
• Ginger is used as a flavoring agent.
• No effects are expected on the body, either good or bad, when ginger is used in very small amounts to enhance the flavor of food.

Possible Additional Effects

• May treat indigestion
• May treat abdominal discomfort
• May reduce fever
• May treat migraine headache
• May act as an antioxidant
• May reduce pain of arthritis (anti-inflammatory)

Warnings and Precautions

Don't take if you:
• Are pregnant, think you may be pregnant or plan pregnancy in the near future
• Have any chronic disease of the gastrointestinal tract, such as stomach or duodenal ulcers, reflux esophagitis, ulcerative colitis, spastic colitis, diverticulosis or diverticulitis

Consult your doctor if you:
• Take this herb for any medical problem that doesn't improve in 2 weeks (There may be safer, more effective treatments.)
• Take any medicinal drugs or herbs including aspirin, laxatives, cold and cough remedies, antacids, vitamins, minerals, amino acids, supplements, other prescription or nonprescription drugs
• Have stomach or intestinal diseases

Pregnancy:
• Problems in pregnant women taking small or usual amounts have not been proved, but the chance of problems does exist. Don't use unless prescribed by your doctor.
• Do not use for morning sickness during pregnancy.

Breastfeeding:
Problems in breastfed infants of lactating mothers taking small or usual amounts have not been proved, but the chance of problems does exist. Don't use unless prescribed by your doctor.

Infants and children:
Treating infants or children under 2 with any herbal preparation is hazardous.

Others:
No problems expected if you are beyond childhood, under 45, not pregnant, basically healthy, take it for only a short time and do not exceed manufacturer's recommended dose.

Storage:
• Store in cool, dry area away from direct light, but don't freeze.
• Store safely out of reach of children.
• Don't store in bathroom medicine cabinet. Heat and moisture may change the action of the herb.

Safe dosage:
Consult your doctor for the appropriate dose for your condition.

Toxicity

Comparative-toxicity rating is not available from standard references.

For symptoms of toxicity: See *Adverse Reactions, Side Effects or Overdose Symptoms* section below.

Adverse Reactions, Side Effects or Overdose Symptoms

Signs and symptoms	What to do
Diarrhea	Discontinue. Call doctor immediately.
Heartburn	Discontinue. Call doctor immediately.
Nausea or vomiting	Discontinue. Call doctor immediately.

Ginkgo Biloba

 Basic Information

Biological name (genus and species):
Ginkgoaceae, Ginkgo biloba

Parts used for medicinal purposes:
Leaf extract

Chemicals this herb contains:
- Bilobalide
- Ginkgolic acids
- Glycosides (quercetin and kaempferol) (see Glossary)
- Isorhamnetin
- Terpene lactones (ginkgolides A, B and C)

 Known Effects

- Increases circulation to the brain and lower extremities
- Aids in treatment of memory loss associated with Alzheimer's disease
- Treats loss of concentration and emotional fatigue in the elderly

 Possible Additional Effects

- May treat tinnitus and vertigo
- May reduce vision loss due to aging
- May reduce symptoms associated with Raynaud's disease
- Potential aid in the treatment of peripheral vascular disease

 Warnings and Precautions

Don't take if you:
Have had a stroke or are prone to them.

Consult your doctor if you:
- Take this herb for any medical problem that doesn't improve in 2 weeks (There may be safer, more effective treatments.)
- Take any medicinal drugs or herbs including aspirin, laxatives, cold and cough remedies, antacids, vitamins, minerals, amino acids, supplements, other prescription or nonprescription drugs

➜

Pregnancy:

Don't use unless prescribed by your doctor.

Breastfeeding:

Don't use unless prescribed by your doctor.

Infants and children:

Treating infants or children under 2 with any herbal preparation is hazardous.

Storage:

- Store in cool, dry area away from direct light, but don't freeze.
- Store safely out of reach of children.
- Don't store in bathroom medicine cabinet. Heat and moisture may change the action of the herb.

Safe dosage:

Consult your doctor for the appropriate dose for your condition.

Toxicity

Comparative-toxicity rating is not available from standard references.

For symptoms of toxicity: See *Adverse Reactions, Side Effects or Overdose Symptoms* section below.

Adverse Reactions, Side Effects or Overdose Symptoms

Signs and symptoms	What to do
Diarrhea	Discontinue. Call doctor immediately.
Headache	Discontinue. Call doctor immediately.
Irritability, restlessness	Discontinue. Call doctor when convenient.
Nausea	Discontinue. Call doctor immediately.

Ginseng

Basic Information

Ginseng is also known as *Asian ginseng; panax ginseng*; and *American, Korean* or *Chinese ginseng.*

Biological name (genus and species): *Panax quinquefolius*

Parts used for medicinal purposes: Roots

Chemicals this herb contains:

- Arabinose
- Camphor
- Ginsenosides
- Mucilage (see Glossary)
- Panaxosides
- Resin (see Glossary)
- Saponins (see Glossary)
- Starch

Known Effects

- Stimulates brain, heart, blood vessels
- Reduces stress and fatigue
- Increases secretion of histamine (see Glossary)
- Improves appetite and digestion
- Stimulant
- Antioxidant

Miscellaneous information:
- A favorite Chinese remedy used for almost everything
- A native plant in the U.S. state of Georgia

Possible Additional Effects

- Used as an aphrodisiac
- May increase mental and physical stamina
- May treat symptoms of menopause
- May reduce effects of radiation exposure
- May reduce blood glucose in diabetics
- May alleviate insomnia

Warnings and Precautions

Don't take if you:
- Are pregnant, think you may be pregnant or plan pregnancy in the near future
- Have any chronic disease of the gastrointestinal tract, such as stomach or duodenal ulcers, reflux esophagitis, ulcerative colitis, spastic colitis, diverticulosis or diverticulitis
- Have been diagnosed with cystic breast disease, breast cancer, heart disease or high blood pressure

Consult your doctor if you:
- Take this herb for any medical problem that doesn't improve in 2 weeks (There may be safer, more effective treatments.)
- Take any medicinal drugs or herbs including aspirin, laxatives, cold and cough remedies, antacids, vitamins, minerals, amino acids, supplements, other prescription or nonprescription drugs

Pregnancy:
Don't use unless prescribed by your doctor.

Breastfeeding:
Don't use unless prescribed by your doctor.

Infants and children:
Treating infants or children under 2 with any herbal preparation is hazardous.

Others:
No problems expected if you are beyond childhood, under 45, not pregnant, basically healthy, take it for only a short time and do not exceed manufacturer's recommended dose.

Storage:
- Store in cool, dry area away from direct light, but don't freeze.
- Store safely out of reach of children.
- Don't store in bathroom medicine cabinet. Heat and moisture may change the action of the herb.

Safe dosage:
Consult your doctor for the appropriate dose for your condition.

Toxicity

Generally regarded as safe when taken in appropriate quantities for short periods of time

For symptoms of toxicity: See *Adverse Reactions, Side Effects or Overdose Symptoms* section below.

Adverse Reactions, Side Effects or Overdose Symptoms

Signs and symptoms	What to do
Diarrhea	Discontinue. Call doctor immediately.
Nausea or vomiting	Discontinue. Call doctor immediately.

Goldenseal

 Basic Information

Biological name (genus and species):
Hydrastis canadensis

Parts used for medicinal purposes:
- Rhizomes
- Roots

Chemicals this herb contains:
- Albumin
- Berberine
- Candine
- Fats
- Hydrastine
- Lignin
- Resin (see Glossary)
- Starch
- Sugar
- Volatile oils (see Glossary)

 Known Effects

- Antibiotic
- Decreases bleeding
- Large amounts stimulate central nervous system
- Depresses muscle tone of small blood vessels
- Laxative

Miscellaneous information:
Goldenseal has a very bitter taste.

 Possible Additional Effects

- May strengthen the immune system
- May treat trachoma
- May treat disorders of the liver
- May treat dyspepsia
- May increase appetite
- May treat and relieve sinusitis
- May treat infectious diarrhea

 Warnings and Precautions

Don't take if you:
- Are pregnant, think you may be pregnant or plan pregnancy in the near future
- Have any chronic disease of the gastrointestinal tract, such as stomach or duodenal ulcers, reflux esophagitis, ulcerative colitis, spastic colitis, diverticulosis or diverticulitis
- Have heart disease, diabetes, glaucoma or high blood pressure
- Are taking coumadin, warfarin

Consult your doctor if you:
- Take this herb for any medical problem that doesn't improve in 2 weeks (There may be safer, more effective treatments.)
- Take any medicinal drugs or herbs including aspirin, laxatives, cold and cough remedies, antacids, vitamins, minerals, amino acids, supplements, other prescription or nonprescription drugs

Pregnancy:
Dangers outweigh any possible benefits. Don't use.

Breastfeeding:
Dangers outweigh any possible benefits. Don't use.

Infants and children:
Treating infants or children under 2 with any herbal preparation is hazardous.

Others:
No problems expected if you are beyond childhood, under 45, not pregnant, basically healthy, take it for only a short time and do not exceed manufacturer's recommended dose.

Storage:
- Store in cool, dry area away from direct light, but don't freeze.
- Store safely out of reach of children.
- Don't store in bathroom medicine cabinet. Heat and moisture may change the action of the herb.

Safe dosage:
Consult your doctor for the appropriate dose for your condition.

 Toxicity

Rated slightly dangerous, particularly in children, persons over 55 and those who take larger than appropriate quantities for extended periods of time

For symptoms of toxicity: See *Adverse Reactions, Side Effects or Overdose Symptoms* section below.

 Adverse Reactions, Side Effects or Overdose Symptoms

Signs and symptoms	What to do
Breathing difficulties	Seek emergency treatment.
Convulsions	Seek emergency treatment.
Depression	Discontinue. Call doctor immediately.
Diarrhea	Discontinue. Call doctor immediately.
Mouth and throat irritation	Discontinue. Call doctor immediately.
Nausea or vomiting	Discontinue. Call doctor immediately.
Numbness of hands and feet	Discontinue. Call doctor immediately.
Weakness leading to paralysis of muscles	Seek emergency treatment.

Gotu Kola (Kola)

 Basic Information

Biological name (genus and species):
Centella asiatica

Parts used for medicinal purposes:
- Nuts
- Roots
- Seeds

Chemicals this herb contains:
- Caffeine
- Catechol
- Epicatechol
- Flavonoids (see Glossary)
- Resins (see Glossary)
- Theobromine
- Triterpenoid compounds

 Known Effects

- Stimulates central nervous system
- Helps body dispose of excess fluid by increasing amount of urine produced
- Anti-inflammatory
- Treats skin disorders (burns, cellulite, scleroderma)

Miscellaneous information:
No effects are expected on the body, either good or bad, when this herb is used in very small amounts to enhance the flavor of food.

➜

Possible Additional Effects

- May decrease fatigue
- May decrease anxiety
- May increase circulation in the legs
- May improve memory
- May help leprosy
- May lessen night cramps
- May decrease tingling/numbness of extremities
- May speed wound healing
- May treat eczema

Warnings and Precautions

Don't take if you:

- Are pregnant, think you may be pregnant or plan pregnancy in the near future
- Have any chronic disease of the gastrointestinal tract, such as stomach or duodenal ulcers, reflux esophagitis, ulcerative colitis, spastic colitis, diverticulosis or diverticulitis

Consult your doctor if you:

- Take this herb for any medical problem that doesn't improve in 2 weeks (There may be safer, more effective treatments.)
- Take any medicinal drugs or herbs including aspirin, laxatives, cold and cough remedies, antacids, vitamins, minerals, amino acids, supplements, other prescription or nonprescription drugs

Pregnancy:
Don't use.

Breastfeeding:
Don't use.

Infants and children:
Treating infants or children under 2 with any herbal preparation is hazardous.

Others:
May cause contact dermatitis when applied topically.

Storage:

- Store in cool, dry area away from direct light, but don't freeze.
- Store safely out of reach of children.
- Don't store in bathroom medicine cabinet. Heat and moisture may change the action of the herb.

Safe dosage:
Consult your doctor for the appropriate dose for your condition.

Toxicity

Rated relatively safe when taken in appropriate quantities for short periods of time

For symptoms of toxicity: See *Adverse Reactions, Side Effects or Overdose Symptoms* section below.

Adverse Reactions, Side Effects or Overdose Symptoms

Signs and symptoms	What to do
Aggravated peptic ulcers in stomach, duodenum or esophagus	Discontinue. Call doctor immediately.
Inability to sleep	Discontinue. Call doctor when convenient.
Increased cholesterol	Discontinue. Call doctor immediately.
Nervousness	Discontinue. Call doctor when convenient.
Photosensitivity	Discontinue. Call doctor immediately.

Grape Hyacinth

Basic Information

Biological name (genus and species):
Muscari racemosum, M. comosum

Parts used for medicinal purposes:
Bulb

Chemicals this herb contains:
• Comisic acid
• Saponins (see Glossary)

Known Effects

Irritates gastrointestinal tract

Possible Additional Effects

• May treat constipation
• May stimulate central nervous system
• May help body dispose of excess
  fluid by increasing amount of
  urine produced

Warnings and Precautions

Don't take if you:
• Are pregnant, think you may be
  pregnant or plan pregnancy in the
  near future
• Have any chronic disease of the
  gastrointestinal tract, such as
  stomach or duodenal ulcers, reflux
  esophagitis, ulcerative colitis, spastic
  colitis, diverticulosis or diverticulitis

Consult your doctor if you:
• Take this herb for any medical
  problem that doesn't improve in
  2 weeks (There may be safer, more
  effective treatments.)

• Take any medicinal drugs or
  herbs including aspirin, laxatives,
  cold and cough remedies, antacids,
  vitamins, minerals, amino acids,
  supplements, other prescription
  or nonprescription drugs

Pregnancy:
Dangers outweigh any possible
benefits. Don't use.

Breastfeeding:
Dangers outweigh any possible
benefits. Don't use.

Infants and children:
Treating infants or children under
2 with any herbal preparation
is hazardous.

Others:
No evidence of any useful therapeutic
effect exists. Don't use.

Storage:
• Store in cool, dry area away from
  direct light, but don't freeze.
• Store safely out of reach of children.
• Don't store in bathroom medicine
  cabinet. Heat and moisture may
  change the action of the herb.

Safe dosage:
Consult your doctor for the
appropriate dose for your condition.

Toxicity

Comparative-toxicity rating is not
available from standard references.

For symptoms of toxicity: See
*Adverse Reactions, Side Effects or
Overdose Symptoms* section below.

➡

Adverse Reactions,
Side Effects or
Overdose Symptoms

Signs and symptoms	What to do
Diarrhea	Discontinue. Call doctor immediately.
Nausea or vomiting	Discontinue. Call doctor immediately.

Grape Seed Extract

 Basic Information

Biological name (genus and species):
Vitis vinifera

Parts used for medicinal purposes:
Not applicable

Chemicals this herb contains:
• Essential fatty acids
• Proanthocyanidins
• Tocopherols

 Known Effects

• Powerful antioxidant
• Helps prevent atherosclerosis
• Prevents free-radical (see Glossary) damage
• Improves circulation
• Anti-inflammatory

 Possible Additional Effects

• May protect against effects of radiation
• May prevent retinopathy
• May reduce risk of varicose veins
• May help heal wounds
• May prevent dental cavities

 Warnings and Precautions

Don't take if you:
Have any chronic disease, without consulting your doctor.

Consult your doctor if you:
• Take this herb for any medical problem that doesn't improve in 2 weeks (There may be safer, more effective treatments.)
• Take any medicinal drugs or herbs including aspirin, laxatives, cold and cough remedies, antacids, vitamins, minerals, amino acids, supplements, other prescription or nonprescription drugs

Pregnancy:
Don't use unless prescribed by your doctor.

Breastfeeding:
Don't use unless prescribed by your doctor.

Infants and children:
Treating infants or children under 2 with any herbal preparation is hazardous.

Others:

No problems expected if you are beyond childhood, under 45, not pregnant, basically healthy, take it for only a short time and do not exceed manufacturer's recommended dose.

Storage:

- Store in cool, dry area away from direct light, but don't freeze.
- Store safely out of reach of children.
- Don't store in bathroom medicine cabinet. Heat and moisture may change the action of the herb.

Safe dosage:

Consult your doctor for the appropriate dose for your condition.

Toxicity

Comparative-toxicity rating is not available from standard references.

Adverse Reactions, Side Effects or Overdose Symptoms

None are expected.

Grindelia (Gumweed, Rosinweed)

Basic Information

Biological name (genus and species):
Grindelia camporum, G. squarrosa

Parts used for medicinal purposes:
Leaves

Chemicals this herb contains:
- Balsamic resin
- Grindelol
- Robustic acid
- Saponins (see Glossary)
- Tannins (see Glossary)
- Volatile oils (see Glossary)

Known Effects

- Depresses central nervous system (in high amounts)
- Dilates pupils of eyes
- Decreases heart rate
- Increases blood pressure
- Interferes with absorption of iron and other minerals when taken internally

Miscellaneous information:

Used in poultices (see Glossary) as a means of applying medications.

Possible Additional Effects

- May decrease thickness and increase fluidity of mucus in lungs and bronchial tubes
- Potential sedative
- May treat asthma
- May treat bronchitis
- May soothe and heal burns when applied topically
- May treat vaginitis

Warnings and Precautions

Don't take if you:
Are pregnant, think you may be pregnant or plan pregnancy in the near future.

Consult your doctor if you:
- Take this herb for any medical problem that doesn't improve in 2 weeks (There may be safer, more effective treatments.)
- Take any medicinal drugs or herbs including aspirin, laxatives, cold and cough remedies, antacids, vitamins, minerals, amino acids, supplements, other prescription or nonprescription drugs

Pregnancy:
Dangers outweigh any possible benefits. Don't use.

Breastfeeding:
Dangers outweigh any possible benefits. Don't use.

Infants and children:
Treating infants or children under 2 with any herbal preparation is hazardous.

Storage:
- Store in cool, dry area away from direct light, but don't freeze.
- Store safely out of reach of children.
- Don't store in bathroom medicine cabinet. Heat and moisture may change the action of the herb.

Safe dosage:
Consult your doctor for the appropriate dose for your condition.

Toxicity

Rated slightly dangerous, particularly in children, persons over 55 and those who take larger than appropriate quantities for extended periods of time

For symptoms of toxicity: See *Adverse Reactions, Side Effects or Overdose Symptoms* section below.

Adverse Reactions, Side Effects or Overdose Symptoms

Signs and symptoms	What to do
Kidney damage characterized by blood in urine, decreased urine flow, swelling of hands and feet	Seek emergency treatment.

Guaiac

Basic Information

Biological name (genus and species):
Guaiacum officinale, G. sanctum

Parts used for medicinal purposes:
Stems

Chemicals this herb contains:
- Guaiaconic acid
- Guaiaretic acid
- Resin (see Glossary)
- Saponins (see Glossary)
- Vanillin

Known Effects

- Irritates gastrointestinal tract
- Increases perspiration
- Tests for oxidizing enzymes to detect blood in stool or urine

Miscellaneous information:

When added to a stool specimen, hydrogen peroxide and guaiac establish the presence or absence of blood. This test is a useful screening procedure to detect malignant and nonmalignant disorders of the intestinal tract.

Possible Additional Effects

- May treat arthritis
- May treat scrofula
- May treat constipation
- May reduce edema

Warnings and Precautions

Don't take if you:

- Are pregnant, think you may be pregnant or plan pregnancy in the near future
- Have any chronic disease of the gastrointestinal tract, such as stomach or duodenal ulcers, reflux esophagitis, ulcerative colitis, spastic colitis, diverticulosis or diverticulitis

Consult your doctor if you:

- Take this herb for any medical problem that doesn't improve in 2 weeks (There may be safer, more effective treatments.)
- Take any medicinal drugs or herbs including aspirin, laxatives, cold and cough remedies, antacids, vitamins, minerals, amino acids, supplements, other prescription or nonprescription drugs

Pregnancy:

Dangers outweigh any possible benefits. Don't use.

Breastfeeding:

Dangers outweigh any possible benefits. Don't use.

Infants and children:

Treating infants or children under 2 with any herbal preparation is hazardous.

Others:

No problems expected if you are beyond childhood, under 45, not pregnant, basically healthy, take it for only a short time and do not exceed manufacturer's recommended dose.

Storage:

- Store in cool, dry area away from direct light, but don't freeze.
- Store safely out of reach of children.
- Don't store in bathroom medicine cabinet. Heat and moisture may change the action of the herb.

Safe dosage:

Consult your doctor for the appropriate dose for your condition.

Toxicity

Comparative-toxicity rating is not available from standard references.

For symptoms of toxicity: See *Adverse Reactions, Side Effects or Overdose Symptoms* section below.

Adverse Reactions, Side Effects or Overdose Symptoms

Signs and symptoms	What to do
Nausea or vomiting	Discontinue. Call doctor immediately.

Harmel (African Rue, Syrian Rue, Wild Rue)

Basic Information

Biological name (genus and species):
Peganum harmala

Parts used for medicinal purposes:
Various parts of the entire plant,
frequently differing by country
and culture

Chemicals this herb contains:
- Harmaline
- Harmalol
- Harmine
- Peganine

Known Effects

- Causes hallucinations
- Destroys bacteria (germs) and
  suppresses their growth or
  reproduction

Miscellaneous information:
Wild rue is often abused where it
grows in Arizona, New Mexico
and Texas.

Possible Additional Effects

- May destroy intestinal worms
- May decrease pain

Warnings and Precautions

Don't take if you:
Are pregnant, think you may be
pregnant or plan pregnancy in the
near future.

Consult your doctor if you:
- Take this herb for any medical
  problem that doesn't improve in
  2 weeks (There may be safer, more
  effective treatments.)
- Take any medicinal drugs or
  herbs including aspirin, laxatives,
  cold and cough remedies, antacids,
  vitamins, minerals, amino acids,
  supplements, other prescription
  or nonprescription drugs

Pregnancy:
Dangers outweigh any possible
benefits. Don't use.

Breastfeeding:
Dangers outweigh any possible
benefits. Don't use.

Infants and children:
Treating infants or children under
2 with any herbal preparation
is hazardous.

Others:
Dangers outweigh any possible
benefits. Do use.

Storage:
- Store in cool, dry area away from
  direct light, but don't freeze.
- Store safely out of reach of children.
- Don't store in bathroom medicine
  cabinet. Heat and moisture may
  change the action of the herb.

Safe dosage:
Consult your doctor for the
appropriate dose for your condition.

Toxicity

Rated slightly dangerous, particularly in
children, persons over 55 and those
who take larger than appropriate
quantities for extended periods of time

For symptoms of toxicity: See *Adverse Reactions, Side Effects or Overdose Symptoms* section below.

 Adverse Reactions, Side Effects or Overdose Symptoms

Signs and symptoms	What to do
Hallucinations	Seek emergency treatment.
Muscle weakness	Discontinue. Call doctor immediately.

Hawthorn

 Basic Information

Biological name (genus and species): *Crataegus oxyacantha*

Parts used for medicinal purposes:
- Berries
- Blossoms
- Leaves

Chemicals this herb contains:
- Acetylcholine
- Anthocyanin-type pigments
- Cardiotonic amines
- Choline
- Cratagolic acid
- Flavonoids (see Glossary)
- Glycosides (see Glossary)
- Pectins
- Purines
- Saponins (see Glossary)
- Triterpene acids

 Known Effects

- Can depress respiration
- Increases blood flow to the heart
- Can depress heart rate
- Antiarrhythmic
- Coronary vasodilator (widens coronary blood vessels)

 Possible Additional Effects

- May treat high blood pressure
- May treat atherosclerosis
- May help treat circulatory disorders
- May lower cholesterol

 Warnings and Precautions

Don't take if you:
- Are pregnant, think you may be pregnant or plan pregnancy in the near future
- Have heart disease

Consult your doctor if you:
- Take this herb for any medical problem that doesn't improve in 2 weeks (There may be safer, more effective treatments.)

- Take any medicinal drugs or herbs including aspirin, laxatives, cold and cough remedies, antacids, vitamins, minerals, amino acids, supplements, other prescription or nonprescription drugs

Pregnancy:
Don't use.

Breastfeeding:
Don't use.

Infants and children:
Treating infants or children under 2 with any herbal preparation is hazardous.

Others:
Do not attempt to self medicate. If you think you have heart problems, consult a physician immediately.

Storage:
- Store in cool, dry area away from direct light, but don't freeze.
- Store safely out of reach of children.
- Don't store in bathroom medicine cabinet. Heat and moisture may change the action of the herb.

Safe dosage:
Consult your doctor for the appropriate dose for your condition.

 Toxicity

Comparative-toxicity rating is not available from standard references.

For symptoms of toxicity: See *Adverse Reactions, Side Effects or Overdose Symptoms* section below.

 Adverse Reactions, Side Effects or Overdose Symptoms

Signs and symptoms	What to do
Breathing difficulties	Seek emergency treatment.
Heartbeat irregularities	Seek emergency treatment..

Heliotrope (Turnsole)

 Basic Information

Biological name (genus and species):
Heliotropium europaeum

Parts used for medicinal purposes:
- Juice
- Leaves
- Seeds

Chemicals this herb contains:
- Heliotrine
- Lasiocarpine

 Known Effects

- Kills liver cells
- Stimulates production of bile

Miscellaneous information:
Heliotrope is a common weed.

 Possible Additional Effects

Leaves and juice may treat ulcers, warts, polyps and tumors.

Warnings and Precautions

Don't take if you:
Are pregnant, think you may be pregnant or plan pregnancy in the near future.

Consult your doctor if you:
- Take this herb for any medical problem that doesn't improve in 2 weeks (There may be safer, more effective treatments.)
- Take any medicinal drugs or herbs including aspirin, laxatives, cold and cough remedies, antacids, vitamins, minerals, amino acids, supplements, other prescription or nonprescription drugs

Pregnancy:
Dangers outweigh any possible benefits. Don't use.

Breastfeeding:
Dangers outweigh any possible benefits. Don't use.

Infants and children:
Treating infants or children under 2 with any herbal preparation is hazardous.

Storage:
- Store in cool, dry area away from direct light, but don't freeze.
- Store safely out of reach of children.
- Don't store in bathroom medicine cabinet. Heat and moisture may change the action of the herb.

Safe dosage:
Consult your doctor for the appropriate dose for your condition.

Toxicity

Rated slightly dangerous, particularly in children, persons over 55 and those who take larger than appropriate quantities for extended periods of time

For symptoms of toxicity: See *Adverse Reactions, Side Effects or Overdose Symptoms* section below.

Adverse Reactions, Side Effects or Overdose Symptoms

Signs and symptoms	What to do
Jaundice (yellow skin and eyes)	Discontinue. Call doctor immediately.

Hellebore (American Hellebore, Green Hellebore)

Basic Information

Biological name (genus and species):
Veratrum viride

Parts used for medicinal purposes:
- Rhizomes
- Root

Chemicals this herb contains:
- Germidine
- Germitrine
- Jervine
- Pseudojervine
- Rubijervine
- Veratrum alkaloids

➔

Known Effects

- Decreases blood pressure
- Decreases heart rate
- Depresses central nervous system

Possible Additional Effects

- May treat hypertension
- May treat toxemia of pregnancy
- May irritate gastrointestinal system

Warnings and Precautions

Don't take if you:
- Are pregnant, think you may be pregnant or plan pregnancy in the near future
- Have any chronic disease of the gastrointestinal tract, such as stomach or duodenal ulcers, reflux esophagitis, ulcerative colitis, spastic colitis, diverticulosis or diverticulitis

Consult your doctor if you:
- Take this herb for any medical problem that doesn't improve in 2 weeks (There may be safer, more effective treatments.)
- Take any medicinal drugs or herbs including aspirin, laxatives, cold and cough remedies, antacids, vitamins, minerals, amino acids, supplements, other prescription or nonprescription drugs

Pregnancy:
Dangers outweigh any possible benefits. Don't use.

Breastfeeding:
Dangers outweigh any possible benefits. Don't use.

Infants and children:
Treating infants or children under 2 with any herbal preparation is hazardous.

Others:
All parts of the plant may be toxic.

Storage:
- Store in cool, dry area away from direct light, but don't freeze.
- Store safely out of reach of children.
- Don't store in bathroom medicine cabinet. Heat and moisture may change the action of the herb.

Safe dosage:
Consult your doctor for the appropriate dose for your condition.

Toxicity

Rated dangerous, particularly in children, persons over 55 and those who take larger than appropriate quantities for extended periods of time

For symptoms of toxicity: See *Adverse Reactions, Side Effects or Overdose Symptoms* section below.

Adverse Reactions, Side Effects or Overdose Symptoms

Signs and symptoms	What to do
Abdominal pain	Discontinue. Call doctor immediately.
Burning sensation in mouth	Discontinue. Call doctor when convenient.
Diarrhea	Discontinue. Call doctor immediately.
Headache	Discontinue. Call doctor when convenient.
Nausea or vomiting	Discontinue. Call doctor immediately.
Precipitous blood-pressure drop: symptoms include faintness, cold sweat, paleness, rapid pulse	Seek emergency treatment.

Helonias (Fairy Wand, False Unicorn Root)

Basic Information

Biological name (genus and species):
Chamaelirium luteum

Parts used for medicinal purposes:
Roots

Chemicals this herb contains:
- Chamaelirin
- Saponins (see Glossary)

Known Effects

- Irritates gastrointestinal system
- Helps body dispose of excess fluid by increasing amount of urine produced
- Produces puckering

Possible Additional Effects

- May prevent miscarriage
- May treat menopause symptoms
- May increase appetite
- Potential vigorous laxative

Warnings and Precautions

Don't take if you:
- Are pregnant, think you may be pregnant or plan pregnancy in the near future
- Have any chronic disease of the gastrointestinal tract, such as stomach or duodenal ulcers, reflux esophagitis, ulcerative colitis, spastic colitis, diverticulosis or diverticulitis

Consult your doctor if you:
- Take this herb for any medical problem that doesn't improve in 2 weeks (There may be safer, more effective treatments.)
- Take any medicinal drugs or herbs including aspirin, laxatives, cold and cough remedies, antacids, vitamins, minerals, amino acids, supplements, other prescription or nonprescription drugs

Pregnancy:
Dangers outweigh any possible benefits. Don't use.

Breastfeeding:
Dangers outweigh any possible benefits. Don't use.

Infants and children:
Treating infants or children under 2 with any herbal preparation is hazardous.

Others:
No problems expected if you are beyond childhood, under 45, not pregnant, basically healthy, take it for only a short time and do not exceed manufacturer's recommended dose.

Storage:
- Store in cool, dry area away from direct light, but don't freeze.
- Store safely out of reach of children.
- Don't store in bathroom medicine cabinet. Heat and moisture may change the action of the herb.

Safe dosage:
Consult your doctor for the appropriate dose for your condition.

Toxicity

Comparative-toxicity rating is not available from standard references.

For symptoms of toxicity: See *Adverse Reactions, Side Effects or Overdose Symptoms* section below.

Adverse Reactions, Side Effects or Overdose Symptoms

Signs and symptoms	What to do
Diarrhea	Discontinue. Call doctor immediately.
Nausea	Discontinue. Call doctor immediately.

Henbane (Hyoscyamus)

Basic Information

Biological name (genus and species): *Hyoscyamus niger*

Parts used for medicinal purposes:
- Berries/fruits
- Leaves
- Roots

Chemicals this herb contains:
- Hyoscyamine
- Scopolamine

Known Effects

Blocks effects of parasympathetic nervous system, causing increased heart rate, dilated pupils, dry mouth, hallucinations, urinary retention, reduced contractions of gastrointestinal tract

Miscellaneous information:
- Henbane is poisonous, especially to children!
- It's used as a mouthwash and painkiller.

Possible Additional Effects

- May treat whooping cough
- May treat asthma
- Potential sedative

Warnings and Precautions

Don't take if you:
- Are pregnant, think you may be pregnant or plan pregnancy in the near future
- Have any chronic disease of the gastrointestinal tract, such as stomach or duodenal ulcers, reflux esophagitis, ulcerative colitis, spastic colitis, diverticulosis or diverticulitis

Consult your doctor if you:
- Take this herb for any medical problem that doesn't improve in 2 weeks (There may be safer, more effective treatments.)
- Take any medicinal drugs or herbs including aspirin, laxatives, cold and cough remedies, antacids, vitamins, minerals, amino acids, supplements, other prescription or nonprescription drugs

Pregnancy:
Dangers outweigh any possible benefits. Don't use.

Breastfeeding:
Dangers outweigh any possible benefits. Don't use.

Infants and children:
Don't use!

Others:
No problems expected if you are beyond childhood, under 45, not pregnant, basically healthy, take it for only a short time and do not exceed manufacturer's recommended dose.

Storage:
• Store in cool, dry area away from direct light, but don't freeze.
• Store safely out of reach of children.
• Don't store in bathroom medicine cabinet. Heat and moisture may change the action of the herb.

Safe dosage:
Consult your doctor for the appropriate dose for your condition.

 Toxicity

Comparative-toxicity rating is not available from standard references.

For symptoms of toxicity: See *Adverse Reactions, Side Effects or Overdose Symptoms* section below.

 Adverse Reactions, Side Effects or Overdose Symptoms

Signs and symptoms	What to do
Delirium	Seek emergency treatment.
Hallucinations	Seek emergency treatment.
Rapid heartbeat	Seek emergency treatment.

Hop, Common

 Basic Information

Biological name (genus and species): *Humulus lupulus*

Parts used for medicinal purposes: Berries/fruits

Chemicals this herb contains:

• Humulene
• Lupulinic acid
• Lupulone

 Known Effects

Inhibits growth and development of germs

Miscellaneous information:
• If fruit is not fresh, it smells bad.
• Hops are used extensively in the brewing industry.
• It produces odors because it evaporates at room temperature.

Possible Additional Effects

Potential tonic

 ## Warnings and Precautions

Don't take if you:
Are pregnant, think you may be pregnant or plan pregnancy in the near future.

Consult your doctor if you:
• Take this herb for any medical problem that doesn't improve in 2 weeks (There may be safer, more effective treatments.)
• Take any medicinal drugs or herbs including aspirin, laxatives, cold and cough remedies, antacids, vitamins, minerals, amino acids, supplements, other prescription or nonprescription drugs

Pregnancy:
Don't use unless prescribed by your doctor.

Breastfeeding:
Don't use unless prescribed by your doctor.

Infants and children:
Treating infants or children under 2 with any herbal preparation is hazardous.

Others:
No problems expected if you are beyond childhood, under 45, not pregnant, basically healthy, take it for only a short time and do not exceed manufacturer's recommended dose.

Storage:
• Store in cool, dry area away from direct light, but don't freeze.
• Store safely out of reach of children.
• Don't store in bathroom medicine cabinet. Heat and moisture may change the action of the herb.

Safe dosage:
Consult your doctor for the appropriate dose for your condition.

 ## Toxicity

Rated relatively safe when taken in appropriate quantities for short periods of time

For symptoms of toxicity: See *Adverse Reactions, Side Effects or Overdose Symptoms* section below.

 ## Adverse Reactions, Side Effects or Overdose Symptoms

Signs and symptoms	What to do
Diarrhea	Discontinue. Call doctor immediately.
Upset stomach	Discontinue. Call doctor immediately.

Horehound

Basic Information

Biological name (genus and species):
Marrubium vulgare

Parts used for medicinal purposes:
- Flowers
- Leaves

Chemicals this herb contains:
- Marrubiin
- Resin (see Glossary)
- Tannins (see Glossary)
- Volatile oils (see Glossary)

Known Effects

- Helps expel gas from intestinal tract
- Decreases thickness and increases fluidity of mucus in lungs and bronchial tubes

Miscellaneous information:
- Leaves and flowers are used to make tincture.
- It's also available as tea and lozenges.

Possible Additional Effects

- Potential cough and cold remedy
- May treat whooping cough

Warnings and Precautions

Don't take if you:
- Are pregnant, think you may be pregnant or plan pregnancy in the near future
- Have any chronic disease of the gastrointestinal tract, such as stomach or duodenal ulcers, reflux esophagitis, ulcerative colitis, spastic colitis, diverticulosis or diverticulitis

Consult your doctor if you:
- Take this herb for any medical problem that doesn't improve in 2 weeks (There may be safer, more effective treatments.)
- Take any medicinal drugs or herbs including aspirin, laxatives, cold and cough remedies, antacids, vitamins, minerals, amino acids, supplements, other prescription or nonprescription drugs
- Have heart disease
- Are over 65

Pregnancy:
Don't use unless prescribed by your doctor.

Breastfeeding:
Don't use unless prescribed by your doctor.

Infants and children:
Treating infants or children under 2 with any herbal preparation is hazardous.

Others:
No problems expected if you are beyond childhood, under 45, not pregnant, basically healthy, take it for only a short time and do not exceed manufacturer's recommended dose.

Storage:
- Store in cool, dry area away from direct light, but don't freeze.
- Store safely out of reach of children.
- Don't store in bathroom medicine cabinet. Heat and moisture may change the action of the herb.

Safe dosage:
Consult your doctor for the appropriate dose for your condition.

Toxicity

Comparative-toxicity rating is not available from standard references.

For symptoms of toxicity: See *Adverse Reactions, Side Effects or Overdose Symptoms* section below.

Adverse Reactions, Side Effects or Overdose Symptoms

Signs and symptoms	What to do
Diarrhea	Discontinue. Call doctor immediately.
Nausea or vomiting	Discontinue. Call doctor immediately.

Horse Chestnut

Basic Information

Biological name (genus and species): *Aesculus hippocastanum*

Parts used for medicinal purposes:
• Bark
• Leaves
• Seeds/nuts

Chemicals this herb contains:
• Aescin
• Coumarins
• Flavonoids (quercetin, kaempferol) (see Glossary)
• Saponins (see Glossary)

Known Effects

• Increases bleeding time (a laboratory test for blood clotting)
• Irritates mucous membrane
• Restricts edema
• Increases blood return to heart
• Diuretic

Miscellaneous information:
• There are more reliable, safer anticoagulants approved by the FDA. Eating even a few nuts can cause toxic symptoms.

• Superstitious adults carry seeds in their pockets to cure arthritis.

Possible Additional Effects

• Potential anticoagulant
• Potential sunscreen (4% solution)
• May help treat varicose veins

Warnings and Precautions

Don't take if you:
• Are pregnant, think you may be pregnant or plan pregnancy in the near future
• Have any chronic disease of the gastrointestinal tract, such as stomach or duodenal ulcers, reflux esophagitis, ulcerative colitis, spastic colitis, diverticulosis or diverticulitis

Consult your doctor if you:
• Take this herb for any medical problem that doesn't improve in 2 weeks (There may be safer, more effective treatments.)
• Take any medicinal drugs or herbs including aspirin, laxatives, cold and cough remedies, antacids, vitamins, minerals, amino acids,

supplements, other prescription or nonprescription drugs

Pregnancy:
Dangers outweigh any possible benefits. Don't use.

Breastfeeding:
Dangers outweigh any possible benefits. Don't use.

Infants and children:
Treating infants or children under 2 with any herbal preparation is hazardous.

Storage:
• Store in cool, dry area away from direct light, but don't freeze.
• Store safely out of reach of children.
• Don't store in bathroom medicine cabinet. Heat and moisture may change the action of the herb.

Safe dosage:
Consult your doctor for the appropriate dose for your condition.

Toxicity

Rated slightly dangerous, particularly in children, persons over 55 and those who take larger than appropriate quantities for extended periods of time

For symptoms of toxicity: See *Adverse Reactions, Side Effects or Overdose Symptoms* section below.

Adverse Reactions, Side Effects or Overdose Symptoms

Signs and symptoms	What to do
Gastrointestinal upset	Discontinue. Call doctor immediately.
Lack of coordination	Discontinue. Call doctor immediately.
Nausea or vomiting	Discontinue. Call doctor immediately.
Unusual bleeding	Discontinue. Call doctor immediately.

Horsemint

Basic Information

Biological name (genus and species):
Monarda punctata

Parts used for medicinal purposes:
• Leaves
• Stems

Chemicals this herb contains:
• Carvacrol
• Cymene
• D-limonene
• Linalool
• Monarda oil
• Thymol

Known Effects

• Irritates tissues and mucous membranes
• Kills germs when used on the skin for external infections

Possible
Additional Effects

Internal use:
- May kill intestinal parasites
- May help expel gas from intestinal tract
- May treat abdominal cramps
- May treat nausea

External use:
- May kill fungal infections on skin
- May kill bacterial infections on skin

 Warnings and
Precautions

Don't take if you:
- Are pregnant, think you may be pregnant or plan pregnancy in the near future
- Have any chronic disease of the gastrointestinal tract, such as stomach or duodenal ulcers, reflux esophagitis, ulcerative colitis, spastic colitis, diverticulosis or diverticulitis

Consult your doctor if you:
- Take this herb for any medical problem that doesn't improve in 2 weeks (There may be safer, more effective treatments.)
- Take any medicinal drugs or herbs including aspirin, laxatives, cold and cough remedies, antacids, vitamins, minerals, amino acids, supplements, other prescription or nonprescription drugs

Pregnancy:
Don't use unless prescribed by your doctor.

Breastfeeding:
Don't use unless prescribed by your doctor.

Infants and children:
Treating infants or children under 2 with any herbal preparation is hazardous.

Others:
No problems expected if you are beyond childhood, under 45, not pregnant, basically healthy, take it for only a short time and do not exceed manufacturer's recommended dose.

Storage:
- Store in cool, dry area away from direct light, but don't freeze.
- Store safely out of reach of children.
- Don't store in bathroom medicine cabinet. Heat and moisture may change the action of the herb.

Safe dosage:
Consult your doctor for the appropriate dose for your condition.

 Toxicity

Comparative-toxicity rating is not available from standard references.

For symptoms of toxicity: See *Adverse Reactions, Side Effects or Overdose Symptoms* section below.

 Adverse Reactions,
Side Effects or
Overdose Symptoms

Signs and symptoms	What to do
Diarrhea	Discontinue. Call doctor immediately.
Nausea or vomiting	Discontinue. Call doctor immediately.
Skin rash when used on skin	Discontinue. Call doctor when convenient.

Horseradish

Basic Information

Biological name (genus and species):
Armoracia lapathifolia, Cochlearia armoracia

Parts used for medicinal purposes:
Roots

Chemicals this herb contains:
• Allyl isothiocyanate
• Sinigrin

Known Effects

External use:
• Irritates skin
• Helps clear sinuses

Internal use:
Irritates gastrointestinal tract

Miscellaneous information:
• Horseradish is used to add flavor to foods.
• No effects are expected on the body, either good or bad, when this herb is used in very small amounts to enhance the flavor of food.

Possible Additional Effects

No additional effects are known.

Warnings and Precautions

Don't take if you:
• Are pregnant, think you may be pregnant or plan pregnancy in the near future

• Have any chronic disease of the gastrointestinal tract, such as stomach or duodenal ulcers, reflux esophagitis, ulcerative colitis, spastic colitis, diverticulosis or diverticulitis

Consult your doctor if you:
• Take this herb for any medical problem that doesn't improve in 2 weeks (There may be safer, more effective treatments.)
• Take any medicinal drugs or herbs including aspirin, laxatives, cold and cough remedies, antacids, vitamins, minerals, amino acids, supplements, other prescription or nonprescription drugs

Pregnancy:
Don't use unless prescribed by your doctor.

Breastfeeding:
Don't use unless prescribed by your doctor.

Infants and children:
Treating infants or children under 2 with any herbal preparation is hazardous.

Others:
Eating large amounts of raw root can be toxic.

Storage:
• Store in cool, dry area away from direct light, but don't freeze.
• Store safely out of reach of children.
• Don't store in bathroom medicine cabinet. Heat and moisture may change the action of the herb.

Safe dosage:
Consult your doctor for the appropriate dose for your condition.

Toxicity

Comparative-toxicity rating is not available from standard references.

For symptoms of toxicity: See *Adverse Reactions, Side Effects or Overdose Symptoms* section below.

Adverse Reactions, Side Effects or Overdose Symptoms

Signs and symptoms	What to do
Diarrhea, with blood	Discontinue. Call doctor immediately.
Nausea or vomiting	Discontinue. Call doctor immediately.
Vomiting, with blood	Seek emergency treatment.

Horsetails (Bottle Brush, Field Horsetail, Shave Grass)

Basic Information

Biological name (genus and species): *Equisetum arvense*

Parts used for medicinal purposes: Stems

Chemicals this herb contains:
• Alkaloids
• Flavonoids (see Glossary)
• Phenolic acids
• Silicates
• Silicic acid
• Sterols

Known Effects

No proven medicinal effects are known.

Possible Additional Effects

• May treat bladder infections
• May treat prostatitis
• May help body dispose of excess fluid by increasing amount of urine produced
• May help heal sores on skin

Warnings and Precautions

Don't take if you:
• Are pregnant, think you may be pregnant or plan pregnancy in the near future
• Have heart disease or high blood pressure—use only under doctor's care

Consult your doctor if you:
• Take this herb for any medical problem that doesn't improve in 2 weeks (There may be safer, more effective treatments.)
• Take any medicinal drugs or herbs including aspirin, laxatives, cold and cough remedies, antacids, vitamins, minerals, amino acids, supplements, other prescription or nonprescription drugs

Pregnancy:
Dangerous. Don't use.

Breastfeeding:
Dangerous. Don't use.

Infants and children:
Treating infants or children under 2 with any herbal preparation is hazardous.

Others:
No problems expected if you are beyond childhood, under 45, not pregnant, basically healthy, take it for only a short time and do not exceed manufacturer's recommended dose.

Storage:
• Store in cool, dry area away from direct light, but don't freeze.
• Store safely out of reach of children.
• Don't store in bathroom medicine cabinet. Heat and moisture may change the action of the herb.

Safe dosage:
Consult your doctor for the appropriate dose for your condition.

Toxicity

Rated slightly dangerous, particularly in children, persons over 55 and those who take larger than appropriate quantities for extended periods of time

For symptoms of toxicity: See *Adverse Reactions, Side Effects or Overdose Symptoms* section below.

Adverse Reactions, Side Effects or Overdose Symptoms

Signs and symptoms	What to do
Cold hands and feet	Discontinue. Call doctor when convenient.
Fever	Discontinue. Call doctor immediately.
Heartbeat irregularities	Seek emergency treatment.
Muscle weakness	Discontinue. Call doctor immediately.
Trouble walking	Discontinue. Call doctor immediately.
Weight loss	Discontinue. Call doctor when convenient.

Houseleek (Jupiter's Eye, Thor's Beard)

Basic Information

Biological name (genus and species):
Sempervivum tectorum

Parts used for medicinal purposes:
Leaves

Chemicals this herb contains:
Malic acid

Known Effects

• Shrinks tissues
• Prevents secretion of fluids

Possible Additional Effects

- May help body dispose of excess fluid by increasing amount of urine produced
- May treat insect bites, burns, bruises, skin disease when used as a poultice (see Glossary)

Warnings and Precautions

Don't take if you:

- Are pregnant, think you may be pregnant or plan pregnancy in the near future
- Have any chronic disease of the gastrointestinal tract, such as stomach or duodenal ulcers, reflux esophagitis, ulcerative colitis, spastic colitis, diverticulosis or diverticulitis

Consult your doctor if you:

- Take this herb for any medical problem that doesn't improve in 2 weeks (There may be safer, more effective treatments.)
- Take any medicinal drugs or herbs including aspirin, laxatives, cold and cough remedies, antacids, vitamins, minerals, amino acids, supplements, other prescription or nonprescription drugs

Pregnancy:

Don't use unless prescribed by your doctor.

Breastfeeding:

Don't use unless prescribed by your doctor.

Infants and children:

Treating infants or children under 2 with any herbal preparation is hazardous.

Others:

No problems expected if you are beyond childhood, under 45, not pregnant, basically healthy, take it for only a short time and do not exceed manufacturer's recommended dose.

Storage:

- Store in cool, dry area away from direct light, but don't freeze.
- Store safely out of reach of children.
- Don't store in bathroom medicine cabinet. Heat and moisture may change the action of the herb.

Safe dosage:

Consult your doctor for the appropriate dose for your condition.

Toxicity

Comparative-toxicity rating is not available from standard references.

For symptoms of toxicity: See *Adverse Reactions, Side Effects or Overdose Symptoms* section below.

Adverse Reactions, Side Effects or Overdose Symptoms

Signs and symptoms	What to do
Diarrhea, watery, explosive	Discontinue. Call doctor immediately.
Vomiting	Discontinue. Call doctor immediately.

Huckleberry

 Basic Information

Biological name (genus and species):
Gaylussacia baccata

Parts used for medicinal purposes:
Entire plant

Chemicals this herb contains:
- Fatty acids
- Hydroquinone
- Loeanolic acid
- Neomyrtillin
- Tannins (see Glossary)
- Ursolic acid

 Known Effects

- Decreases blood sugar
- Helps body dispose of excess fluid by increasing amount of urine produced
- Interferes with absorption of iron and other minerals when taken internally

 Possible Additional Effects

- May treat diarrhea
- May treat gastroenteritis
- May treat and prevent scurvy

 Warnings and Precautions

Don't take if you:
Are allergic to blueberries or huckleberries.

Consult your doctor if you:
- Take this herb for any medical problem that doesn't improve in 2 weeks (There may be safer, more effective treatments.)
- Take any medicinal drugs or herbs including aspirin, laxatives, cold and cough remedies, antacids, vitamins, minerals, amino acids, supplements, other prescription or nonprescription drugs

Pregnancy:
Pregnant women should experience no problems taking usual amounts as part of a balanced diet. Other products extracted from this herb have not been proved to cause problems.

Breastfeeding:
Breastfed infants of lactating mothers should experience no problems when mother takes usual amounts as part of a balanced diet. Other products extracted from this herb have not been proved to cause problems.

Infants and children:
Treating infants or children under 2 with any herbal preparation is hazardous.

Others:
No problems expected if you are beyond childhood, under 45, basically healthy, take it for only a short time and do not exceed manufacturer's recommended dose.

Storage:
- Store in cool, dry area away from direct light, but don't freeze.
- Store safely out of reach of children.
- Don't store in bathroom medicine cabinet. Heat and moisture may change the action of the herb.

Safe dosage:
Consult your doctor for the appropriate dose for your condition.

 Toxicity

Generally regarded as safe when taken in appropriate quantities for short periods of time

 Adverse Reactions, Side Effects or Overdose Symptoms

None are expected.

Hydrangea (Peegee, Seven Barks)

 Basic Information

Biological name (genus and species):
Hydrangea paniculata

Parts used for medicinal purposes:
Roots

Chemicals this herb contains:
• Hydrangin (can change to cyanide)
• Resin (see Glossary)
• Saponins (see Glossary)
• Volatile oils (see Glossary)

 Known Effects

• Helps expel gas from intestinal tract
• Shrinks tissues
• Prevents secretion of fluids

Miscellaneous information:
• Leaves contain cyanide.
• Smoking this herb can cause mind-altering effects and toxicity.

 Possible Additional Effects

• May treat cystitis
• May treat bladder stones
• May treat dyspepsia

 Warnings and Precautions

Don't take if you:
• Are pregnant, think you may be pregnant or plan pregnancy in the near future
• Have any chronic disease of the gastrointestinal tract, such as stomach or duodenal ulcers, reflux esophagitis, ulcerative colitis, spastic colitis, diverticulosis or diverticulitis

Consult your doctor if you:
• Take this herb for any medical problem that doesn't improve in 2 weeks (There may be safer, more effective treatments.)
• Take any medicinal drugs or herbs including aspirin, laxatives, cold and cough remedies, antacids, vitamins, minerals, amino acids, supplements, other prescription or nonprescription drugs

Pregnancy:
Dangers outweigh any possible benefits. Don't use.

Breastfeeding:
Dangers outweigh any possible benefits. Don't use.

Infants and children:
Treating infants or children under 2 with any herbal preparation is hazardous.

Storage:
- Store in cool, dry area away from direct light, but don't freeze.
- Store safely out of reach of children.
- Don't store in bathroom medicine cabinet. Heat and moisture may change the action of the herb.

Safe dosage:
Consult your doctor for the appropriate dose for your condition.

 Toxicity

Rated relatively safe when taken in appropriate quantities for short periods of time

For symptoms of toxicity: See *Adverse Reactions, Side Effects or Overdose Symptoms* section below.

 Adverse Reactions, Side Effects or Overdose Symptoms

Signs and symptoms	What to do
Dizziness	Discontinue. Call doctor immediately.
Heavy feeling in chest	Discontinue. Call doctor immediately.
Nausea or vomiting	Discontinue. Call doctor immediately.

Hyssop

 Basic Information

Biological name (genus and species):
Hyssopus officinalis

Parts used for medicinal purposes:
Aerial parts (those above ground)
- Essential oils (see Glossary)
- Flowers
- Leaves

Chemicals this herb contains:
- Diosmine
- Flavonoids (see Glossary)
- Hyssopin
- Isolic acid
- Marrubiin
- Oleonolic acid
- Resin (see Glossary)
- Tannins (see Glossary)
- Volatile oils (see Glossary)

 Known Effects

Expectorant: stimulates coughing, relieves congestion

Miscellaneous information:
Available as tea, compress, tincture, dried or fresh.

 Possible Additional Effects

- May treat bronchitis
- May have a mild sedative effect (antianxiety)

→

- Potential muscle relaxant
- Potential antiseptic: used externally, may treat small wounds and herpes simplex
- May have antiviral properties
- May reduce indigestion
- May help heal cold sores
- May decrease gastrointestinal gas production

 ## Warnings and Precautions

Don't take if you:
Are pregnant, think you may be pregnant or are considering pregnancy.

Consult your doctor if you:
- Take this herb for any medical problem that doesn't improve in 2 weeks (There may be safer, more effective treatments.)
- Take any medicinal drugs or herbs including aspirin, laxatives, cold and cough remedies, antacids, vitamins, minerals, amino acids, supplements, other prescription or nonprescription drugs
- Plan to take hyssop at all—use only under medical supervision!

Pregnancy:
Don't use.

Breastfeeding:
Don't use unless prescribed by your doctor.

Infants and children:
Treating infants or children under 2 with any herbal preparation is hazardous.

Storage:
- Store in cool, dry area away from direct light, but don't freeze.
- Store safely out of reach of children.
- Don't store in bathroom medicine cabinet. Heat and moisture may change the action of the herb.

Safe dosage:
Consult your doctor for the appropriate dose for your condition.

 ## Toxicity

Comparative-toxicity rating is not available from standard references.

For symptoms of toxicity: See *Adverse Reactions, Side Effects or Overdose Symptoms* section below.

 ## Adverse Reactions, Side Effects or Overdose Symptoms

Signs and symptoms	What to do
Diarrhea	Discontinue. Call doctor if it persists.
Nausea	Discontinue. Call doctor if it persists.

Indian Nettle

 ## Basic Information

Indian nettle is also called *kuppi, mercury weed, Indian acalypha* and *hierba del cancer*.

Biological name (genus and species): *Acalypha indica, A. virginica*

Parts used for medicinal purposes: Leaves

Chemicals this herb contains:
- Acalyphine
- Cyanogenic glycoside (see Glossary)
- Inositol methylether
- Resin (see Glossary)
- Triacetomamine
- Volatile oils (see Glossary)

Known Effects

- Irritates stomach lining
- Decreases thickness and increases fluidity of mucus in lungs and bronchial tubes
- Causes vomiting

Miscellaneous information:
- Basic ingredients are similar to ipecac
- Used as a mouthwash and a poultice (see Glossary)

Possible Additional Effects

May stimulate bowel movements

Warnings and Precautions

Don't take if you:
Are pregnant, think you may be pregnant or plan pregnancy in the near future.

Consult your doctor if you:
- Take this herb for any medical problem that doesn't improve in 2 weeks (There may be safer, more effective treatments.)
- Take any medicinal drugs or herbs including aspirin, laxatives, cold and cough remedies, antacids, vitamins, minerals, amino acids, supplements, other prescription or nonprescription drugs

Pregnancy:
Dangers outweigh any possible benefits. Don't use.

Breastfeeding:
Dangers outweigh any possible benefits. Don't use.

Infants and children:
Treating infants or children under 2 with any herbal preparation is hazardous.

Others:
No problems expected if you are beyond childhood, under 45, not pregnant, basically healthy, take it for only a short time and do not exceed manufacturer's recommended dose.

Storage:
- Store in cool, dry area away from direct light, but don't freeze.
- Store safely out of reach of children.
- Don't store in bathroom medicine cabinet. Heat and moisture may change the action of the herb.

Safe dosage:
Consult your doctor for the appropriate dose for your condition.

Toxicity

Rated relatively safe when taken in appropriate quantities for short periods of time

For symptoms of toxicity: See *Adverse Reactions, Side Effects or Overdose Symptoms* section below.

Adverse Reactions, Side Effects or Overdose Symptoms

Signs and symptoms	What to do
Diarrhea	Discontinue. Call doctor immediately.
Nausea or vomiting	Discontinue. Call doctor immediately.

Indian Tobacco (Asthma Weed, Lobelia)

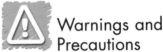

Basic Information

Biological name (genus and species):
Lobelia inflata

Parts used for medicinal purposes:
- Leaves
- Seeds

Chemicals this herb contains:
- Isolobinine
- Lobelanidine
- Lobelanine
- Lobeline
- Norlobelidione
- Norlobelol

Known Effects

- Large amounts stimulate central nervous system
- Small amounts depress central nervous system as blood level drops
- Activates vomiting center in people not accustomed to lobelia
- Effective expectorant

Miscellaneous information:
- Indian tobacco is sometimes advertised as "legal grass." Do not be misled! Toxic effects can be dangerous.
- It is not recommended for medicinal use.

Possible Additional Effects

No additional effects are known.

Warnings and Precautions

Don't take if you:
- Are pregnant, think you may be pregnant or plan pregnancy in the near future
- Have any chronic disease of the gastrointestinal tract, such as stomach or duodenal ulcers, reflux esophagitis, ulcerative colitis, spastic colitis, diverticulosis or diverticulitis

Consult your doctor if you:
- Take this herb for any medical problem that doesn't improve in 2 weeks (There may be safer, more effective treatments.)
- Take any medicinal drugs or herbs including aspirin, laxatives, cold and cough remedies, antacids, vitamins, minerals, amino acids, supplements, other prescription or nonprescription drugs

Pregnancy:
Dangers outweigh any possible benefits. Don't use.

Breastfeeding:
Dangers outweigh any possible benefits. Don't use.

Infants and children:
Treating infants or children under 2 with any herbal preparation is hazardous.

Others:
Dangers outweigh any possible benefits. Don't use.

Storage:
- Store in cool, dry area away from direct light, but don't freeze.
- Store safely out of reach of children.
- Don't store in bathroom medicine cabinet. Heat and moisture may change the action of the herb.

Safe dosage:
Consult your doctor for the appropriate dose for your condition.

 Toxicity

Rated slightly dangerous, particularly in children, persons over 55 and those who take larger than appropriate quantities for extended periods of time.

For symptoms of toxicity: See *Adverse Reactions, Side Effects or Overdose Symptoms* section below.

 Adverse Reactions, Side Effects or Overdose Symptoms

Signs and symptoms	What to do
Coma	Seek emergency treatment.
Diarrhea	Discontinue. Call doctor immediately.
Excess salivation	Discontinue. Call doctor when convenient.
Excess tear formation	Discontinue. Call doctor when convenient.
Giddiness	Discontinue. Call doctor when convenient.
Headache	Discontinue. Call doctor when convenient.
Nausea or vomiting	Discontinue. Call doctor immediately.
Stupor	Seek emergency treatment.
Tremors	Discontinue. Call doctor immediately.

Indigo, Wild

 Basic Information

Biological name (genus and species):
Baptisia tinctoria

Parts used for medicinal purposes:
Roots

Chemicals this herb contains:
- Baptisine
- Baptisol
- Cytisine
- Quinolizidine

 Known Effects

- Irritates gastrointestinal lining
- Causes watery, explosive bowel movements
- Causes vomiting

Miscellaneous information:
Blue dye in wild indigo is inferior to that in domestically grown indigo.

 Possible Additional Effects

- May treat typhoid fever
- May treat amebiasis

Warnings and Precautions

Don't take if you:

- Are pregnant, think you may be pregnant or plan pregnancy in the near future
- Have any chronic disease of the gastrointestinal tract, such as stomach or duodenal ulcers, reflux esophagitis, ulcerative colitis, spastic colitis, diverticulosis or diverticulitis

Consult your doctor if you:

- Take this herb for any medical problem that doesn't improve in 2 weeks (There may be safer, more effective treatments.)
- Take any medicinal drugs or herbs including aspirin, laxatives, cold and cough remedies, antacids, vitamins, minerals, amino acids, supplements, other prescription or nonprescription drugs

Pregnancy:
Dangers outweigh any possible benefits. Don't use.

Breastfeeding:
Dangers outweigh any possible benefits. Don't use.

Infants and children:
Treating infants or children under 2 with any herbal preparation is hazardous.

Others:
No problems expected if you are beyond childhood, under 45, not pregnant, basically healthy, take it for only a short time and do not exceed manufacturer's recommended dose.

Storage:

- Store in cool, dry area away from direct light, but don't freeze.
- Store safely out of reach of children.
- Don't store in bathroom medicine cabinet. Heat and moisture may change the action of the herb.

Safe dosage:
At present no "safe" dosage has been established.

Toxicity

Comparative-toxicity rating is not available from standard references.

For symptoms of toxicity: See *Adverse Reactions, Side Effects or Overdose Symptoms* section below.

Adverse Reactions, Side Effects or Overdose Symptoms

Signs and symptoms	What to do
Diarrhea	Discontinue. Call doctor immediately.
Nausea or vomiting	Discontinue. Call doctor immediately.

Irish Moss

 ## Basic Information

Biological name (genus and species):
Chondrus crispus, Gigartina mamillosa

Parts used for medicinal purposes:
Entire plant

Chemicals this herb contains:
- Bromine
- Calcium
- Carrageenan
- Chlorine
- Protein
- Sodium

 ## Known Effects

- Protects scraped tissues
- Interferes with blood-clotting mechanism

Miscellaneous information:
- Used for hand lotions and as substitute for gelatin in jellies
- Chemically similar to agar, a substance used in laboratories as a base for growing germ cultures

 ## Possible Additional Effects

- May help form bulky stools
- May treat coughs
- May treat diarrhea

 ## Warnings and Precautions

Don't take if you:
- Are pregnant, think you may be pregnant or plan pregnancy in the near future

- Have any chronic disease of the gastrointestinal tract, such as stomach or duodenal ulcers, reflux esophagitis, ulcerative colitis, spastic colitis, diverticulosis or diverticulitis
- Take anticoagulants

Consult your doctor if you:
- Take this herb for any medical problem that doesn't improve in 2 weeks (There may be safer, more effective treatments.)
- Take any medicinal drugs or herbs including aspirin, laxatives, cold and cough remedies, antacids, vitamins, minerals, amino acids, supplements, other prescription or nonprescription drugs

Pregnancy:
Don't use unless prescribed by your doctor.

Breastfeeding:
Don't use unless prescribed by your doctor.

Infants and children:
Treating infants or children under 2 with any herbal preparation is hazardous.

Others:
No problems expected if you are beyond childhood, under 45, not pregnant, basically healthy, take it for only a short time and do not exceed manufacturer's recommended dose.

Storage:
- Store in cool, dry area away from direct light, but don't freeze.
- Store safely out of reach of children.
- Don't store in bathroom medicine cabinet. Heat and moisture may change the action of the herb.

Safe dosage:
Consult your doctor for the appropriate dose for your condition.

Toxicity

Comparative-toxicity rating is not available from standard references.

For symptoms of toxicity: See *Adverse Reactions, Side Effects or Overdose Symptoms* section below.

Adverse Reactions, Side Effects or Overdose Symptoms

Signs and symptoms	What to do
May interact with other anticoagulants to increase anticoagulant effect	Discontinue. Call doctor immediately.
Nausea	Discontinue. Call doctor immediately.

Jalap Root

Basic Information

Jalap root is also known as *conqueror root, high john root, ipomoea* and *turpeth.*

Biological name (genus and species): *Exagonium purga*

Parts used for medicinal purposes: Roots

Chemicals this herb contains:
• Convolvulin
• Gum (see Glossary)
• Jalapin
• Jalapinolic acid
• Starch
• Sugar
• Volatile oils (see Glossary)

Known Effects

• Irritates the gastrointestinal system
• Laxative

Possible Additional Effects

No additional effects are known.

Warnings and Precautions

Don't take if you:
• Are pregnant, think you may be pregnant or plan pregnancy in the near future
• Have any chronic disease of the gastrointestinal tract, such as stomach or duodenal ulcers, reflux esophagitis, ulcerative colitis, spastic colitis, diverticulosis or diverticulitis

Consult your doctor if you:
• Take this herb for any medical problem that doesn't improve in 2 weeks (There may be safer, more effective treatments.)
• Take any medicinal drugs or herbs including aspirin, laxatives, cold and cough remedies, antacids, vitamins, minerals, amino acids, supplements, other prescription or nonprescription drugs

Pregnancy:
Dangers outweigh any possible benefits. Don't use.

Breastfeeding:
Dangers outweigh any possible benefits. Don't use.

Infants and children:
Treating infants or children under 2 with any herbal preparation is hazardous.

Others:
No problems expected if you are beyond childhood, under 45, not pregnant, basically healthy, take it for only a short time and do not exceed manufacturer's recommended dose.

Storage:
• Store in cool, dry area away from direct light, but don't freeze.
• Store safely out of reach of children.
• Don't store in bathroom medicine cabinet. Heat and moisture may change the action of the herb.

Safe dosage:
Consult your doctor for the appropriate dose for your condition.

Toxicity

Comparative-toxicity rating is not available from standard references.

For symptoms of toxicity: See *Adverse Reactions, Side Effects or Overdose Symptoms* section below.

Adverse Reactions, Side Effects or Overdose Symptoms

Signs and symptoms	What to do
Diarrhea, explosive, watery, with possible fluid and electrolyte depletion, leading to weakness and possible heartbeat irregularities	Discontinue. Call doctor immediately.

Jamaican Dogwood (Fish-Poison Tree)

Basic Information

Biological name (genus and species):
Piscidia piscipula

Parts used for medicinal purposes:
Bark

Chemicals this herb contains:
• Piscidin
• Rotenone

Known Effects

• Causes hallucinations
• Treats painful conditions
• Depresses uterine contractions

Miscellaneous information:
• Poisonous to fish
• Active chemicals in bark have odor similar to opium

Possible
Additional Effects

- May produce euphoria
- May treat dysmenorrhea (painful menstruation)

 Warnings and
Precautions

Don't take if you:

Are pregnant, think you may be pregnant or plan pregnancy in the near future.

Consult your doctor if you:

- Take this herb for any medical problem that doesn't improve in 2 weeks (There may be safer, more effective treatments.)
- Take any medicinal drugs or herbs including aspirin, laxatives, cold and cough remedies, antacids, vitamins, minerals, amino acids, supplements, other prescription or nonprescription drugs

Pregnancy:

Don't use unless prescribed by your doctor.

Breastfeeding:

Don't use unless prescribed by your doctor.

Infants and children:

Treating infants or children under 2 with any herbal preparation is hazardous.

Others:

No problems expected if you are beyond childhood, under 45, not pregnant, basically healthy, take it for only a short time and do not exceed manufacturer's recommended dose.

Storage:

- Store in cool, dry area away from direct light, but don't freeze.
- Store safely out of reach of children.
- Don't store in bathroom medicine cabinet. Heat and moisture may change the action of the herb.

Safe dosage:

Consult your doctor for the appropriate dose for your condition.

 Toxicity

Rated slightly dangerous, particularly in children, persons over 55 and those who take larger than appropriate quantities for extended periods of time

For symptoms of toxicity: See *Adverse Reactions, Side Effects or Overdose Symptoms* section below.

 Adverse Reactions,
Side Effects or
Overdose Symptoms

Signs and symptoms	What to do
Hallucinations	Seek emergency treatment.

Jequirity Bean (Crab's Eyes, Indian Licorice, Rosary Pea)

Basic Information

Biological name (genus and species):
Abrus precatorius

Parts used for medicinal purposes:
Seeds/beans

Chemicals this herb contains:
- Abrin
- Anthocyanins
- Indole alkaloids

Known Effects

Abrin in the seed causes cell destruction.

Miscellaneous information:
- No longer used therapeutically
- Causes toxic reactions with ingestion
- Common weed in Florida, Central America and South America

Possible Additional Effects

Used as drops to potentially treat eye problems

Warnings and Precautions

Don't take if you:
- Are pregnant, think you may be pregnant or plan pregnancy in the near future
- Have any chronic disease of the gastrointestinal tract, such as stomach or duodenal ulcers, reflux esophagitis, ulcerative colitis, spastic colitis, diverticulosis or diverticulitis

Consult your doctor if you:
- Take this herb for any medical problem that doesn't improve in 2 weeks (There may be safer, more effective treatments.)
- Take any medicinal drugs or herbs including aspirin, laxatives, cold and cough remedies, antacids, vitamins, minerals, amino acids, supplements, other prescription or nonprescription drugs

Pregnancy:
Dangers outweigh any possible benefits. Don't use.

Breastfeeding:
Dangers outweigh any possible benefits. Don't use.

Infants and children:
Treating infants or children under 2 with any herbal preparation is hazardous.

Others:
Dangers outweigh any possible benefits for anyone. Don't use. Swallowing even one bean can cause toxic symptoms hours or even days after eating.

Storage:
- Store in cool, dry area away from direct light, but don't freeze.
- Store safely out of reach of children.
- Don't store in bathroom medicine cabinet. Heat and moisture may change the action of the herb.

Safe dosage:
Consult your doctor for the appropriate dose for your condition.

Toxicity

Rated dangerous, particularly in children, persons over 55 and those who take larger than appropriate quantities for extended periods of time

For symptoms of toxicity: See *Adverse Reactions, Side Effects or Overdose Symptoms* section below.

Adverse Reactions, Side Effects or Overdose Symptoms

Signs and symptoms	What to do
Convulsions	Seek emergency treatment.
Diarrhea	Discontinue. Call doctor immediately.
Increased heart rate	Discontinue. Call doctor immediately.
Kidney damage characterized by blood in urine, decreased urine flow, swelling of hands and feet	Seek emergency treatment.
Nausea or vomiting	Discontinue. Call doctor immediately.

Jersey Tea (Red Root)

Basic Information

Biological name (genus and species):
Ceanothus americanus

Parts used for medicinal purposes:
Roots

Chemicals this herb contains:
- Ceanothic acid
- Malonic acid
- Orthophosphoric acid
- Oxalic acid
- Pyrophosphoric acid
- Resin (see Glossary)
- Succinic acid
- Tannins (see Glossary)

Known Effects

- Shrinks tissues
- Prevents secretion of fluids
- Increases blood clotting
- Interferes with absorption of iron and other minerals when taken internally

Possible Additional Effects

- May treat syphilis (archaic)
- May treat "spleen" problems
- May stop mild bleeding from broken capillaries in skin
- May decrease thickness and increase fluidity of mucus in lungs and bronchial tubes

- Potential sedative
- May relieve spasm in skeletal muscle or smooth muscle
- May treat depression

 Warnings and Precautions

Don't take if you:

Are pregnant, think you may be pregnant or plan pregnancy in the near future.

Consult your doctor if you:

- Take this herb for any medical problem that doesn't improve in 2 weeks (There may be safer, more effective treatments.)
- Take any medicinal drugs or herbs including aspirin, laxatives, cold and cough remedies, antacids, vitamins, minerals, amino acids, supplements, other prescription or nonprescription drugs

Pregnancy:

Problems in pregnant women taking small or usual amounts have not been proved, but the chance of problems does exist. Don't use unless prescribed by your doctor.

Breastfeeding:

Don't use unless prescribed by your doctor.

Infants and children:

Treating infants or children under 2 with any herbal preparation is hazardous.

Others:

No problems expected if you are beyond childhood, under 45, not pregnant, basically healthy, take it for only a short time and do not exceed manufacturer's recommended dose.

Storage:

- Store in cool, dry area away from direct light, but don't freeze.
- Store safely out of reach of children.
- Don't store in bathroom medicine cabinet. Heat and moisture may change the action of the herb.

Safe dosage:

Consult your doctor for the appropriate dose for your condition.

 Toxicity

Comparative-toxicity rating is not available from standard references.

For symptoms of toxicity: See *Adverse Reactions, Side Effects or Overdose Symptoms* section below.

 Adverse Reactions, Side Effects or Overdose Symptoms

Signs and symptoms	What to do
Prolonged minor bleeding	Discontinue. Call doctor immediately.

Jimson Weed (Sacred Datura, Stramonium, Thorn Apple)

Basic Information

Biological name (genus and species):
Datura stramonium

Parts used for medicinal purposes:
• Leaves
• Seeds

Chemicals this herb contains:
• Atropine
• Hyoscyamine
• Scopolamine

Known Effects

Negates normal activity of acetylcholine, an important chemical at the synapses (connections between nerve cells) of heart, brain, smooth muscles and glands

Miscellaneous information:
• There are more refined, predictable sources for the active chemicals in jimson weed.
• The highest concentration of toxins are in seeds but toxins may be in all parts of the plant.

Possible Additional Effects

• May treat asthma
• May treat gastrointestinal problems
• May produce hallucinations
• Potential sedative

Warnings and Precautions

Don't take if you:
• Are pregnant, think you may be pregnant or plan pregnancy in the near future
• Have heart disease

Consult your doctor if you:
• Take this herb for any medical problem that doesn't improve in 2 weeks (There may be safer, more effective treatments.)
• Take any medicinal drugs or herbs including aspirin, laxatives, cold and cough remedies, antacids, vitamins, minerals, amino acids, supplements, other prescription or nonprescription drugs

Pregnancy:
Dangers outweigh any possible benefits. Don't use.

Breastfeeding:
Dangers outweigh any possible benefits. Don't use.

Infants and children:
Treating infants or children under 2 with any herbal preparation is hazardous.

Others:
Dangers outweigh any possible benefits. Don't use.

Storage:
• Store in cool, dry area away from direct light, but don't freeze.
• Store safely out of reach of children.
• Don't store in bathroom medicine cabinet. Heat and moisture may change the action of the herb.

Safe dosage:
Consult your doctor for the appropriate dose for your condition.

Toxicity

Rated dangerous, particularly in children, persons over 55 and those who take larger than appropriate quantities for extended periods of time

For symptoms of toxicity: See *Adverse Reactions, Side Effects or Overdose Symptoms* section below.

Adverse Reactions, Side Effects or Overdose Symptoms

Signs and symptoms	What to do
Convulsions	Seek emergency treatment.
Dilated pupils	Discontinue. Call doctor immediately.
Dry mouth	Discontinue. Call doctor when convenient.
Extremely fast heart rate	Seek emergency treatment.
Flushing	Discontinue. Call doctor when convenient.
Hallucinations	Seek emergency treatment.
Increased blood pressure	Discontinue. Call doctor immediately.
Unconsciousness	Seek emergency treatment.

Juniper, Common

Basic Information

Biological name (genus and species):
Juniperus communis

Parts used for medicinal purposes:
Berries/fruits

Chemicals this herb contains:
- Alcohols
- Alpha-pinene
- Cadinene
- Camphene
- Flavone
- Resin (see Glossary)
- Sabinene
- Sugar
- Tannins (see Glossary)
- Terpinene
- Volatile oils (see Glossary)

Known Effects

- Irritates kidneys
- Diuretic
- Can cause uterine contractions

Miscellaneous information:
Provides flavor in gin.

Possible Additional Effects

- May treat chronic kidney disorders
- May help body dispose of excess fluid by increasing amount of urine produced
- May treat digestive problems
- May help reduce high blood pressure by decreasing fluid retention
- Potential anti-inflammatory

Warnings and
Precautions

Don't take if you:

- Are pregnant, think you may be pregnant or plan pregnancy in the near future
- Have any chronic disease of the gastrointestinal tract, such as stomach or duodenal ulcers, reflux esophagitis, ulcerative colitis, spastic colitis, diverticulosis or diverticulitis
- Have kidney disease or infection or a history of kidney problems

Consult your doctor if you:

- Take this herb for any medical problem that doesn't improve in 2 weeks (There may be safer, more effective treatments.)
- Take any medicinal drugs or herbs including aspirin, laxatives, cold and cough remedies, antacids, vitamins, minerals, amino acids, supplements, other prescription or nonprescription drugs

Pregnancy:

Juniper can cause uterine contractions. Don't use.

Breastfeeding:

Dangers outweigh any possible benefits. Don't use.

Infants and children:

Treating infants or children under 2 with any herbal preparation is hazardous.

Others:

- No problems expected if you are beyond childhood, under 45, not pregnant, basically healthy, take it for only a short time and do not exceed manufacturer's recommended dose
- For short-term use only

Storage:

- Store in cool, dry area away from direct light, but don't freeze.
- Store safely out of reach of children.
- Don't store in bathroom medicine cabinet. Heat and moisture may change the action of the herb.

Safe dosage:

Consult your doctor for the appropriate dose for your condition.

 Toxicity

Rated slightly dangerous, particularly in children, persons over 55 and those who take larger than appropriate quantities for extended periods of time

For symptoms of toxicity: See *Adverse Reactions, Side Effects or Overdose Symptoms* section below.

 Adverse Reactions, Side Effects or Overdose Symptoms

Signs and symptoms	What to do
Single dose:	
Allergy symptoms	Discontinue. Call doctor immediately.
Diarrhea, watery, explosive	Discontinue. Call doctor immediately.
Increased heart rate	Discontinue. Call doctor immediately.
Small, repeated doses:	
Convulsions	Seek emergency treatment.
Hallucinations	Seek emergency treatment.
Kidney damage characterized by blood in urine, decreased urine flow, swelling of hands and feet	Discontinue. Call doctor immediately.
Personality changes	Discontinue. Call doctor immediately.

Kava Kava

Basic Information

Biological name (genus and species):
Piper methysticum

Parts used for medicinal purposes:
Roots

Chemicals this herb contains:
- Demethoxyyangonin
- Dihydrokawain
- Dihydromethysticin
- Flavorawin A
- Kawain
- Methysticin
- Starch
- Yangonin

Known Effects

- Depresses the central nervous system
- Antianxiety

Miscellaneous information:
- Used to make a fermented liquor
- Sedative effect is mild
- Available in dry bulk, capsules, tinctures
- Generally requires 3 to 6 weeks before effectiveness can be evaluated

Possible Additional Effects

- May induce restful sleep
- May treat fatigue
- Potential genitourinary antiseptic (see Glossary)
- May treat coughs
- Potential muscle relaxant
- Potential analgesic

Warnings and Precautions

Don't take if you:
- Are pregnant, think you may be pregnant or plan pregnancy in the near future
- Are driving or operating equipment (Large doses cause sedation.)

Consult your doctor if you:
- Take this herb for any medical problem that doesn't improve in 2 weeks (There may be safer, more effective treatments.)
- Take any medicinal drugs or herbs including aspirin, laxatives, cold and cough remedies, antacids, vitamins, minerals, amino acids, supplements, other prescription or nonprescription drugs

Pregnancy:
Problems in pregnant women taking small or usual amounts have not been proved, but the chance of problems does exist. Don't use unless prescribed by your doctor.

Breastfeeding:
Problems in breastfed infants of lactating mothers taking small or usual amounts have not been proved, but the chance of problems does exist. Don't use unless prescribed by your doctor.

Infants and children:
Treating infants or children under 2 with any herbal preparation is hazardous.

Others:
No problems expected if you are beyond childhood, under 45, not pregnant, basically healthy, take it for only a short time and do not exceed manufacturer's recommended dose.

→

Storage:
- Store in cool, dry area away from direct light, but don't freeze.
- Store safely out of reach of children.
- Don't store in bathroom medicine cabinet. Heat and moisture may change the action of the herb.

Safe dosage:
Consult your doctor for the appropriate dose for your condition.

 Toxicity

Rated slightly dangerous, particularly in children, persons over 55 and those who take larger than appropriate quantities for extended periods of time

For symptoms of toxicity: See *Adverse Reactions, Side Effects or Overdose Symptoms* section below.

 Adverse Reactions, Side Effects or Overdose Symptoms

Signs and symptoms	What to do
Allergic skin reaction or shortness of breath	Discontinue. Call doctor immediately.
Gastrointestinal upset	Discontinue. Call doctor immediately.
Oversedation	Discontinue. Call doctor immediately.
Repeated small amounts may lead to undesirable skin and nail coloring, inflammation of the body and eyes	Discontinue. Call doctor immediately.

Kelp

 Basic Information

Biological name (genus and species):
Laminaria, Fucus, Sargassum

Parts used for medicinal purposes:
Leaves

Chemicals this herb contains:
- Alginic acid
- Bromine
- Iodine
- Potassium
- Sodium

 Known Effects

Provides bulk for bowel movements

Miscellaneous information:
- Iodine can interfere with normal thyroid function.
- Iodine is used as a substitute for table salt.

 Possible Additional Effects

- May treat chronic constipation without catharsis
- May soften stools
- May treat ulcers
- May control obesity

Warnings and
Precautions

Don't take if you:
- Are pregnant, think you may be pregnant or plan pregnancy in the near future
- Are allergic to iodine in any form, particularly if you have had an allergic reaction to injected dye used for X-ray studies of the kidney or other organs

Consult your doctor if you:
- Take this herb for any medical problem that doesn't improve in 2 weeks (There may be safer, more effective treatments.)
- Take any medicinal drugs or herbs including aspirin, laxatives, cold and cough remedies, antacids, vitamins, minerals, amino acids, supplements, other prescription or nonprescription drugs

Pregnancy:
Don't use unless prescribed by your doctor.

Breastfeeding:
Don't use unless prescribed by your doctor.

Infants and children:
Treating infants or children under 2 with any herbal preparation is hazardous.

Others:
No problems expected if you are beyond childhood, under 45, not pregnant, basically healthy, take it for only a short time and do not exceed manufacturer's recommended dose.

Storage:
- Store in cool, dry area away from direct light, but don't freeze.
- Store safely out of reach of children.
- Don't store in bathroom medicine cabinet. Heat and moisture may change the action of the herb.

Safe dosage:
Consult your doctor for the appropriate dose for your condition.

 Toxicity

Comparative-toxicity rating is not available from standard references.

 Adverse Reactions,
Side Effects or
Overdose Symptoms

None are expected.

Lemongrass

 Basic Information

Biological name (genus and species):
Cymbopogon citratus

Parts used for medicinal purposes:
Various parts of the entire plant, frequently differing by country and culture

➔

Chemicals this herb contains:
- Citronellal
- Methylneptenone
- Myrcene
- Terpenes (see Glossary)
- Terpene alcohol

Known Effects

Kills insects, but less efficiently than malathion or parathione

Miscellaneous information:
Lemongrass is used in perfumes and sometimes as an insect repellent.

Possible Additional Effects

- May treat constipation
- May treat fever
- Potential pain reducer
- Potential sedative

Warnings and Precautions

Don't take if you:
- Are pregnant, think you may be pregnant or plan pregnancy in the near future
- Have any chronic disease of the gastrointestinal tract, such as stomach or duodenal ulcers, reflux esophagitis, ulcerative colitis, spastic colitis, diverticulosis or diverticulitis

Consult your doctor if you:
- Take this herb for any medical problem that doesn't improve in 2 weeks (There may be safer, more effective treatments.)
- Take any medicinal drugs or herbs including aspirin, laxatives, cold and cough remedies, antacids, vitamins, minerals, amino acids, supplements, other prescription or nonprescription drugs

Pregnancy:
Don't use unless prescribed by your doctor.

Breastfeeding:
Don't use unless prescribed by your doctor.

Infants and children:
Treating infants or children under 2 with any herbal preparation is hazardous.

Others:
No problems expected if you are beyond childhood, under 45, not pregnant, basically healthy, take it for only a short time and do not exceed manufacturer's recommended dose.

Storage:
- Store in cool, dry area away from direct light, but don't freeze.
- Store safely out of reach of children.
- Don't store in bathroom medicine cabinet. Heat and moisture may change the action of the herb.

Safe dosage:
Consult your doctor for the appropriate dose for your condition.

Toxicity

Comparative-toxicity rating is not available from standard references.

For symptoms of toxicity: See *Adverse Reactions, Side Effects or Overdose Symptoms* section below.

Adverse Reactions, Side Effects or Overdose Symptoms

Signs and symptoms	What to do
Diarrhea	Discontinue. Call doctor immediately.
Nausea or vomiting	Discontinue. Call doctor immediately.

Licorice, Common (Licorice Root, Spanish Licorice Root)

Basic Information

Biological name (genus and species): *Glycyrrhiza glabra*

Parts used for medicinal purposes:
- Rhizomes
- Roots

Chemicals this herb contains:
- Asparagine
- Fat
- Glycyrrhizin
- Gum (see Glossary)
- Pentacyclic terpenes
- Protein
- Sugar
- Yellow dye

Known Effects

- Decreases inflammation
- Provides estrogen-like hormone effects
- Decreases spasm of smooth muscle or skeletal muscle (asthma, allergic reactions)
- Decreases thickness and increases fluidity of mucus in lungs and bronchial tubes
- Cough suppressant
- Treats constipation, heartburn, ulcers

Miscellaneous information:
- Warning: Consuming large amounts of licorice may lead to high blood pressure.
- Licorice is available as liquid extract and capsules.
- Most licorice in the United States is anise-flavored candy, not true licorice.

Possible Additional Effects

- May protect scraped tissues (external use)
- May improve liver function

Warnings and Precautions

Don't take if you:
- Are pregnant, think you may be pregnant or plan pregnancy in the near future
- Have heart disease
- Take diuretics

Consult your doctor if you:
- Take this herb for any medical problem that doesn't improve in 2 weeks (There may be safer, more effective treatments.)
- Take any medicinal drugs or herbs including aspirin, laxatives, cold and cough remedies, antacids, vitamins, minerals, amino acids, supplements, other prescription or nonprescription drugs
- Have a history of heart disease
- Are over age 55

Pregnancy:
Dangers outweigh any possible benefits. Don't use.

Breastfeeding:
Dangers outweigh any possible benefits. Don't use.

Infants and children:
Treating infants or children under 2 with any herbal preparation is hazardous.

→

Others:

No problems expected if you are beyond childhood, under 45, not pregnant, basically healthy, take it for only a short time and do not exceed manufacturer's recommended dose.

Storage:

- Store in cool, dry area away from direct light, but don't freeze.
- Store safely out of reach of children.
- Don't store in bathroom medicine cabinet. Heat and moisture may change the action of the herb.

Safe dosage:

Consult your doctor for the appropriate dose for your condition.

 Toxicity

Rated slightly dangerous, particularly in children, persons over 55 and those who take larger than appropriate quantities for extended periods of time

For symptoms of toxicity: See *Adverse Reactions, Side Effects or Overdose Symptoms* section below.

 Adverse Reactions, Side Effects or Overdose Symptoms

Signs and symptoms	What to do
High blood pressure	Discontinue. Call doctor immediately.
Effects of sodium retention:	
Edema	Discontinue. Call doctor immediately.
Lung congestion	Discontinue. Call doctor immediately.
Effects of sodium depletion:	
Heartbeat irregularities	Discontinue. Call doctor immediately.
Nausea	Discontinue. Call doctor immediately.
Weakness	Discontinue. Call doctor immediately.

Liferoot (Golden Groundsel, Squaw Weed)

 Basic Information

Biological name (genus and species): *Senecio vulgaris, S. aureus*

Parts used for medicinal purposes: Roots

Chemicals this herb contains: Pyrrolizidine

 Known Effects

- Increases blood pressure
- Stimulates uterine contractions

Miscellaneous information:

Pyrrolizidine has a high potential for causing liver disorders, including cancer.

 Possible Additional Effects

- May treat menstrual irregularities
- May treat dysmenorrhea (painful menstruation)
- May treat excessive menstrual bleeding (menorrhagia)
- May help relieve vaginal discharge
- May cause overdue labor to begin

Warnings and Precautions

Don't take if you:
Are pregnant, think you may be pregnant or plan pregnancy in the near future.

Consult your doctor if you:
• Take this herb for any medical problem that doesn't improve in 2 weeks (There may be safer, more effective treatments.)
• Take any medicinal drugs or herbs including aspirin, laxatives, cold and cough remedies, antacids, vitamins, minerals, amino acids, supplements, other prescription or nonprescription drugs

Pregnancy:
Dangers outweigh any possible benefits. Don't use.

Breastfeeding:
Dangers outweigh any possible benefits. Don't use.

Infants and children:
Treating infants or children under 2 with any herbal preparation is hazardous.

Others:
No problems expected if you are beyond childhood, under 45, not pregnant, basically healthy, take it for only a short time and do not exceed manufacturer's recommended dose.

Storage:
• Store in cool, dry area away from direct light, but don't freeze.
• Store safely out of reach of children.
• Don't store in bathroom medicine cabinet. Heat and moisture may change the action of the herb.

Safe dosage:
Consult your doctor for the appropriate dose for your condition.

 ## Toxicity

Rated slightly dangerous, particularly in children, persons over 55 and those who take larger than appropriate quantities for extended periods of time

For symptoms of toxicity: See *Adverse Reactions, Side Effects or Overdose Symptoms* section below.

 ## Adverse Reactions, Side Effects or Overdose Symptoms

Signs and symptoms	What to do
Abnormal liver-function tests	Discontinue. Call doctor immediately.
Jaundice (yellow skin and eyes)	Discontinue. Call doctor immediately.

Lily-of-the-Valley

Basic Information

Biological name (genus and species):
Convallaria majalis

Parts used for medicinal purposes:
- Berries/fruits
- Petals/flower
- Roots

Chemicals this herb contains:
- Convallamarin
- Convallarin
- Convallatoxin (highly toxic)

Known Effects

- Increases efficiency of heart-muscle contraction
- Helps body dispose of excess fluid by increasing amount of urine produced

Miscellaneous information:
Although lily-of-the-valley has similar action to digitalis, there are safer, less expensive, more reliable products to use.

Possible Additional Effects

- May treat congestive heart failure
- May treat heartbeat irregularities
- May improve circulation

Warnings and Precautions

Don't take if you:
- Are pregnant, think you may be pregnant or plan pregnancy in the near future
- Have any chronic disease of the gastrointestinal tract, such as stomach or duodenal ulcers, reflux esophagitis, ulcerative colitis, spastic colitis, diverticulosis or diverticulitis

Consult your doctor if you:
- Take this herb for any medical problem that doesn't improve in 2 weeks (There may be safer, more effective treatments.)
- Take any medicinal drugs or herbs including aspirin, laxatives, cold and cough remedies, antacids, vitamins, minerals, amino acids, supplements, other prescription or nonprescription drugs

Pregnancy:
Dangers outweigh any possible benefits. Don't use.

Breastfeeding:
Dangers outweigh any possible benefits. Don't use.

Infants and children:
Treating infants or children under 2 with any herbal preparation is hazardous.

Others:
Dangers outweigh any possible benefits. Don't use.

Storage:
- Store in cool, dry area away from direct light, but don't freeze.
- Store safely out of reach of children.
- Don't store in bathroom medicine cabinet. Heat and moisture may change the action of the herb.

Safe dosage:
Consult your doctor for the appropriate dose for your condition.

Toxicity

Rated dangerous, particularly in children, persons over 55 and those who take larger than appropriate quantities for extended periods of time

For symptoms of toxicity: See *Adverse Reactions, Side Effects or Overdose Symptoms* section below.

 Adverse Reactions, Side Effects or Overdose Symptoms

Signs and symptoms	What to do
Heartbeat irregularities	Seek emergency treatment.
Nausea or vomiting	Discontinue. Call doctor immediately.

Linden Tree

 Basic Information

The linden tree is called a *lime tree* in Europe.

Biological name (genus and species): *Tilia europaea*

Parts used for medicinal purposes: Petals/flower

Chemicals this herb contains:
• Tannins (see Glossary)
• Volatile oils (see Glossary)

 Known Effects

• Decreases spasm of smooth or skeletal muscle
• Increases perspiration
• Clears excess mucus from lungs
• Promotes digestion

 Possible Additional Effects

• May treat coughs
• May decrease thickness and increase fluidity of mucus in lungs and bronchial tubes
• May reduce fever
• May have relaxing effect to help treat insomnia, nervous tension

 Warnings and Precautions

Don't take if you:
Are pregnant, think you may be pregnant or plan pregnancy in the near future.

Consult your doctor if you:
• Take this herb for any medical problem that doesn't improve in 2 weeks (There may be safer, more effective treatments.)
• Take any medicinal drugs or herbs including aspirin, laxatives, cold and cough remedies, antacids, vitamins, minerals, amino acids, supplements, other prescription or nonprescription drugs
• Have a history of heart disease

Pregnancy:
Don't use unless prescribed by your doctor.

Breastfeeding:
Don't use unless prescribed by your doctor.

Infants and children:

Treating infants or children under 2 with any herbal preparation is hazardous.

Others:

No problems expected if you are beyond childhood, under 45, not pregnant, basically healthy, take it for only a short time and do not exceed manufacturer's recommended dose.

Storage:

- Store in cool, dry area away from direct light, but don't freeze.
- Store safely out of reach of children.
- Don't store in bathroom medicine cabinet. Heat and moisture may change the action of the herb.

Safe dosage:

Consult your doctor for the appropriate dose for your condition.

Toxicity

Rated relatively safe when taken in appropriate quantities for short periods of time

For symptoms of toxicity: See *Adverse Reactions, Side Effects or Overdose Symptoms* section below.

Adverse Reactions, Side Effects or Overdose Symptoms

Signs and symptoms	What to do
Drowsiness	Discontinue. Call doctor when convenient.

Mace (Nutmeg)

Basic Information

Biological name (genus and species):
Myristica fragrans

Parts used for medicinal purposes:
- Fibrous covering
- Seeds

Chemicals this herb contains:
- Elemicin
- Eugenol
- Fixed oil (see Glossary)
- Isoeugenol
- Isomethyleugenol
- Methoxyeugenol
- Methyleugenol
- Myristicin
- Protein
- Starch

Known Effects

- Stimulates muscular movement of intestinal tract
- Stimulates central nervous system
- Helps treat diarrhea and indigestion
- Removes excess gas from gastrointestinal tract

Miscellaneous information:

- No effects are expected on the body, either good or bad, when the herb is used in very small amounts to enhance the flavor of food.
- Nutmeg is the seed. Mace is the fibrous covering.
- It is available as a powder and tincture.

Possible Additional Effects

- May produce hallucinations
- May alter mood
- May treat digestive disorders
- May treat cholera

 ## Warnings and Precautions

Don't take if you:

- Are pregnant, think you may be pregnant or plan pregnancy in the near future
- Have any chronic disease of the gastrointestinal tract, such as stomach or duodenal ulcers, reflux esophagitis, ulcerative colitis, spastic colitis, diverticulosis or diverticulitis

Consult your doctor if you:

- Take any medicinal drugs or herbs including aspirin, laxatives, cold and cough remedies, antacids, vitamins, minerals, amino acids, supplements, other prescription or nonprescription drugs
- Are over age 60

Pregnancy:

Dangers outweigh any possible benefits. Don't use.

Breastfeeding:

Dangers outweigh any possible benefits. Don't use.

Infants and children:

Treating infants or children under 2 with any herbal preparation is hazardous.

Others:

Mind-altering and hallucinogenic effects are unpleasant. Do not use nutmeg for these purposes.

Storage:

- Store in cool, dry area away from direct light, but don't freeze.
- Store safely out of reach of children.
- Don't store in bathroom medicine cabinet. Heat and moisture may change the action of the herb.

Safe dosage:

Consult your doctor for the appropriate dose for your condition.

 ## Toxicity

- Mace is rated slightly dangerous, particularly in children, persons over 55 and those who take larger than appropriate quantities for extended periods of time.
- Narcotic properties—known to be toxic in humans—can cause delirium, disorientation and drunkenness.

For symptoms of toxicity: See *Adverse Reactions, Side Effects or Overdose Symptoms* section below.

 ## Adverse Reactions, Side Effects or Overdose Symptoms

Signs and symptoms	What to do
Diarrhea	Discontinue. Call doctor immediately.
Drowsiness	Discontinue. Call doctor when convenient.
Hallucinations	Seek emergency treatment.
Nausea or vomiting	Discontinue. Call doctor immediately.
Reduced body temperature	Discontinue. Call doctor immediately.
Weak, thready, rapid pulse	Seek emergency treatment.

Malabar Nut (Vasaka)

Basic Information

Biological name (genus and species):
Adhatoda vasica

Parts used for medicinal purposes:
Leaves

Chemicals this herb contains:
• Adhatodic acid
• Peganine
• Vasicine

Known Effects

• Dilates bronchial tubes
• Decreases thickness and increases fluidity of mucus in lungs and bronchial tubes

Possible Additional Effects

• May treat coughs and colds
• May treat bronchitis
• May treat asthma

Warnings and Precautions

Don't take if you:
• Are pregnant, think you may be pregnant or plan pregnancy in the near future
• Have any chronic disease of the gastrointestinal tract, such as stomach or duodenal ulcers, reflux esophagitis, ulcerative colitis, spastic colitis, diverticulosis or diverticulitis

Consult your doctor if you:
• Take this herb for any medical problem that doesn't improve in 2 weeks (There may be safer, more effective treatments.)
• Take any medicinal drugs or herbs including aspirin, laxatives, cold and cough remedies, antacids, vitamins, minerals, amino acids, supplements, other prescription or nonprescription drugs

Pregnancy:
Don't use unless prescribed by your doctor.

Breastfeeding:
Don't use unless prescribed by your doctor.

Infants and children:
Treating infants or children under 2 with any herbal preparation is hazardous.

Others:
No problems expected if you are beyond childhood, under 45, not pregnant, basically healthy, take it for only a short time and do not exceed manufacturer's recommended dose.

Storage:
• Store in cool, dry area away from direct light, but don't freeze.
• Store safely out of reach of children.
• Don't store in bathroom medicine cabinet. Heat and moisture may change the action of the herb.

Safe dosage:
Consult your doctor for the appropriate dose for your condition.

Toxicity

Rated slightly dangerous, particularly in children, persons over 55 and those who take larger than appropriate quantities for extended periods of time

For symptoms of toxicity: See *Adverse Reactions, Side Effects or Overdose Symptoms* section below.

Adverse Reactions, Side Effects or Overdose Symptoms

Signs and symptoms	What to do
Diarrhea	Discontinue. Call doctor immediately.
Nausea or vomiting	Discontinue. Call doctor immediately.

Male Fern (Aspidium)

Basic Information

Biological name (genus and species): *Dryopteris filix-mas*

Parts used for medicinal purposes:
• Leaves
• Roots

Chemicals this herb contains:
• Alkanes
• Oleoresin (see Glossary)
• Resin (see Glossary)
• Triterpenes
• Volatile oils (see Glossary)

Known Effects

• Destroys intestinal worms
• Decreases normal muscle function
• Interferes with absorption of iron and other minerals when taken internally

Possible Additional Effects

No additional effects are known.

Warnings and Precautions

Don't take if you:
• Are pregnant, think you may be pregnant or plan pregnancy in the near future
• Have any chronic disease of the gastrointestinal tract, such as stomach or duodenal ulcers, reflux esophagitis, ulcerative colitis, spastic colitis, diverticulosis or diverticulitis
• Are over age 55
• Have heart disease
• Have kidney disease

Consult your doctor if you:
• Take this herb for any medical problem that doesn't improve in 2 weeks (There may be safer, more effective treatments.)
• Take any medicinal drugs or herbs including aspirin, laxatives, cold and cough remedies, antacids, vitamins, minerals, amino acids, supplements, other prescription or nonprescription drugs

Pregnancy:
Dangers outweigh any possible benefits. Don't use.

➔

Breastfeeding:
Dangers outweigh any possible benefits. Don't use.

Infants and children:
Treating infants or children under 2 with any herbal preparation is hazardous.

Others:
Dangers outweigh any possible benefits. Don't use.

Storage:
- Store in cool, dry area away from direct light, but don't freeze.
- Store safely out of reach of children.
- Don't store in bathroom medicine cabinet. Heat and moisture may change the action of the herb.

Safe dosage:
Consult your doctor for the appropriate dose for your condition.

 Toxicity

Rated dangerous, particularly in children, persons over 55 and those who take larger than appropriate quantities for extended periods of time

For symptoms of toxicity: See *Adverse Reactions, Side Effects or Overdose Symptoms* section below.

 Adverse Reactions, Side Effects or Overdose Symptoms

Signs and symptoms	What to do
Abdominal cramping	Discontinue. Call doctor when convenient.
Breathing difficulty	Seek emergency treatment.
Coma	Seek emergency treatment.
Convulsions	Seek emergency treatment.
Diarrhea	Discontinue. Call doctor immediately.
Headache	Discontinue. Call doctor when convenient.
Heartbeat irregularities	Seek emergency treatment.
Nausea or vomiting	Discontinue. Call doctor immediately.
Vision impairment	Discontinue. Call doctor when convenient.

Mandrake (Love Apple, Satan's Apple)

 Basic Information

Biological name (genus and species):
Mandragora officinarum

Parts used for medicinal purposes:
Roots

Chemicals this herb contains:
- Hyoscyamine
- Mandragorin
- Scopolamine

 Known Effects
- Increases heart rate
- Dilates pupils
- Causes dry mouth
- Causes urinary retention
- Causes hallucinations
- Reduces muscular movements of intestinal tract

Possible Additional Effects

- May relieve pain
- Potential sedative
- Potential aphrodisiac
- May treat ulcers
- May treat skin diseases
- May treat hemorrhoids
- May cause explosive, watery diarrhea
- Potential anesthetic

 ## Warnings and Precautions

Don't take if you:

- Are pregnant, think you may be pregnant or plan pregnancy in the near future
- Have heart disease

Consult your doctor if you:

- Take this herb for any medical problem that doesn't improve in 2 weeks (There may be safer, more effective treatments.)
- Take any medicinal drugs or herbs including aspirin, laxatives, cold and cough remedies, antacids, vitamins, minerals, amino acids, supplements, other prescription or nonprescription drugs

Pregnancy:

Dangers outweigh any possible benefits. Don't use.

Breastfeeding:

Dangers outweigh any possible benefits. Don't use.

Infants and children:

Treating infants or children under 2 with any herbal preparation is hazardous.

Others:

No problems expected if you are beyond childhood, under 45, not pregnant, basically healthy, take it for only a short time and do not exceed manufacturer's recommended dose.

Storage:

- Store in cool, dry area away from direct light, but don't freeze.
- Store safely out of reach of children.
- Don't store in bathroom medicine cabinet. Heat and moisture may change the action of the herb.

Safe dosage:

Consult your doctor for the appropriate dose for your condition.

 ## Toxicity

Rated dangerous, particularly in children, persons over 55 and those who take larger than appropriate quantities for extended periods of time

For symptoms of toxicity: See
Adverse Reactions, Side Effects or Overdose Symptoms section below.

 ## Adverse Reactions, Side Effects or Overdose Symptoms

Signs and symptoms	What to do
Coma	Seek emergency treatment.
Confusion	Discontinue. Call doctor immediately.
Irregular heartbeat	Seek emergency treatment.

Marshmallow Plant

Basic Information

Biological name (genus and species):
Althaea officinalis

Parts used for medicinal purposes:
• Leaves
• Roots

Chemicals this herb contains:
• Asparagine
• Fat
• Mucilage (see Glossary)
• Pectin
• Starch
• Sugar

Known Effects

• Softens or soothes skin
• Helps treat sore throat, cough, colds, sinusitis

Miscellaneous information:
• Marshmallow plant is used as a "filler" in a variety of pills.
• It is available in dried bulk, capsules, tincture and is used as a poultice (see Glossary) for applying medications.

Possible Additional Effects

• May protect injured or scraped skin
• May treat kidney stones
• May treat indigestion

Warnings and Precautions

Don't take if you:
• Are pregnant, think you may be pregnant or plan pregnancy in the near future

• Have any chronic disease of the gastrointestinal tract, such as stomach or duodenal ulcers, reflux esophagitis, ulcerative colitis, spastic colitis, diverticulosis or diverticulitis

Consult your doctor if you:
• Take this herb for any medical problem that doesn't improve in 2 weeks (There may be safer, more effective treatments.)
• Take any medicinal drugs or herbs including aspirin, laxatives, cold and cough remedies, antacids, vitamins, minerals, amino acids, supplements, other prescription or nonprescription drugs

Pregnancy:
Don't use unless prescribed by your doctor.

Breastfeeding:
Don't use unless prescribed by your doctor.

Infants and children:
Treating infants or children under 2 with any herbal preparation is hazardous.

Others:
No problems expected if you are beyond childhood, under 45, not pregnant, basically healthy, take it for only a short time and do not exceed manufacturer's recommended dose.

Storage:
• Store in cool, dry area away from direct light, but don't freeze.
• Store safely out of reach of children.
• Don't store in bathroom medicine cabinet. Heat and moisture may change the action of the herb.

Safe dosage:
Consult your doctor for the appropriate dose for your condition.

Toxicity

Comparative-toxicity rating is not available from standard references.

Adverse Reactions, Side Effects or Overdose Symptoms

None are expected.

Mayapple (American Mandrake, Podophyllum)

Basic Information

Biological name (genus and species): *Podophyllum peltatum*

Parts used for medicinal purposes: Roots

Chemicals this herb contains:
- Alpha-peltatin
- Beta-peltatin
- Podophyllotoxin

Known Effects

- Inhibits or prevents cell division
- Stimulates gastrointestinal tract
- Induces vomiting

Possible Additional Effects

- May treat constipation and recurrent fecal impactions
- May cause testicular cancer (Certain components are under study.)

Warnings and Precautions

Don't take if you:
- Are pregnant, think you may be pregnant or plan pregnancy in the near future

- Have any chronic disease of the gastrointestinal tract, such as stomach or duodenal ulcers, reflux esophagitis, ulcerative colitis, spastic colitis, diverticulosis or diverticulitis

Consult your doctor if you:
- Take this herb for any medical problem that doesn't improve in 2 weeks (There may be safer, more effective treatments.)
- Take any medicinal drugs or herbs including aspirin, laxatives, cold and cough remedies, antacids, vitamins, minerals, amino acids, supplements, other prescription or nonprescription drugs

Pregnancy:
Don't use unless prescribed by your doctor.

Breastfeeding:
Don't use unless prescribed by your doctor.

Infants and children:
Treating infants or children under 2 with any herbal preparation is hazardous.

Others:
No problems expected if you are beyond childhood, under 45, not pregnant, basically healthy, take it for only a short time and do not exceed manufacturer's recommended dose.

Storage:
- Store in cool, dry area away from direct light, but don't freeze.
- Store safely out of reach of children.
- Don't store in bathroom medicine cabinet. Heat and moisture may change the action of the herb.

Safe dosage:

Consult your doctor for the appropriate dose for your condition.

 Toxicity

Rated slightly dangerous, particularly in children, persons over 55 and those who take larger than appropriate quantities for extended periods of time

For symptoms of toxicity: See *Adverse Reactions, Side Effects or Overdose Symptoms* section below.

 Adverse Reactions, Side Effects or Overdose Symptoms

Signs and symptoms	What to do
Diarrhea	Discontinue. Call doctor immediately.
Drowsiness	Discontinue. Call doctor when convenient.
Lethargy	Discontinue. Call doctor when convenient.
Nausea or vomiting	Discontinue. Call doctor immediately.
Unconsciousness	Seek emergency treatment.

Meadowsweet (Queen-of-the-Meadow, Spirea)

 Basic Information

Biological name (genus and species):
Filipendula ulmaria

Parts used for medicinal purposes:
- Petals/flower
- Roots

Chemicals this herb contains:
- Gallic acid
- Methyl salicylate
- Salicylic acid
- Salicylic aldehyde
- Tannic acid
- Volatile oils (see Glossary)

 Known Effects
- Helps treat gastrointestinal upset
- Helps treat headaches

 Possible Additional Effects
- May help body dispose of excess fluid by increasing amount of urine produced
- May treat diarrhea
- May reduce pain
- May relieve menstrual cramps

Warnings and Precautions

Don't take if you:
- Are pregnant, think you may be pregnant or plan pregnancy in the near future
- Have chronic kidney problems

Consult your doctor if you:
- Take this herb for any medical problem that doesn't improve in 2 weeks (There may be safer, more effective treatments.)
- Take any medicinal drugs or herbs including aspirin, laxatives, cold and cough remedies, antacids, vitamins, minerals, amino acids, supplements, other prescription or nonprescription drugs

Pregnancy:
Don't use unless prescribed by your doctor—contains salicylates.

Breastfeeding:
Don't use unless prescribed by your doctor—contains salicylates.

Infants and children:
Treating infants or children under 2 with any herbal preparation is hazardous.

Others:
No problems expected if you are beyond childhood, under 45, not pregnant, basically healthy, take it for only a short time and do not exceed manufacturer's recommended dose.

Storage:
- Store in cool, dry area away from direct light, but don't freeze.
- Store safely out of reach of children.
- Don't store in bathroom medicine cabinet. Heat and moisture may change the action of the herb.

Safe dosage:
Consult your doctor for the appropriate dose for your condition.

 ## Toxicity

Generally regarded as safe when taken in appropriate quantities for short periods of time

For symptoms of toxicity: See *Adverse Reactions, Side Effects or Overdose Symptoms* section below.

 ## Adverse Reactions, Side Effects or Overdose Symptoms

Signs and symptoms	What to do
Coma	Seek emergency treatment.
Kidney damage characterized by blood in urine, decreased urine flow, swelling of hands and feet	Seek emergency treatment.
Lethargy	Discontinue. Call doctor when convenient.
Unconsciousness	Seek emergency treatment.
Upset stomach	Discontinue. Call doctor when convenient.

Mexican Sarsaparilla

 Basic Information

Biological name (genus and species):
Smilax aristolochiaefolia, S. regelii, S. febrifuga, S. ornata

Parts used for medicinal purposes:
• Bark
• Berries
• Roots

Chemicals this herb contains:
• Resin (see Glossary)
• Sarsasapogenin
• Smilagenin
• Starch
• Stigmasterol
• Volatile oils (see Glossary)

 Known Effects

• Irritates mucous membranes
• Irritates gastrointestinal tract

Miscellaneous information:
• Berries are edible.
• Berries, bark and other parts of plant are used to make the soft drink of the same name.

 Possible Additional Effects

• May relieve toothache
• May temporarily relieve constipation

 Warnings and Precautions

Don't take if you:
Are pregnant, think you may be pregnant or plan pregnancy in the near future.

Consult your doctor if you:
• Take this herb for any medical problem that doesn't improve in 2 weeks (There may be safer, more effective treatments.)
• Take any medicinal drugs or herbs including aspirin, laxatives, cold and cough remedies, antacids, vitamins, minerals, amino acids, supplements, other prescription or nonprescription drugs

Pregnancy:
Don't use unless prescribed by your doctor.

Breastfeeding:
Don't use unless prescribed by your doctor.

Infants and children:
Treating infants or children under 2 with any herbal preparation is hazardous.

Others:
No problems expected if you are beyond childhood, under 45, not pregnant, basically healthy, take it for only a short time and do not exceed manufacturer's recommended dose.

Storage:
• Store in cool, dry area away from direct light, but don't freeze.
• Store safely out of reach of children.
• Don't store in bathroom medicine cabinet. Heat and moisture may change the action of the herb.

Safe dosage:
Consult your doctor for the appropriate dose for your condition.

Toxicity

Rated relatively safe when taken in appropriate quantities for short periods of time

 Adverse Reactions, Side Effects or Overdose Symptoms

None are expected.

Milk Thistle (Mary Thistle, Wild Artichoke)

 Basic Information

Biological name (genus and species):
Silybum marianum

Parts used for medicinal purposes:
- Fruit
- Leaves
- Seeds

Chemicals this herb contains:
Silymarin

 Known Effects

- Protects the liver from chemical damage
- Increases the secretion and flow of bile
- Antioxidant
- Helps treat chronic inflammatory liver disease (hepatitis)

 Possible Additional Effects

- May reduce jaundice
- May reduce inflammation associated with hepatitis and cirrhosis
- May reduce gallbladder inflammation
- May help treat psoriasis

 Warnings and Precautions

Don't take if you:
No proven contraindications (see Glossary) exist.

Consult your doctor if you:
- Take this herb for any medical problem that doesn't improve in 2 weeks (There may be safer, more effective treatments.)
- Take any medicinal drugs or herbs including aspirin, laxatives, cold and cough remedies, antacids, vitamins, minerals, amino acids, supplements, other prescription or nonprescription drugs
- Have liver disease

Pregnancy:
Don't use unless prescribed by your doctor.

Breastfeeding:
Don't use unless prescribed by your doctor.

Infants and children:
Treating infants or children under 2 with any herbal preparation is hazardous.

Others:
You may develop loose stools during the first few days of use.

➜

Storage:
- Store in cool, dry area away from direct light, but don't freeze.
- Store safely out of reach of children.
- Don't store in bathroom medicine cabinet. Heat and moisture may change the action of the herb.

Safe dosage:

Consult your doctor for the appropriate dose for your condition.

Toxicity

Comparative-toxicity rating is not available from standard references.

For symptoms of toxicity: See *Adverse Reactions, Side Effects or Overdose Symptoms* section below.

Adverse Reactions, Side Effects or Overdose Symptoms

Signs and symptoms	What to do
Loose stools	Discontinue. Call doctor when convenient.

Milkweed, Common (Blood-Flower)

Basic Information

Biological name (genus and species):
Asclepias syriaca

Parts used for medicinal purposes:
Roots

Chemicals this herb contains:
- Asclepiadin
- Asclepione (a bitter—see Glossary)
- Galitoxin

Known Effects

- Irritates and stimulates gastrointestinal tract
- Decreases thickness and increases fluidity of mucus in lungs and bronchial tubes
- Increases perspiration

Miscellaneous information:

All parts of milkweed may be toxic.

Possible Additional Effects

- May treat bronchitis
- May treat arthritis

Warnings and Precautions

Don't take if you:
- Are pregnant, think you may be pregnant or plan pregnancy in the near future
- Have any chronic disease of the gastrointestinal tract, such as stomach or duodenal ulcers, reflux esophagitis, ulcerative colitis, spastic colitis, diverticulosis or diverticulitis

Consult your doctor if you:
- Take this herb for any medical problem that doesn't improve in 2 weeks (There may be safer, more effective treatments.)

- Take any medicinal drugs or herbs including aspirin, laxatives, cold and cough remedies, antacids, vitamins, minerals, amino acids, supplements, other prescription or nonprescription drugs

Pregnancy:
Dangers outweigh any possible benefits. Don't use.

Breastfeeding:
Dangers outweigh any possible benefits. Don't use.

Infants and children:
Treating infants or children under 2 with any herbal preparation is hazardous.

Others:
Dangers outweigh any possible benefits. Don't use.

Storage:
- Store in cool, dry area away from direct light, but don't freeze.
- Store safely out of reach of children.
- Don't store in bathroom medicine cabinet. Heat and moisture may change the action of the herb.

Safe dosage:
Consult your doctor for the appropriate dose for your condition.

Toxicity

Rated slightly dangerous, particularly in children, persons over 55 and those who take larger than appropriate quantities for extended periods of time

For symptoms of toxicity: See *Adverse Reactions, Side Effects or Overdose Symptoms* section below.

Adverse Reactions, Side Effects or Overdose Symptoms

Signs and symptoms	What to do
Coma	Seek emergency treatment.
Diarrhea	Discontinue. Call doctor immediately.
Drowsiness	Discontinue. Call doctor when convenient.
Jaundice (yellow skin and eyes)	Discontinue. Call doctor immediately.
Kidney damage characterized by blood in urine, decreased urine flow, swelling of hands and feet	Seek emergency treatment.
Lethargy	Discontinue. Call doctor when convenient.
Loss of appetite	Discontinue. Call doctor when convenient.
Nausea or vomiting	Discontinue. Call doctor immediately.
Seizures	Seek emergency treatment.
Unsteady walk	Discontinue. Call doctor immediately.

Milkwort

Basic Information

Biological name (genus and species):
Polygala vulgaris, P. senega

Parts used for medicinal purposes:
Roots

Chemicals this herb contains:
Saponins (see Glossary)

Known Effects

- Increases secretions from bronchial tubes
- Irritates intestinal tract
- Decreases thickness and increases fluidity of mucus in lungs and bronchial tubes
- Helps body dispose of excess fluid by increasing amount of urine produced
- Increases perspiration

Possible Additional Effects

- May treat croup
- May treat arthritis
- May treat hives
- May treat gout
- May treat pleurisy
- May treat constipation
- May increase milk production in lactating women

Warnings and Precautions

Don't take if you:
- Are pregnant, think you may be pregnant or plan pregnancy in the near future
- Have any chronic disease of the gastrointestinal tract, such as stomach or duodenal ulcers, reflux esophagitis, ulcerative colitis, spastic colitis, diverticulosis or diverticulitis

Consult your doctor if you:
- Take this herb for any medical problem that doesn't improve in 2 weeks (There may be safer, more effective treatments.)
- Take any medicinal drugs or herbs including aspirin, laxatives, cold and cough remedies, antacids, vitamins, minerals, amino acids, supplements, other prescription or nonprescription drugs

Pregnancy:
Dangers outweigh any possible benefits. Don't use.

Breastfeeding:
Dangers outweigh any possible benefits. Don't use.

Infants and children:
Treating infants or children under 2 with any herbal preparation is hazardous.

Others:
No problems expected if you are beyond childhood, under 45, not pregnant, basically healthy, take it for only a short time and do not exceed manufacturer's recommended dose.

Storage:
- Store in cool, dry area away from direct light, but don't freeze.
- Store safely out of reach of children.
- Don't store in bathroom medicine cabinet. Heat and moisture may change the action of the herb.

Safe dosage:
Consult your doctor for the appropriate dose for your condition.

Toxicity

Comparative-toxicity rating is not available from standard references.

For symptoms of toxicity: See *Adverse Reactions, Side Effects or Overdose Symptoms* section below.

 Adverse Reactions, Side Effects or Overdose Symptoms

Signs and symptoms	What to do
Coma	Seek emergency treatment.
Diarrhea	Discontinue. Call doctor immediately.
Drowsiness	Discontinue. Call doctor when convenient.
Lethargy	Discontinue. Call doctor when convenient.
Nausea, violent	Discontinue. Call doctor immediately.
Vomiting	Discontinue. Call doctor immediately.

Mistletoe

 Basic Information

Biological name (genus and species):
Phoradendron serotinum, Viscum album

Parts used for medicinal purposes:
• Berries/fruits
• Leaves
• Stems

Chemicals this herb contains:
• Beta-phenylethylamine
• Tyramine
• Viscotoxins

 Known Effects

• Stimulates central nervous system
• Causes contraction of smooth muscle

Miscellaneous information:
Mistletoe is particularly dangerous for people taking monoamine-oxidase medications to treat high blood pressure.

 Possible Additional Effects

• May relieve nervousness
• May reduce high blood pressure

 Warnings and Precautions

Don't take if you:
• Are pregnant, think you may be pregnant or plan pregnancy in the near future

- Have any chronic disease of the gastrointestinal tract, such as stomach or duodenal ulcers, reflux esophagitis, ulcerative colitis, spastic colitis, diverticulosis or diverticulitis

Consult your doctor if you:
- Take this herb for any medical problem that doesn't improve in 2 weeks (There may be safer, more effective treatments.)
- Take any medicinal drugs or herbs including aspirin, laxatives, cold and cough remedies, antacids, vitamins, minerals, amino acids, supplements, other prescription or nonprescription drugs
- Wish to use this herb—it is considered poisonous

Pregnancy:
Dangers outweigh any possible benefits. Don't use.

Breastfeeding:
Dangers outweigh any possible benefits. Don't use.

Infants and children:
Treating infants or children under 2 with any herbal preparation is hazardous.

Others:
Do not allow children to eat the berries of this popular Christmas plant. As few as one or two berries may cause toxic symptoms.

Storage:
- Store in cool, dry area away from direct light, but don't freeze.
- Store safely out of reach of children.
- Don't store in bathroom medicine cabinet. Heat and moisture may change the action of the herb.

Safe dosage:
Consult your doctor for the appropriate dose for your condition.

Toxicity

Rated slightly dangerous, particularly in children, persons over 55 and those who take larger than appropriate quantities for extended periods of time

For symptoms of toxicity: See *Adverse Reactions, Side Effects or Overdose Symptoms* section below.

Adverse Reactions, Side Effects or Overdose Symptoms

Signs and symptoms	What to do
Convulsions	Seek emergency treatment.
Diarrhea	Discontinue. Call doctor immediately.
Hallucinations	Seek emergency treatment.
Headache	Discontinue. Call doctor immediately.
Increased blood pressure	Discontinue. Call doctor immediately.
Muscle spasms	Discontinue. Call doctor immediately.
Nausea or vomiting	Discontinue. Call doctor immediately.
Slow heartbeat	Seek emergency treatment.

Mormon Tea (Brigham Tea, Nevada Jointfir)

Basic Information

Biological name (genus and species):
Ephedra nevadensis, E. trifurca

Parts used for medicinal purposes:
Stems

Chemicals this herb contains:
Ephedrine

Known Effects

- Stimulates central nervous system
- Increases blood pressure
- Increases heart rate

Miscellaneous information:
Mormon tea has no value in treating bronchial asthma.

Possible Additional Effects

- May elevate mood
- May reduce symptoms of congestive heart failure, kidney failure, liver failure
- May decrease appetite
- May stimulate energy
- May reduce symptoms of fatigue

Warnings and Precautions

Don't take if you:
- Are pregnant, think you may be pregnant or plan pregnancy in the near future
- Have diabetes mellitus, because it impedes control with diet and insulin
- Have heart disease

Consult your doctor if you:
- Take this herb for any medical problem that doesn't improve in 2 weeks (There may be safer, more effective treatments.)
- Take any medicinal drugs or herbs including aspirin, laxatives, cold and cough remedies, antacids, vitamins, minerals, amino acids, supplements, other prescription or nonprescription drugs

Pregnancy:
Dangers outweigh any possible benefits. Don't use.

Breastfeeding:
Dangers outweigh any possible benefits. Don't use.

Infants and children:
Treating infants or children under 2 with any herbal preparation is hazardous.

Others:
No problems expected if you are beyond childhood, under 45, not pregnant, basically healthy, take it for only a short time and do not exceed manufacturer's recommended dose.

Storage:
- Store in cool, dry area away from direct light, but don't freeze.
- Store safely out of reach of children.
- Don't store in bathroom medicine cabinet. Heat and moisture may change the action of the herb.

Safe dosage:
Consult your doctor for the appropriate dose for your condition.

➡

Toxicity

Rated slightly dangerous, particularly in children, persons over 55 and those who take larger than appropriate quantities for extended periods of time

For symptoms of toxicity: See *Adverse Reactions, Side Effects or Overdose Symptoms* section below.

 Adverse Reactions, Side Effects or Overdose Symptoms

Signs and symptoms	What to do
Excessively high blood pressure	Seek emergency treatment.
Irregular heartbeat	Seek emergency treatment.
Rapid heartbeat	Discontinue. Call doctor immediately.

Morning Glory

 Basic Information

Biological name (genus and species):
Ipomoea purpurea

Parts used for medicinal purposes:
Seeds

Chemicals this herb contains:
- Cetyl alcohol
- Dihydroxycinnamic acid
- Lysergic acid
- Scopoletin

 Known Effects

- Stimulates central nervous system
- Stimulates gastrointestinal tract

 Possible Additional Effects

- May cause hallucinations
- Potential purgative for constipation
- May elevate mood

 Warnings and Precautions

Don't take if you:
- Are pregnant, think you may be pregnant or plan pregnancy in the near future
- Have any chronic disease of the gastrointestinal tract, such as stomach or duodenal ulcers, reflux esophagitis, ulcerative colitis, spastic colitis, diverticulosis or diverticulitis

Consult your doctor if you:
- Take this herb for any medical problem that doesn't improve in 2 weeks (There may be safer, more effective treatments.)
- Take any medicinal drugs or herbs including aspirin, laxatives, cold and cough remedies, antacids, vitamins, minerals, amino acids, supplements, other prescription or nonprescription drugs

Pregnancy:
Don't use unless prescribed by your doctor.

Breast-feeding:
Don't use unless prescribed by
your doctor.

Infants and children:
Treating infants or children under
2 with any herbal preparation
is hazardous.

Others:
No problems expected if you are
beyond childhood, under 45, not
pregnant, basically healthy, take it for
only a short time and do not exceed
manufacturer's recommended dose.

Storage:
• Store in cool, dry area away from
  direct light, but don't freeze.
• Store safely out of reach of children.
• Don't store in bathroom medicine
  cabinet. Heat and moisture may
  change the action of the herb.

Safe dosage:
Consult your doctor for the
appropriate dose for your condition.

Toxicity

Rated slightly dangerous, particularly in
children, persons over 55 and those
who take larger than appropriate
quantities for extended periods of time

For symptoms of toxicity: See
*Adverse Reactions, Side Effects or
Overdose Symptoms* section below.

Adverse Reactions, Side Effects or Overdose Symptoms

Signs and symptoms	What to do
Confusion	Discontinue. Call doctor immediately.
Diarrhea, explosive and watery	Discontinue. Call doctor immediately.
Disturbed vision	Discontinue. Call doctor immediately.
Hallucinations	Seek emergency treatment.
Nausea or vomiting	Discontinue. Call doctor immediately.

Mountain Ash (Rowan Tree)

Basic Information

Biological name (genus and species):
Sorbus aucuparia

Parts used for medicinal purposes:
• Berries/fruits
• Seeds

Chemicals this herb contains:
• Fixed oil (see Glossary)
• Malic acid
• Sorbic acid
• Sorbitol
• Sorbose

Known Effects

• Irritates and stimulates
  gastrointestinal tract
• Helps body dispose of excess fluid
  by increasing amount of
  urine produced

→

Miscellaneous information:
Used as a sweetener.

Possible Additional Effects

• May prevent scurvy
• May treat hemorrhoids
• May treat stomach and duodenal ulcers

Warnings and Precautions

Don't take if you:
Are pregnant, think you may be pregnant or plan pregnancy in the near future.

Consult your doctor if you:
• Take this herb for any medical problem that doesn't improve in 2 weeks (There may be safer, more effective treatments.)
• Take any medicinal drugs or herbs including aspirin, laxatives, cold and cough remedies, antacids, vitamins, minerals, amino acids, supplements, other prescription or nonprescription drugs

Pregnancy:
Don't use unless prescribed by your doctor.

Breastfeeding:
Problems in breastfed infants of lactating mothers taking small or usual amounts have not been proved, but the chance of problems does exist. Don't use unless prescribed by your doctor.

Infants and children:
Treating infants or children under 2 with any herbal preparation is hazardous.

Others:
No problems expected if you are beyond childhood, under 45, not pregnant, basically healthy, take it for only a short time and do not exceed manufacturer's recommended dose.

Storage:
• Store in cool, dry area away from direct light, but don't freeze.
• Store safely out of reach of children.
• Don't store in bathroom medicine cabinet. Heat and moisture may change the action of the herb.

Safe dosage:
Consult your doctor for the appropriate dose for your condition.

Toxicity

Comparative-toxicity rating is not available from standard references.

For symptoms of toxicity: See *Adverse Reactions, Side Effects or Overdose Symptoms* section below.

Adverse Reactions, Side Effects or Overdose Symptoms

Signs and symptoms	What to do
Diarrhea	Discontinue. Call doctor immediately.

Mountain Tobacco (Leopard's Bane, Wolf's Bane)

Basic Information

Biological name (genus and species):
Arnica montana

Parts used for medicinal purposes:
Petals/flower

Chemicals this herb contains:
- Angelic acid
- Arnidiol
- Choline
- Fatty acids
- Formic acid
- Thymohydroquinone

Known Effects

- Provides counterirritation (see Glossary) when applied to skin overlying an inflamed or irritated joint
- Depresses central nervous system
- Irritates gastrointestinal tract

Possible Additional Effects

May relieve discomfort of sprains, strains, bruises when applied to skin over injury

Warnings and Precautions

Don't take if you:
- Are pregnant, think you may be pregnant or plan pregnancy in the near future
- Have any chronic disease of the gastrointestinal tract, such as stomach or duodenal ulcers, reflux esophagitis, ulcerative colitis, spastic colitis, diverticulosis or diverticulitis

Consult your doctor if you:
- Take this herb for any medical problem that doesn't improve in 2 weeks (There may be safer, more effective treatments.)
- Take any medicinal drugs or herbs including aspirin, laxatives, cold and cough remedies, antacids, vitamins, minerals, amino acids, supplements, other prescription or nonprescription drugs

Pregnancy:
Dangers outweigh any possible benefits. Don't use.

Breastfeeding:
Dangers outweigh any possible benefits. Don't use.

Infants and children:
Treating infants or children under 2 with any herbal preparation is hazardous.

Others:
Don't take internally. Probably safe for application to skin.

Storage:
- Store in cool, dry area away from direct light, but don't freeze.
- Store safely out of reach of children.
- Don't store in bathroom medicine cabinet. Heat and moisture may change the action of the herb.

Safe dosage:
Consult your doctor for the appropriate dose for your condition.

→

Toxicity

Rated slightly dangerous, particularly in children, persons over 55 and those who take larger than appropriate quantities for extended periods of time

For symptoms of toxicity: See *Adverse Reactions, Side Effects or Overdose Symptoms* section below.

Adverse Reactions, Side Effects or Overdose Symptoms

Signs and symptoms	What to do
Diarrhea, explosive, watery	Discontinue. Call doctor immediately.
Heartbeat irregularities	Seek emergency treatment.
Muscle weakness	Discontinue. Call doctor immediately.
Nausea or vomiting	Discontinue. Call doctor immediately.
Precipitous blood-pressure drop: symptoms include faintness, cold sweat, paleness, rapid pulse	Seek emergency treatment.

Mulberry

Basic Information

Biological name (genus and species):
Morus rubra

Parts used for medicinal purposes:
• Bark
• Berries/fruits

Chemicals this herb contains:
Unidentified

Known Effects

• Stimulates gastrointestinal tract
• Depresses central nervous system

Possible Additional Effects

• May reduce fever
• May induce drowsiness
• Potential mild laxative

Warnings and Precautions

Don't take if you:
• Are pregnant, think you may be pregnant or plan pregnancy in the near future
• Have any chronic disease of the gastrointestinal tract, such as stomach or duodenal ulcers, reflux esophagitis, ulcerative colitis, spastic colitis, diverticulosis or diverticulitis

Consult your doctor if you:
- Take this herb for any medical problem that doesn't improve in 2 weeks (There may be safer, more effective treatments.)
- Take any medicinal drugs or herbs including aspirin, laxatives, cold and cough remedies, antacids, vitamins, minerals, amino acids, supplements, other prescription or nonprescription drugs

Pregnancy:
Dangers outweigh any possible benefits. Don't use.

Breastfeeding:
Dangers outweigh any possible benefits. Don't use.

Infants and children:
Treating infants or children under 2 with any herbal preparation is hazardous.

Others:
This product will not help you and may cause toxic symptoms.

Storage:
- Store in cool, dry area away from direct light, but don't freeze.
- Store safely out of reach of children.
- Don't store in bathroom medicine cabinet. Heat and moisture may change the action of the herb.

Safe dosage:
Consult your doctor for the appropriate dose for your condition.

 Toxicity

Comparative-toxicity rating is not available from standard references.

For symptoms of toxicity: See *Adverse Reactions, Side Effects or Overdose Symptoms* section below.

 Adverse Reactions, Side Effects or Overdose Symptoms

Signs and symptoms	What to do
Diarrhea	Discontinue. Call doctor immediately.
Hallucinations	Seek emergency treatment.
Nausea or vomiting	Discontinue. Call doctor immediately.

Mullein

 Basic Information

Biological name (genus and species):
Verbascum thapsiforme, V. phlomoides, V. thapsus

Parts used for medicinal purposes:
- Flowers
- Leaves

Chemicals this herb contains:
Saponin (see Glossary)

 Known Effects

- Covers and protects scraped tissues
- Softens and soothes irritated skin
- Treats throat irritations and coughs

Miscellaneous information:
Available as tea, compress and inhalant.

→

Possible Additional Effects

- May relieve bronchial irritation when smoked
- May treat sunburn, hemorrhoids, injured skin and mucous membranes when applied topically
- May treat stomach cramps
- May treat diarrhea

Warnings and Precautions

Don't take if you:

Are pregnant, think you may be pregnant or plan pregnancy in the near future.

Consult your doctor if you:

- Take this herb for any medical problem that doesn't improve in 2 weeks (There may be safer, more effective treatments.)
- Take any medicinal drugs or herbs including aspirin, laxatives, cold and cough remedies, antacids, vitamins, minerals, amino acids, supplements, other prescription or nonprescription drugs

Pregnancy:

Don't use unless prescribed by your doctor.

Breastfeeding:

Don't use unless prescribed by your doctor.

Infants and children:

Treating infants or children under 2 with any herbal preparation is hazardous.

Others:

No problems expected if you are beyond childhood, under 45, not pregnant, basically healthy, take it for only a short time and do not exceed manufacturer's recommended dose.

Storage:

- Store in cool, dry area away from direct light, but don't freeze.
- Store safely out of reach of children.
- Don't store in bathroom medicine cabinet. Heat and moisture may change the action of the herb.

Safe dosage:

Consult your doctor for the appropriate dose for your condition.

Toxicity

Comparative-toxicity rating is not available from standard references.

For symptoms of toxicity: See *Adverse Reactions, Side Effects or Overdose Symptoms* section below.

Adverse Reactions, Side Effects or Overdose Symptoms

Signs and symptoms	What to do
Mild stomach upset	Discontinue. Call doctor when convenient.

Myrrh

Basic Information

Biological name (genus and species):
Commiphora molmol

Parts used for medicinal purposes:
- Leaves
- Resin from stems

Chemicals this herb contains:
- Acetic acid
- Formic acid
- Myrrholic acids
- Resin (see Glossary)
- Volatile oils (see Glossary)

Known Effects

Helps expel gas from intestinal tract

Miscellaneous information:
Primary use of myrrh is in perfumes and incense.

Possible Additional Effects

- May treat dyspepsia
- Used as mouthwash
- May treat bronchitis
- May treat sore and strep throat
- May treat canker sores
- May treat eczema

Warnings and Precautions

Don't take if you:
Are pregnant, think you may be pregnant or plan pregnancy in the near future.

Consult your doctor if you:
- Take this herb for any medical problem that doesn't improve in 2 weeks (There may be safer, more effective treatments.)
- Take any medicinal drugs or herbs including aspirin, laxatives, cold and cough remedies, antacids, vitamins, minerals, amino acids, supplements, other prescription or nonprescription drugs

Pregnancy:
Don't use unless prescribed by your doctor.

Breastfeeding:
Don't use unless prescribed by your doctor.

Infants and children:
Treating infants or children under 2 with any herbal preparation is hazardous.

Others:
No problems expected if you are beyond childhood, under 45, not pregnant, basically healthy, take it for only a short time and do not exceed manufacturer's recommended dose.

Storage:
- Store in cool, dry area away from direct light, but don't freeze.
- Store safely out of reach of children.
- Don't store in bathroom medicine cabinet. Heat and moisture may change the action of the herb.

Safe dosage:
Consult your doctor for the appropriate dose for your condition.

→

Toxicity

Comparative-toxicity rating is not available from standard references. Myrrh may be toxic in high concentrations.

For symptoms of toxicity: See *Adverse Reactions, Side Effects or Overdose Symptoms* section below.

Adverse Reactions, Side Effects or Overdose Symptoms

Signs and symptoms	What to do
Convulsions	Seek emergency treatment.
Drowsiness	Discontinue. Call doctor when convenient.
Lethargy	Discontinue. Call doctor when convenient.

Myrtle

Basic Information

Biological name (genus and species): *Myrtus communis*

Parts used for medicinal purposes: Leaves

Chemicals this herb contains:
- D-pinene
- Eucalyptol
- Myrtenol

Known Effects

- Myrtle irritates mucous membranes.
- Large amounts may depress central nervous system.

Miscellaneous information:
Myrtle is used as a condiment, flavoring, perfume essence and gargle.

Possible Additional Effects

- May treat stomach irritations
- May treat bronchitis
- May treat cystitis

Warnings and Precautions

Don't take if you:
- Are pregnant, think you may be pregnant or plan pregnancy in the near future
- Have chronic kidney disease

Consult your doctor if you:
- Take this herb for any medical problem that doesn't improve in 2 weeks (There may be safer, more effective treatments.)
- Take any medicinal drugs or herbs including aspirin, laxatives, cold and cough remedies, antacids, vitamins, minerals, amino acids, supplements, other prescription or nonprescription drugs

Pregnancy:
Don't use unless prescribed by your doctor.

Breastfeeding:
Don't use unless prescribed by your doctor.

Infants and children:
Treating infants or children under 2 with any herbal preparation is hazardous.

Others:

No problems expected if you are beyond childhood, under 45, not pregnant, basically healthy, take it for only a short time and do not exceed manufacturer's recommended dose.

Storage:

• Store in cool, dry area away from direct light, but don't freeze.
• Store safely out of reach of children.
• Don't store in bathroom medicine cabinet. Heat and moisture may change the action of the herb.

Safe dosage:

Consult your doctor for the appropriate dose for your condition.

 Toxicity

Comparative-toxicity rating is not available from standard references.

For symptoms of toxicity: See *Adverse Reactions, Side Effects or Overdose Symptoms* section below.

 Adverse Reactions, Side Effects or Overdose Symptoms

Signs and symptoms	What to do
Coma	Seek emergency treatment.
Convulsions	Seek emergency treatment.
Kidney damage characterized by blood in urine, decreased urine flow, swelling of hands and feet	Seek emergency treatment.

Oak Bark

 Basic Information

Biological name (genus and species):
Quercus

Parts used for medicinal purposes:
• Bark
• Seeds

Chemicals this herb contains:
Quercitannic acid

 Known Effects

• Anti-inflammatory
• Relieves sore throats when used as a gargle
• Helps treat strains

 Possible Additional Effects

• May treat hemorrhoids
• May treat diarrhea
• Potential mouthwash for inflammation

 Warnings and Precautions

Don't take if you:

• Are pregnant, think you may be pregnant or plan pregnancy in the near future
• Have any chronic disease of the gastrointestinal tract, such as stomach or duodenal ulcers, reflux

➜

esophagitis, ulcerative colitis, spastic colitis, diverticulosis or diverticulitis

Consult your doctor if you:
• Take this herb for any medical problem that doesn't improve in 2 weeks (There may be safer, more effective treatments.)
• Take any medicinal drugs or herbs including aspirin, laxatives, cold and cough remedies, antacids, vitamins, minerals, amino acids, supplements, other prescription or nonprescription drugs

Pregnancy:
Dangers outweigh any possible benefits. Don't use.

Breastfeeding:
Dangers outweigh any possible benefits. Don't use.

Infants and children:
Treating infants or children under 2 with any herbal preparation is hazardous.

Others:
No problems expected if you are beyond childhood, under 45, not pregnant, basically healthy, take it for only a short time and do not exceed manufacturer's recommended dose.

Storage:
• Store in cool, dry area away from direct light, but don't freeze.
• Store safely out of reach of children.
• Don't store in bathroom medicine cabinet. Heat and moisture may change the action of the herb.

Safe dosage:
Consult your doctor for the appropriate dose for your condition.

Toxicity

Comparative-toxicity rating is not available from standard references.

For symptoms of toxicity: See *Adverse Reactions, Side Effects or Overdose Symptoms* section below.

Adverse Reactions, Side Effects or Overdose Symptoms

Signs and symptoms	What to do
Constipation	Discontinue. Call doctor when convenient.
Dry mouth	Discontinue. Call doctor when convenient.
Increased urination	Discontinue. Call doctor when convenient.
Jaundice (yellow skin and eyes)	Discontinue. Call doctor immediately.
Kidney damage characterized by blood in urine, decreased urine flow, swelling of hands and feet	Seek emergency treatment.
Skin eruptions	Discontinue. Call doctor when convenient.
Thirst	Discontinue. Call doctor when convenient.

Oats (Oat Beard)

 Basic Information

Biological name (genus and species):
Avena sativa

Parts used for medicinal purposes:
Seeds

Chemicals this herb contains:
- Albumin
- Gluten
- Gum oil
- Protein compound
- Salts
- Saponins (see Glossary)
- Starch
- Sugar

 Known Effects

- Aids sleep
- Decreases cholesterol
- Helps dry skin

Miscellaneous information:

- "Feeling his oats" refers to the stimulant effect of this herb on some animals, particularly horses.
- Fiber intake should be increased gradually.

 Possible Additional Effects

- May decrease depression
- May relieve indigestion

 Warnings and Precautions

Don't take if you:

No proven contraindications (see Glossary) exist.

Consult your doctor if you:

- Take this herb for any medical problem that doesn't improve in 2 weeks (There may be safer, more effective treatments.)
- Take any medicinal drugs or herbs including aspirin, laxatives, cold and cough remedies, antacids, vitamins, minerals, amino acids, supplements, other prescription or nonprescription drugs

Pregnancy:

Pregnant women should experience no problems taking usual amounts as part of a balanced diet.

Breastfeeding:

Breastfed infants of lactating mothers should experience no problems when mother takes usual amounts as part of a balanced diet.

Infants and children:

Treating infants or children under 2 with any herbal preparation is hazardous.

Others:

No problems expected if you are beyond childhood and under 45, basically healthy and take for only a short time.

Storage:
- Store in cool, dry area away from direct light, but don't freeze.
- Store safely out of reach of children.
- Don't store in bathroom medicine cabinet. Heat and moisture may change the action of the herb.

Safe dosage:
Consult your doctor for the appropriate dose for your condition.

 Toxicity

Comparative-toxicity rating is not available from standard references.

 Adverse Reactions, Side Effects or Overdose Symptoms

None are expected.

Orris Root (Black Flag)

 Basic Information

Biological name (genus and species):
Iris versicolor

Parts used for medicinal purposes:
Roots

Chemicals this herb contains:
- Gum (see Glossary)
- Oleoresin (see Glossary)
- Tannins (see Glossary)

 Known Effects

- Depresses central nervous system
- Causes vomiting
- Interferes with absorption of iron and other minerals when taken internally

 Possible Additional Effects

- May treat skin disorders
- May treat arthritis
- May treat tumors

 Warnings and Precautions

Don't take if you:
- Are pregnant, think you may be pregnant or plan pregnancy in the near future
- Have any chronic disease of the gastrointestinal tract, such as stomach or duodenal ulcers, reflux esophagitis, ulcerative colitis, spastic colitis, diverticulosis or diverticulitis

Consult your doctor if you:
- Take this herb for any medical problem that doesn't improve in 2 weeks (There may be safer, more effective treatments.)
- Take any medicinal drugs or herbs including aspirin, laxatives, cold and cough remedies, antacids, vitamins, minerals, amino acids, supplements, other prescription or nonprescription drugs

Pregnancy:
Don't use unless prescribed by your doctor.

Breastfeeding:
Don't use unless prescribed by your doctor.

Infants and children:
Treating infants or children under 2 with any herbal preparation is hazardous.

Others:
Don't use. This product will not help you and may cause toxic symptoms.

Storage:
- Store in cool, dry area away from direct light, but don't freeze.
- Store safely out of reach of children.
- Don't store in bathroom medicine cabinet. Heat and moisture may change the action of the herb.

Safe dosage:
Consult your doctor for the appropriate dose for your condition.

Toxicity

Rated relatively safe when taken in appropriate quantities for short periods of time

For symptoms of toxicity: See *Adverse Reactions, Side Effects or Overdose Symptoms* section below.

Adverse Reactions, Side Effects or Overdose Symptoms

Signs and symptoms	What to do
Burning sensation in throat and mouth	Discontinue. Call doctor when convenient.
Cramping, abdominal pain	Discontinue. Call doctor when convenient.
Diarrhea, watery	Discontinue. Call doctor immediately.
Nausea or vomiting	Discontinue. Call doctor immediately.

Papaya

Basic Information

Biological name (genus and species):
Carica papaya

Parts used for medicinal purposes:
- Berries/fruits
- Inner bark
- Stems

Chemicals this herb contains:
- Amylolytic enzyme
- Caricin
- Myrosin
- Peptidase
- Vitamins C and E

Known Effects

- Stimulates stomach to increase secretions
- Releases histamine from body tissues
- Depresses central nervous system
- Kills some intestinal parasites

Miscellaneous information:
- No problems expected when eaten as a common food
- Used as a meat tenderizer

Possible Additional Effects

- May aid digestion
- May liquify excessive mucus in mouth and stomach
- May treat sore teeth (inner bark)

 ## Warnings and Precautions

Don't take if you:

Have any chronic disease of the gastrointestinal tract, such as stomach or duodenal ulcers, reflux esophagitis, ulcerative colitis, spastic colitis, diverticulosis or diverticulitis.

Consult your doctor if you:

- Take this herb for any medical problem that doesn't improve in 2 weeks (There may be safer, more effective treatments.)
- Take any medicinal drugs or herbs including aspirin, laxatives, cold and cough remedies, antacids, vitamins, minerals, amino acids, supplements, other prescription or nonprescription drugs

Pregnancy:

Pregnant women should experience no problems taking usual amounts as part of a balanced diet. Other products extracted from this herb have not been proved to cause problems.

Breastfeeding:

Breastfed infants of lactating mothers should experience no problems when mother takes usual amounts as part of a balanced diet. Other products extracted from this herb have not been proved to cause problems.

Infants and children:

Treating infants or children under 2 with any herbal preparation is hazardous.

Others:

No problems expected if you are beyond childhood, under 45, basically healthy, take it for only a short time and do not exceed manufacturer's recommended dose.

Storage:

- Store in cool, dry area away from direct light, but don't freeze.
- Store safely out of reach of children.
- Don't store in bathroom medicine cabinet. Heat and moisture may change the action of the herb.

Safe dosage:

Consult your doctor for the appropriate dose for your condition.

 ## Toxicity

Generally regarded as safe when taken in appropriate quantities for short periods of time

For symptoms of toxicity: See *Adverse Reactions, Side Effects or Overdose Symptoms* section below.

 ## Adverse Reactions, Side Effects or Overdose Symptoms

Signs and symptoms	What to do
Heartburn caused by irritation of lower part of esophagus	Discontinue. Call doctor when convenient.

Parsley

 Basic Information

Biological name (genus and species): *Petroselinum crispum*

Parts used for medicinal purposes:
- Berries/fruits
- Leaves
- Roots
- Stems

Chemicals this herb contains:
- Apiin (also called *parsley camphor*)
- Apiol
- Pinene
- Vitamins A and C
- Volatile oils (see Glossary)

 Known Effects

- Reduces urinary tract inflammation
- Uterine stimulant
- Aids digestion
- Increases renal (see Glossary) function—helps body dispose of excess fluid by increasing amounts of urine produced

Miscellaneous information:
- When fresh sprigs are eaten, no problems are expected.
- Parsley is available as tincture, leaves, seeds, stems and roots.
- It is a good source of vitamins C and A.

 Possible Additional Effects

- May treat painful menstruation and premenstrual syndrome (PMS)
- May treat dyspepsia
- May relieve gas
- May facilitate passage of kidney stones

 Warnings and Precautions

Don't take if you:
- Are pregnant, think you may be pregnant or plan pregnancy in the near future
- Have any chronic disease of the gastrointestinal tract, such as stomach or duodenal ulcers, reflux esophagitis, ulcerative colitis, spastic colitis, diverticulosis or diverticulitis

Consult your doctor if you:
- Take this herb for any medical problem that doesn't improve in 2 weeks (There may be safer, more effective treatments.)
- Take any medicinal drugs or herbs including aspirin, laxatives, cold and cough remedies, antacids, vitamins, minerals, amino acids, supplements, other prescription or nonprescription drugs

Pregnancy:
- Dangers outweigh any possible benefits. Avoid taking any herbal medication made from parsley.
- Fresh parsley as a condiment is all right to eat.

Breastfeeding:
- Dangers outweigh any possible benefits. Avoid taking any herbal medication made from parsley.
- Fresh parsley as a condiment is all right to eat.

Infants and children:
Treating infants or children under 2 with any herbal preparation is hazardous.

Others:
No problems expected if you are beyond childhood, under 45, not

→

pregnant, basically healthy, take it for only a short time and do not exceed manufacturer's recommended dose.

Storage:
- Store in cool, dry area away from direct light, but don't freeze.
- Store safely out of reach of children.
- Don't store in bathroom medicine cabinet. Heat and moisture may change the action of the herb.

Safe dosage:
Consult your doctor for the appropriate dose for your condition.

 Toxicity

Rated relatively safe when taken in appropriate quantities for short periods of time

For symptoms of toxicity: See *Adverse Reactions, Side Effects or Overdose Symptoms* section below.

 Adverse Reactions, Side Effects or Overdose Symptoms

Signs and symptoms	What to do
Dizziness	Discontinue. Call doctor immediately.
Jaundice (yellow skin and eyes)	Discontinue. Call doctor immediately.
Nausea or vomiting	Discontinue. Call doctor immediately.
Photosensitivity	Avoid high sunlight exposure.

Partridgeberry (Squawvine)

 Basic Information

Biological name (genus and species):
Mitchella repens

Parts used for medicinal purposes:
Stems

Chemicals this herb contains:
- Dextrin
- Mucilage (see Glossary)
- Saponins (see Glossary)
- Wax (see Glossary)

 Known Effects

- Helps body dispose of excess fluid by increasing amount of urine produced

- Shrinks tissues
- Prevents secretion of fluids

 Possible Additional Effects

- May make labor less difficult
- May help flow of milk in lactating women
- May treat insomnia
- May decrease diarrhea
- May treat congestive heart failure, kidney failure, liver failure

 Warnings and Precautions

Don't take if you:
Are pregnant, think you may be pregnant or plan pregnancy in the near future.

Consult your doctor if you:

- Take this herb for any medical problem that doesn't improve in 2 weeks (There may be safer, more effective treatments.)
- Take any medicinal drugs or herbs including aspirin, laxatives, cold and cough remedies, antacids, vitamins, minerals, amino acids, supplements, other prescription or nonprescription drugs

Pregnancy:

Don't use unless prescribed by your doctor.

Breastfeeding:

Don't use unless prescribed by your doctor.

Infants and children:

Treating infants or children under 2 with any herbal preparation is hazardous.

Others:

No problems expected if you are beyond childhood, under 45, not pregnant, basically healthy, take it for only a short time and do not exceed manufacturer's recommended dose.

Storage:

- Store in cool, dry area away from direct light, but don't freeze.
- Store safely out of reach of children.
- Don't store in bathroom medicine cabinet. Heat and moisture may change the action of the herb.

Safe dosage:

Consult your doctor for the appropriate dose for your condition.

 Toxicity

Rated relatively safe when taken in appropriate quantities for short periods of time

 Adverse Reactions, Side Effects or Overdose Symptoms

None are expected.

Pasque Flower (May Flower, Pulsatilla)

 Basic Information

Biological name (genus and species):
Anemone pulsatilla

Parts used for medicinal purposes:
- Petals/flower
- Roots

Chemicals this herb contains:
- Anemone camphor
- Ranunculin
- Tannins (see Glossary)
- Volatile oils (see Glossary)

 Known Effects

- Irritates mucous membranes
- Shrinks tissues
- Prevents secretion of fluids
- Decreases thickness and increases fluidity of mucus in lungs and bronchial tubes
- Interferes with absorption of iron and other minerals when taken internally

➔

Possible Additional Effects

- May treat menstrual disorders
- May depress sexual excitement
- May increase sexual strength

Warnings and Precautions

Don't take if you:

- Are pregnant, think you may be pregnant or plan pregnancy in the near future
- Have any chronic disease of the gastrointestinal tract, such as stomach or duodenal ulcers, reflux esophagitis, ulcerative colitis, spastic colitis, diverticulosis or diverticulitis

Consult your doctor if you:

- Take this herb for any medical problem that doesn't improve in 2 weeks (There may be safer, more effective treatments.)
- Take any medicinal drugs or herbs including aspirin, laxatives, cold and cough remedies, antacids, vitamins, minerals, amino acids, supplements, other prescription or nonprescription drugs

Pregnancy:

Dangers outweigh any possible benefits. Don't use.

Breastfeeding:

Dangers outweigh any possible benefits. Don't use.

Infants and children:

Treating infants or children under 2 with any herbal preparation is hazardous.

Others:

No problems expected if you are beyond childhood, under 45, not pregnant, basically healthy, take it for only a short time and do not exceed manufacturer's recommended dose.

Storage:

- Store in cool, dry area away from direct light, but don't freeze.
- Store safely out of reach of children.
- Don't store in bathroom medicine cabinet. Heat and moisture may change the action of the herb.

Safe dosage:

Consult your doctor for the appropriate dose for your condition.

Toxicity

Rated slightly dangerous, particularly in children, persons over 55 and those who take larger than appropriate quantities for extended periods of time

For symptoms of toxicity: See *Adverse Reactions, Side Effects or Overdose Symptoms* section below.

Adverse Reactions, Side Effects or Overdose Symptoms

Signs and symptoms	What to do
Abdominal pain	Discontinue. Call doctor when convenient.
Diarrhea	Discontinue. Call doctor immediately.
Kidney damage characterized by blood in urine, decreased urine flow, swelling of hands and feet	Seek emergency treatment.
Nausea or vomiting	Discontinue. Call doctor immediately.

Passion Flower (Maypop)

Basic Information

Biological name (genus and species):
Passiflora incarnata

Parts used for medicinal purposes:
• Flowers
• Fruit

Chemicals this herb contains:
• Cyanogenic glycosides (see Glossary)
• Harmaline
• Harman
• Harmine
• Harmol

Known Effects

• Depresses nerve transfer in spinal cord and brain
• Increases respiratory rate
• Slightly depresses central nervous system
• Causes hallucinations

Miscellaneous information:
• Smoking passion flower reportedly causes mental changes similar to marijuana.
• It's available in capsules, herbal remedies or tinctures.
• No good human studies of clinical effectiveness exist.

Possible Additional Effects

• May reduce headaches
• May aid against convulsions
• May help treat insomnia
• Potential "nerve tonic" for Parkinson's

Warnings and Precautions

Don't take if you:
Are pregnant, think you may be pregnant or plan pregnancy in the near future.

Consult your doctor if you:
• Take this herb for any medical problem that doesn't improve in 2 weeks (There may be safer, more effective treatments.)
• Take any medicinal drugs or herbs including aspirin, laxatives, cold and cough remedies, antacids, vitamins, minerals, amino acids, supplements, other prescription or nonprescription drugs
• Are using sleeping pills

Pregnancy:
Dangers outweigh any possible benefits. Don't use.

Breastfeeding:
Dangers outweigh any possible benefits. Don't use.

Infants and children:
Treating infants or children under 2 with any herbal preparation is hazardous.

Others:
This product will not help you. It may cause toxic symptoms.

Storage:
• Store in cool, dry area away from direct light, but don't freeze.
• Store safely out of reach of children.
• Don't store in bathroom medicine cabinet. Heat and moisture may change the action of the herb.

➜

Safe dosage:
Consult your doctor for the appropriate dose for your condition.

Toxicity

Rated relatively safe when taken in appropriate quantities for short periods of time

For symptoms of toxicity: See *Adverse Reactions, Side Effects or Overdose Symptoms* section below.

Adverse Reactions, Side Effects or Overdose Symptoms

Signs and symptoms	What to do
Convulsions	Seek emergency treatment.
Decreased body temperature	Discontinue. Call doctor immediately.
Diarrhea	Discontinue. Call doctor immediately.
Hallucinations	Seek emergency treatment.
Muscle paralysis, including muscles used in breathing	Seek emergency treatment.
Nausea, vomiting, upset stomach	Discontinue. Call doctor immediately.
Sleepiness	Do not operate machinery or drive.

Pau D'Arco (Lapacho, Taheebo)

Basic Information

Biological name (genus and species): *Tabebuia* (several species exist, including *avellanedae* and *impetiginosa*)

Parts used for medicinal purposes: Inner bark

Chemicals this herb contains:
- Bioflavonoids
- Naphthoquinones, especially lapachol

Known Effects

- Antibiotic
- Antifungal
- Antiparasitic
- Relieves indigestion

Miscellaneous information:
- Prescribed as a cancer cure but no proven effects on cancer exist at this time.
- Pau d'arco is available as capsules, tinctures, tea and dried bark.

Possible Additional Effects

- Potential anti-inflammatory
- May treat rheumatism

Warnings and Precautions

Don't take if you:
Are pregnant, think you may be pregnant or plan pregnancy in the near future.

Consult your doctor if you:
- Take this herb for any medical problem that doesn't improve in 2 weeks (There may be safer, more effective treatments.)
- Take any medicinal drugs or herbs including aspirin, laxatives, cold and cough remedies, antacids, vitamins, minerals, amino acids, supplements, other prescription or nonprescription drugs

Pregnancy:
Don't use unless prescribed by your doctor.

Breastfeeding:
Don't use unless prescribed by your doctor.

Infants and children:
Treating infants or children under 2 with any herbal preparation is hazardous.

Others:
Extended use of this herb (more than 7-10 days) should be done only under the advice of your doctor.

Storage:
- Store in cool, dry area away from direct light, but don't freeze.
- Store safely out of reach of children.
- Don't store in bathroom medicine cabinet. Heat and moisture may change the action of the herb.

Safe dosage:
Consult your doctor for the appropriate dose for your condition. 250mg to 1g per day is average.

Toxicity

Comparative-toxicity rating is not available from standard references.

Adverse Reactions, Side Effects or Overdose Symptoms

None are expected.

Peach

Basic Information

Biological name (genus and species):
Prunus persica or other *Prunus* species

Parts used for medicinal purposes:
- Bark
- Leaves
- Roots
- Seeds

Chemicals this herb contains:
- Cyanide, especially in kernels
- Phloretin
- Volatile oils (see Glossary)

Known Effects

Irritates and stimulates gastrointestinal tract

Miscellaneous information:
- North American Indians made tea from the bark.
- The fruit, except for the peach pit, is safe.

➜

Possible Additional Effects

• May treat constipation (leaves)
• May treat systemic infections (bark and roots)

Warnings and Precautions

Don't take if you:
• Are pregnant, think you may be pregnant or plan pregnancy in the near future
• Have any chronic disease of the gastrointestinal tract, such as stomach or duodenal ulcers, reflux esophagitis, ulcerative colitis, spastic colitis, diverticulosis or diverticulitis

Consult your doctor if you:
• Take this herb for any medical problem that doesn't improve in 2 weeks (There may be safer, more effective treatments.)
• Take any medicinal drugs or herbs including aspirin, laxatives, cold and cough remedies, antacids, vitamins, minerals, amino acids, supplements, other prescription or nonprescription drugs

Pregnancy:
The dangers of taking this as a medicinal herb outweigh any possible benefits. Avoid pits! There should be no problems with the fruit.

Breastfeeding:
The dangers of taking this as a medicinal herb outweigh any possible benefits. Avoid pits! There should be no problems with the fruit.

Infants and children:
Treating infants or children under 2 with any herbal preparation is hazardous.

Others:
Pits will not help you and may cause toxic symptoms.

Storage:
• Store in cool, dry area away from direct light, but don't freeze.
• Store safely out of reach of children.
• Don't store in bathroom medicine cabinet. Heat and moisture may change the action of the herb.

Safe dosage:
Consult your doctor for the appropriate dose for your condition.

Toxicity

Comparative-toxicity rating is not available from standard references.

For symptoms of toxicity: See *Adverse Reactions, Side Effects or Overdose Symptoms* section below.

Adverse Reactions, Side Effects or Overdose Symptoms

Signs and symptoms	What to do
Diarrhea	Discontinue. Call doctor immediately.
Nausea or vomiting	Discontinue. Call doctor immediately.

Pellitory

Basic Information

Biological name (genus and species):
Anacyclus pyrethrum

Parts used for medicinal purposes:
Various parts of the entire plant,
frequently differing by country
and culture

Chemicals this herb contains:
Pellitorine

Known Effects

Kills insects

Miscellaneous information:
Tastes bitter.

Possible Additional Effects

- May relieve pain from toothache or gum infections
- May relieve facial pain
- May increase saliva flow

Warnings and Precautions

Don't take if you:
- Are pregnant, think you may be pregnant or plan pregnancy in the near future
- Have any chronic disease of the gastrointestinal tract, such as stomach or duodenal ulcers, reflux esophagitis, ulcerative colitis, spastic colitis, diverticulosis or diverticulitis

Consult your doctor if you:
- Take this herb for any medical problem that doesn't improve in 2 weeks (There may be safer, more effective treatments.)
- Take any medicinal drugs or herbs including aspirin, laxatives, cold and cough remedies, antacids, vitamins, minerals, amino acids, supplements, other prescription or nonprescription drugs

Pregnancy:
Don't use unless prescribed by your doctor.

Breastfeeding:
Don't use unless prescribed by your doctor.

Infants and children:
Treating infants or children under 2 with any herbal preparation is hazardous.

Others:
No problems expected if you are beyond childhood, under 45, not pregnant, basically healthy, take it for only a short time and do not exceed manufacturer's recommended dose.

Storage:
- Store in cool, dry area away from direct light, but don't freeze.
- Store safely out of reach of children.
- Don't store in bathroom medicine cabinet. Heat and moisture may change the action of the herb.

Safe dosage:
Consult your doctor for the appropriate dose for your condition.

Toxicity

Comparative-toxicity rating is not available from standard references.

For symptoms of toxicity: See *Adverse Reactions, Side Effects or Overdose Symptoms* section below.

 Adverse Reactions, Side Effects or Overdose Symptoms

Signs and symptoms	What to do
Diarrhea	Discontinue. Call doctor immediately.
Nausea or vomiting	Discontinue. Call doctor immediately.

Pennyroyal

 Basic Information

Biological name (genus and species):
Mentha pulegium, Hedeoma pulegioides

Parts used for medicinal purposes:
Entire plant

Chemicals this herb contains:
Pulegone (yellow or green-yellow oil)

 Known Effects

- Stimulates uterine contractions
- Depresses central nervous system
- Irritates mucous membranes
- Reddens skin by increasing blood supply to it
- Decongestant
- Can cause severe liver and kidney damage

Miscellaneous information:
- Pennyroyal is used as a flavoring agent.
- As little as 2 ounces of the essential oil can cause severe liver and kidney damage.

- It's also available as tinctures, dried leaves and flowers.
- The oil is toxic. Do not ingest.

 Possible Additional Effects

- May decrease intestinal cramps and flatulence
- May help treat colds, coughs
- May regulate menstruation
- May reduce gas, indigestion

 Warnings and Precautions

Don't take if you:
Are pregnant, think you may be pregnant or plan pregnancy in the near future.

Consult your doctor if you:
- Take this herb for any medical problem that doesn't improve in 2 weeks (There may be safer, more effective treatments.)
- Take any medicinal drugs or herbs including aspirin, laxatives, cold and cough remedies, antacids, vitamins, minerals, amino acids, supplements, other prescription or nonprescription drugs

Pregnancy:
Dangers outweigh any possible benefits. Don't use.

Breastfeeding:
Dangers outweigh any possible benefits. Don't use.

Infants and children:
Treating infants or children under 2 with any herbal preparation is hazardous.

Others:
Don't use in an attempt to induce abortion. Pennyroyal can be deadly.

Storage:
• Store in cool, dry area away from direct light, but don't freeze.
• Store safely out of reach of children.
• Don't store in bathroom medicine cabinet. Heat and moisture may change the action of the herb.

Safe dosage:
Consult your doctor for the appropriate dose for your condition.

Toxicity

Rated relatively safe when taken in appropriate quantities for short periods of time

For symptoms of toxicity: See *Adverse Reactions, Side Effects or Overdose Symptoms* section below.

Adverse Reactions, Side Effects or Overdose Symptoms

Signs and symptoms	What to do
Bleeding from gastrointestinal tract	Seek emergency treatment.
Blood in urine	Seek emergency treatment.
Jaundice (yellow skin and eyes)	Discontinue. Call doctor immediately.
Seizures	Seek emergency treatment.
Unusual vaginal bleeding	Seek emergency treatment.

Peppermint

Basic Information

Biological name (genus and species):
Mentha piperita

Parts used for medicinal purposes:
• Flowering tops
• Leaves

Chemicals this herb contains:
• Menthol
• Menthone
• Methyl acetate
• Tannic acid
• Terpenes (see Glossary)
• Volatile oils (see Glossary)

Known Effects

• Treats stomach discomfort
• Increases bile-acid flow for normal gallbladder function
• Stimulates gastrointestinal tract

Miscellaneous information:
• Peppermint is used to add flavor to medical and nonmedical preparations.

- No effects are expected on the body, either good or bad, when the herb is used in very small amounts to enhance the flavor of food.

Possible Additional Effects

- May aid in expelling gas from intestinal tract
- May reduce insomnia
- Potential antibacterial

Warnings and Precautions

Don't take if you:
- Are pregnant, think you may be pregnant or plan pregnancy in the near future
- Have any chronic disease of the gastrointestinal tract, such as stomach or duodenal ulcers, reflux esophagitis, ulcerative colitis, spastic colitis, diverticulosis or diverticulitis
- Have epilepsy or other neural disorders

Consult your doctor if you:
- Take this herb for any medical problem that doesn't improve in 2 weeks (There may be safer, more effective treatments.)
- Take any medicinal drugs or herbs including aspirin, laxatives, cold and cough remedies, antacids, vitamins, minerals, amino acids, supplements, other prescription or nonprescription drugs

Pregnancy:
Problems in pregnant women taking small or usual amounts have not been proved, but the chance of problems does exist. Don't use unless prescribed by your doctor.

Breastfeeding:
Problems in breastfed infants of lactating mothers taking small or usual amounts have not been proved, but the chance of problems does exist. Don't use unless prescribed by your doctor.

Infants and children:
Treating infants or children under 2 with any herbal preparation is hazardous.

Others:
No problems expected if you are beyond childhood, under 45, not pregnant, basically healthy, take it for only a short time and do not exceed manufacturer's recommended dose.

Storage:
- Store in cool, dry area away from direct light, but don't freeze.
- Store safely out of reach of children.
- Don't store in bathroom medicine cabinet. Heat and moisture may change the action of the herb.

Safe dosage:
Consult your doctor for the appropriate dose for your condition.

Toxicity

Comparative-toxicity rating is not available from standard references.

For symptoms of toxicity: See *Adverse Reactions, Side Effects or Overdose Symptoms* section below.

Adverse Reactions, Side Effects or Overdose Symptoms

Signs and symptoms	What to do
Drowsiness	Discontinue. Call doctor when convenient.
Vomiting	Discontinue. Call doctor immediately.

Periwinkle (Madagascar or Cape Periwinkle, Old Maid)

Basic Information

Biological name (genus and species):
Catharanthus roseus, Vinca rosea

Parts used for medicinal purposes:
Leaves

Chemicals this herb contains:
• Vinblastine
• Vincristine
• Vinleurosine
• Vinrosidine

Known Effects

• Inhibits growth and development of germs
• Depresses bone-marrow production, damaging body's blood cell-manufacturing processes
• Effective in treatment of several different types of malignant tumors
• Reduces granulocytes (white blood cells) in body

Miscellaneous information:
When purified, derivatives of *Vinca* (vincristine sulfate, vinblastine sulfate) are used to treat cancer under rigidly controlled supervision.

Possible Additional Effects

• May decrease inflammation when used as ointment
• May treat sore throats and inflamed tonsils
• May treat diabetes mellitus
• May cause hallucinations when smoked

Warnings and Precautions

Don't take if you:
• Are pregnant, think you may be pregnant or plan pregnancy in the near future
• Have any chronic disease of the gastrointestinal tract, such as stomach or duodenal ulcers, reflux esophagitis, ulcerative colitis, spastic colitis, diverticulosis or diverticulitis

Consult your doctor if you:
• Take this herb for any medical problem that doesn't improve in 2 weeks (There may be safer, more effective treatments.)
• Take any medicinal drugs or herbs including aspirin, laxatives, cold and cough remedies, antacids, vitamins, minerals, amino acids, supplements, other prescription or nonprescription drugs

Pregnancy:
Dangers outweigh any possible benefits. Don't use.

Breastfeeding:
Dangers outweigh any possible benefits. Don't use.

Infants and children:
Treating infants or children under 2 with any herbal preparation is hazardous.

Others:
This product will not help you and may cause toxic symptoms.

Storage:
• Store in cool, dry area away from direct light, but don't freeze.
• Store safely out of reach of children.

- Don't store in bathroom medicine cabinet. Heat and moisture may change the action of the herb.

Safe dosage:

Consult your doctor for the appropriate dose for your condition.

Toxicity

Rated slightly dangerous, particularly in children, persons over 55 and those who take larger than appropriate quantities for extended periods of time

For symptoms of toxicity: See *Adverse Reactions, Side Effects or Overdose Symptoms* section below.

Adverse Reactions, Side Effects or Overdose Symptoms

Signs and symptoms	What to do
Drowsiness	Discontinue. Call doctor when convenient.
Hair loss	Discontinue. Call doctor when convenient.
Nausea	Discontinue. Call doctor immediately.
Seizures	Seek emergency treatment.
Yellow eyes, dark urine and yellow skin resulting from destruction of some liver cells	Seek emergency treatment.

Pipsissewa

Basic Information

Biological name (genus and species): *Chimaphila umbellata*

Parts used for medicinal purposes: Leaves

Chemicals this herb contains:
- Arbutin
- Chimaphilin
- Chlorophyll
- Ericolin
- Minerals
- Pectic acid
- Tannins (see Glossary)
- Ursolic acid

Known Effects

- Helps body dispose of excess fluid by increasing amount of urine produced

- Interferes with absorption of iron and other minerals when taken internally

Possible Additional Effects

- May treat indigestion or mild stomach upsets
- May treat irritations of urinary tract (kidney, bladder, urethra)

Warnings and Precautions

Don't take if you:

- Are pregnant, think you may be pregnant or plan pregnancy in the near future
- Have any chronic disease of the gastrointestinal tract, such as stomach or duodenal ulcers, reflux esophagitis, ulcerative colitis, spastic colitis, diverticulosis or diverticulitis

Consult your doctor if you:
• Take this herb for any medical problem that doesn't improve in 2 weeks (There may be safer, more effective treatments.)
• Take any medicinal drugs or herbs including aspirin, laxatives, cold and cough remedies, antacids, vitamins, minerals, amino acids, supplements, other prescription or nonprescription drugs

Pregnancy:
Dangers outweigh any possible benefits. Don't use.

Breastfeeding:
Dangers outweigh any possible benefits. Don't use.

Infants and children:
Treating infants or children under 2 with any herbal preparation is hazardous.

Others:
No problems expected if you are beyond childhood, under 45, not pregnant, basically healthy, take it for only a short time and do not exceed manufacturer's recommended dose.

Storage:
• Store in cool, dry area away from direct light, but don't freeze.
• Store safely out of reach of children.
• Don't store in bathroom medicine cabinet. Heat and moisture may change the action of the herb.

Safe dosage:
Consult your doctor for the appropriate dose for your condition.

Toxicity

Comparative-toxicity rating is not available from standard references.

For symptoms of toxicity: See *Adverse Reactions, Side Effects or Overdose Symptoms* section below.

Adverse Reactions, Side Effects or Overdose Symptoms

Signs and symptoms	What to do
Diarrhea	Discontinue. Call doctor immediately.
Nausea or vomiting	Discontinue. Call doctor immediately.
Skin eruptions	Discontinue. Call doctor when convenient.

Pitcher Plant

Basic Information

Biological name (genus and species):
Sarracenia

Parts used for medicinal purposes:
Roots

Chemicals this herb contains:
• Resin (see Glossary)
• Yellow dye

Known Effects

• Irritates gastrointestinal tract
• Has diuretic properties

Possible
Additional Effects

• May treat constipation
• May treat indigestion

 Warnings and
Precautions

Don't take if you:
Are pregnant, think you may be pregnant or plan pregnancy in the near future.

Consult your doctor if you:
• Take this herb for any medical problem that doesn't improve in 2 weeks (There may be safer, more effective treatments.)
• Take any medicinal drugs or herbs including aspirin, laxatives, cold and cough remedies, antacids, vitamins, minerals, amino acids, supplements, other prescription or nonprescription drugs

Pregnancy:
Don't use unless prescribed by your doctor.

Breastfeeding:
Don't use unless prescribed by your doctor.

Infants and children:
Treating infants or children under 2 with any herbal preparation is hazardous.

Others:
No problems expected if you are beyond childhood, under 45, not pregnant, basically healthy, take it for only a short time and do not exceed manufacturer's recommended dose.

Storage:
• Store in cool, dry area away from direct light, but don't freeze.
• Store safely out of reach of children.
• Don't store in bathroom medicine cabinet. Heat and moisture may change the action of the herb.

Safe dosage:
Consult your doctor for the appropriate dose for your condition.

 Toxicity

Comparative-toxicity rating is not available from standard references.

 Adverse Reactions,
Side Effects or
Overdose Symptoms

None are expected.

Pleurisy Root (Butterfly Weed)

 Basic Information

Biological name (genus and species):
Asclepias tuberosa

Parts used for medicinal purposes:
Roots

Chemicals this herb contains:
• Asclepiadin
• Asclepione
• Galitoxin
• Volatile oils (see Glossary)

Known Effects

- Decreases thickness and increases fluidity of mucus in lungs and bronchial tubes
- Irritates mucous membranes
- Stimulates and irritates gastrointestinal tract

Possible Additional Effects

- Potential mild laxative to cause watery, explosive bowel movements
- May increase perspiration
- May help treat pleurisy

Warnings and Precautions

Don't take if you:
- Are pregnant, think you may be pregnant or plan pregnancy in the near future
- Have any chronic disease of the gastrointestinal tract, such as stomach or duodenal ulcers, reflux esophagitis, ulcerative colitis, spastic colitis, diverticulosis or diverticulitis

Consult your doctor if you:
- Take this herb for any medical problem that doesn't improve in 2 weeks (There may be safer, more effective treatments.)
- Take any medicinal drugs or herbs including aspirin, laxatives, cold and cough remedies, antacids, vitamins, minerals, amino acids, supplements, other prescription or nonprescription drugs

Pregnancy:
Dangers outweigh any possible benefits. Don't use.

Breastfeeding:
Dangers outweigh any possible benefits. Don't use.

Infants and children:
Treating infants or children under 2 with any herbal preparation is hazardous.

Others:
Dangers outweigh any possible benefits. Don't use.

Storage:
- Store in cool, dry area away from direct light, but don't freeze.
- Store safely out of reach of children.
- Don't store in bathroom medicine cabinet. Heat and moisture may change the action of the herb.

Safe dosage:
Consult your doctor for the appropriate dose for your condition.

Toxicity

Comparative-toxicity rating is not available from standard references.

For symptoms of toxicity: See *Adverse Reactions, Side Effects or Overdose Symptoms* section below.

Adverse Reactions, Side Effects or Overdose Symptoms

Signs and symptoms	What to do
Appetite loss	Discontinue. Call doctor when convenient.
Coma	Seek emergency treatment.
Diarrhea	Discontinue. Call doctor immediately.
Lethargy	Discontinue. Call doctor when convenient.
Muscle weakness	Discontinue. Call doctor immediately.
Nausea or vomiting	Discontinue. Call doctor immediately.

Poke (Pokeweed, Stoke)

Basic Information

Biological name (genus and species):
Phytolacca americana

Parts used for medicinal purposes:
- Leaves
- Roots
- Seeds

Chemicals this herb contains:
- Asparagine
- Mitogen
- Phytolaccagenin
- Resin (see Glossary)
- Saponins (see Glossary)

Known Effects

Stimulates and irritates
gastrointestinal tract

Miscellaneous information:
- All parts of native plants are poisonous. Don't take it. Children are especially vulnerable to toxic effects.
- Leaves are boiled and eaten as flavoring in some areas, particularly the southern United States. Used this way, pokeweed may be toxic. Don't use!

Possible Additional Effects

- May treat chronic arthritis
- May treat constipation

Warnings and Precautions

Don't take if you:
- Are pregnant, think you may be pregnant or plan pregnancy in the near future

- Have any chronic disease of the gastrointestinal tract, such as stomach or duodenal ulcers, reflux esophagitis, ulcerative colitis, spastic colitis, diverticulosis or diverticulitis

Consult your doctor if you:
- Take this herb for any medical problem that doesn't improve in 2 weeks (There may be safer, more effective treatments.)
- Take any medicinal drugs or herbs including aspirin, laxatives, cold and cough remedies, antacids, vitamins, minerals, amino acids, supplements, other prescription or nonprescription drugs

Pregnancy:
Dangers outweigh any possible benefits. Don't use.

Breastfeeding:
Dangers outweigh any possible benefits. Don't use.

Infants and children:
Treating infants or children under 2 with any herbal preparation is hazardous.

Others:
Handling roots may cause skin abrasions.

Storage:
- Store in cool, dry area away from direct light, but don't freeze.
- Store safely out of reach of children.
- Don't store in bathroom medicine cabinet. Heat and moisture may change the action of the herb.

Safe dosage:
Consult your doctor for the appropriate dose for your condition.

Toxicity

Comparative-toxicity rating is not available from standard references.

For symptoms of toxicity: See *Adverse Reactions, Side Effects or Overdose Symptoms* section below.

 Adverse Reactions, Side Effects or Overdose Symptoms

Signs and symptoms	What to do
Decreased heart rate	Seek emergency treatment.
Diarrhea	Discontinue. Call doctor immediately.
Nausea or vomiting	Discontinue. Call doctor immediately.
Skin eruptions	Discontinue. Call doctor when convenient.

Pomegranate

 Basic Information

Biological name (genus and species): *Punica granatum*

Parts used for medicinal purposes:
• Bark
• Berries/fruits, including rind

Chemicals this herb contains:
• Isopelletierine
• Methyl-isopelletierine
• Pelletierine
• Pseudo-pelletierine
• Tannins (see Glossary)

 Known Effects

Rind and bark:
• Shrinks tissues
• Prevents secretion of fluids
• Destroys intestinal worms
• Interferes with absorption of iron and other minerals when taken internally

Miscellaneous information:
• Fruits are edible and nontoxic.
• Bark and rind contain herbal-medicinal properties.

 Possible Additional Effects

May treat stasis ulcers and bed sores

 Warnings and Precautions

Don't take if you:
• Are pregnant, think you may be pregnant or plan pregnancy in the near future
• Have any chronic disease of the gastrointestinal tract, such as stomach or duodenal ulcers, reflux esophagitis, ulcerative colitis, spastic colitis, diverticulosis or diverticulitis

Consult your doctor if you:
• Take this herb for any medical problem that doesn't improve in 2 weeks (There may be safer, more effective treatments.)

• Take any medicinal drugs or herbs including aspirin, laxatives, cold and cough remedies, antacids, vitamins, minerals, amino acids, supplements, other prescription or nonprescription drugs

Pregnancy:
Taken internally as a medicinal herb, dangers outweigh any possible benefits. Don't use. Eating fruit as part of your diet will not cause problems.

Breastfeeding:
Taken internally as a medicinal herb, dangers outweigh any possible benefits. Don't use. Eating fruit as part of your diet will not cause problems.

Infants and children:
Treating infants or children under 2 with any herbal preparation is hazardous.

Others:
Taken internally, dangers outweigh any possible benefits. Don't use.

Storage:
• Store in cool, dry area away from direct light, but don't freeze.
• Store safely out of reach of children.
• Don't store in bathroom medicine cabinet. Heat and moisture may change the action of the herb.

Safe dosage:
Consult your doctor for the appropriate dose for your condition.

 Toxicity

Comparative-toxicity rating is not available from standard references.

For symptoms of toxicity: See *Adverse Reactions, Side Effects or Overdose Symptoms* section below.

 Adverse Reactions, Side Effects or Overdose Symptoms

Signs and symptoms	What to do
Diarrhea	Discontinue. Call doctor immediately.
Dilated pupils	Seek emergency treatment.
Dizziness	Discontinue. Call doctor immediately.
Double vision	Seek emergency treatment.
Nausea or vomiting	Discontinue. Call doctor immediately.
Weakness	Discontinue. Call doctor immediately.

Poplar Bud

 Basic Information

Biological name (genus and species):
Populus candicans

Parts used for medicinal purposes:
Leaf bud

Chemicals this herb contains:
• Chrysin
• Gallic acid
• Humulene
• Malic acid
• Mannite
• Populin
• Resin (see Glossary)
• Salicin
• Tectochrysin

Known Effects

- Blocks pain impulses to brain
- Changes fever-control "thermostat" in brain
- Antioxidant

Miscellaneous information:
- Antioxidant effect helps prevent rancidity in ointments.
- Poplar bud is used as an additive in several pharmaceutical preparations.

Possible Additional Effects

- May reduce pain of sprains and bruises when applied to skin
- May treat coughs and colds when taken internally
- May reduce fever

Warnings and Precautions

Don't take if you:
- Are pregnant, think you may be pregnant or plan pregnancy in the near future
- Have any chronic disease of the gastrointestinal tract, such as stomach or duodenal ulcers, reflux esophagitis, ulcerative colitis, spastic colitis, diverticulosis or diverticulitis

Consult your doctor if you:
- Take this herb for any medical problem that doesn't improve in 2 weeks (There may be safer, more effective treatments.)
- Take any medicinal drugs or herbs including aspirin, laxatives, cold and cough remedies, antacids, vitamins, minerals, amino acids, supplements, other prescription or nonprescription drugs

Pregnancy:
Don't use unless prescribed by your doctor.

Breastfeeding:
Don't use unless prescribed by your doctor.

Infants and children:
Treating infants or children under 2 with any herbal preparation is hazardous.

Others:
No problems expected if you are beyond childhood, under 45, not pregnant, basically healthy, take it for only a short time and do not exceed manufacturer's recommended dose.

Storage:
- Store in cool, dry area away from direct light, but don't freeze.
- Store safely out of reach of children.
- Don't store in bathroom medicine cabinet. Heat and moisture may change the action of the herb.

Safe dosage:
Consult your doctor for the appropriate dose for your condition.

Toxicity

Comparative-toxicity rating is not available from standard references.

For symptoms of toxicity: See *Adverse Reactions, Side Effects or Overdose Symptoms* section below.

Adverse Reactions, Side Effects or Overdose Symptoms

Signs and symptoms	What to do
Itching and redness of skin, rash	Apply hydrocortisone ointment, available without prescription.

Prickly Ash

Basic Information

Biological name (genus and species):
Zanthoxylum americanum
(northern), *Zanthoxylum clava-*
herculus (southern)

Parts used for medicinal purposes:
• Bark
• Berries/fruits

Chemicals this herb contains:
• Acid amide
• Asarinin
• Berberine
• Herculin
• Xanthoxyletin
• Xanthyletin

Known Effects

• Stimulates and irritates
  gastrointestinal tract
• Increases perspiration

Possible Additional Effects

• May stimulate appetite
• May treat arthritis
• May decrease flatulence

Warnings and Precautions

Don't take if you:
• Are pregnant, think you may be
  pregnant or plan pregnancy in the
  near future
• Have any chronic disease of the
  gastrointestinal tract, such as stomach
  or duodenal ulcers, reflux
  esophagitis, ulcerative colitis, spastic
  colitis, diverticulosis or diverticulitis

Consult your doctor if you:
• Take this herb for any medical
  problem that doesn't improve in
  2 weeks (There may be safer, more
  effective treatments.)
• Take any medicinal drugs or
  herbs including aspirin, laxatives,
  cold and cough remedies, antacids,
  vitamins, minerals, amino acids,
  supplements, other prescription
  or nonprescription drugs

Pregnancy:
Don't use unless prescribed by
your doctor.

Breastfeeding:
Don't use unless prescribed by
your doctor.

Infants and children:
Treating infants or children under
2 with any herbal preparation
is hazardous.

Others:
No problems expected if you are
beyond childhood, under 45, not
pregnant, basically healthy, take it for
only a short time and do not exceed
manufacturer's recommended dose.

Storage:
• Store in cool, dry area away from
  direct light, but don't freeze.
• Store safely out of reach of children.
• Don't store in bathroom medicine
  cabinet. Heat and moisture may
  change the action of the herb.

Safe dosage:
Consult your doctor for the
appropriate dose for your condition.

Toxicity

Comparative-toxicity rating is not
available from standard references.

For symptoms of toxicity: See
*Adverse Reactions, Side Effects or
Overdose Symptoms* section below.

Adverse Reactions, Side Effects or Overdose Symptoms

Signs and symptoms	What to do
Diarrhea	Discontinue. Call doctor immediately.
Nausea or vomiting	Discontinue. Call doctor immediately.

Prickly Poppy (Mexican Poppy, Thistle Poppy)

Basic Information

Biological name (genus and species):
Argemone mexicana

Parts used for medicinal purposes:
Seeds

Chemicals this herb contains:
• Berberine
• Dihydrosanguinarine
• Protopine
• Sanguinarine

Known Effects

Mildly depresses central
nervous system

Miscellaneous information:
This poppy is not the origin of
morphine, codeine or other narcotics.

Possible Additional Effects

Smoking prickly poppy may produce
euphoria and reduce pain.

Warnings and Precautions

Don't take if you:
• Are pregnant, think you may be
pregnant or plan pregnancy in the
near future
• Have any chronic disease of the
gastrointestinal tract, such as stomach
or duodenal ulcers, reflux
esophagitis, ulcerative colitis, spastic
colitis, diverticulosis or diverticulitis

Consult your doctor if you:
• Take this herb for any medical
problem that doesn't improve in
2 weeks (There may be safer, more
effective treatments.)

• Take any medicinal drugs or herbs including aspirin, laxatives, cold and cough remedies, antacids, vitamins, minerals, amino acids, supplements, other prescription or nonprescription drugs

Pregnancy:
Dangers outweigh any possible benefits. Don't use.

Breastfeeding:
Dangers outweigh any possible benefits. Don't use.

Infants and children:
Treating infants or children under 2 with any herbal preparation is hazardous.

Others:
Dangers outweigh any possible benefits. Don't use.

Storage:
• Store in cool, dry area away from direct light, but don't freeze.
• Store safely out of reach of children.
• Don't store in bathroom medicine cabinet. Heat and moisture may change the action of the herb.

Safe dosage:
Consult your doctor for the appropriate dose for your condition.

 Toxicity

Rated slightly dangerous, particularly in children, persons over 55 and those who take larger than appropriate quantities for extended periods of time.

For symptoms of toxicity: See *Adverse Reactions, Side Effects or Overdose Symptoms* section below.

 Adverse Reactions, Side Effects or Overdose Symptoms

Signs and symptoms	What to do
Diarrhea	Discontinue. Call doctor immediately.
Dizziness	Discontinue. Call doctor immediately.
Fluid retention	Discontinue. Call doctor when convenient.
Loss of consciousness	Seek emergency treatment.
Nausea or vomiting	Discontinue. Call doctor immediately.
Swollen abdomen	Discontinue. Call doctor when convenient.
Vision disturbances	Discontinue. Call doctor immediately.

Prostrate Knotweed (Pigweed)

 Basic Information

Biological name (genus and species):
Polygonum aviculare

Parts used for medicinal purposes:

Various parts of the entire plant, frequently differing by country and culture

Chemicals this herb contains:
• Avicularin
• Emodin
• Quercetin 3-arabinoside

Known Effects

- Reduces capillary fragility
- Reduces capillary permeability
- Retards destruction of epinephrine

Possible Additional Effects

- May cause watery, explosive bowel movements
- May treat kidney and bladder stones

Warnings and Precautions

Don't take if you:
- Are pregnant, think you may be pregnant or plan pregnancy in the near future
- Have any chronic disease of the gastrointestinal tract, such as stomach or duodenal ulcers, reflux esophagitis, ulcerative colitis, spastic colitis, diverticulosis or diverticulitis

Consult your doctor if you:
- Take this herb for any medical problem that doesn't improve in 2 weeks (There may be safer, more effective treatments.)
- Take any medicinal drugs or herbs including aspirin, laxatives, cold and cough remedies, antacids, vitamins, minerals, amino acids, supplements, other prescription or nonprescription drugs

Pregnancy:
Don't use unless prescribed by your doctor.

Breastfeeding:
Don't use unless prescribed by your doctor.

Infants and children:
Treating infants or children under 2 with any herbal preparation is hazardous.

Others:
No problems expected if you are beyond childhood, under 45, not pregnant, basically healthy, take it for only a short time and do not exceed manufacturer's recommended dose.

Storage:
- Store in cool, dry area away from direct light, but don't freeze.
- Store safely out of reach of children.
- Don't store in bathroom medicine cabinet. Heat and moisture may change the action of the herb.

Safe dosage:
Consult your doctor for the appropriate dose for your condition.

Toxicity

Rated relatively safe when taken in appropriate quantities for short periods of time

For symptoms of toxicity: See *Adverse Reactions, Side Effects or Overdose Symptoms* section below.

Adverse Reactions, Side Effects or Overdose Symptoms

Signs and symptoms	What to do
Abdominal pain	Discontinue. Call doctor when convenient.
Diarrhea	Discontinue. Call doctor immediately.
Nausea or vomiting	Discontinue. Call doctor immediately.
Skin eruptions	Discontinue. Call doctor when convenient.

Psyllium

 Basic Information

Biological name (genus and species):
Plantago psyllium

Parts used for medicinal purposes:
Seeds

Chemicals this herb contains:
• Glycosides (see Glossary)
• Mucilage (see Glossary)

 Known Effects

• Produces bulky bowel movements
• Softens stools
• Reduces risk of heart disease by removing excess cholesterol from blood

Miscellaneous information:
Psyllium is a popular product and available over-the-counter without prescription.

 Possible Additional Effects

No additional effects are known.

 Warnings and Precautions

Don't take if you:
Are pregnant, think you may be pregnant or plan pregnancy in the near future.

Consult your doctor if you:
• Take this herb for any medical problem that doesn't improve in 2 weeks (There may be safer, more effective treatments.)
• Take any medicinal drugs or herbs including aspirin, laxatives, cold and cough remedies, antacids, vitamins, minerals, amino acids, supplements, other prescription or nonprescription drugs

Pregnancy:
Problems in pregnant women taking small or usual amounts have not been proved, but the chance of problems does exist. Don't use unless prescribed by your doctor.

Breastfeeding:
Problems in breastfed infants of lactating mothers taking small or usual amounts have not been proved, but the chance of problems does exist. Don't use unless prescribed by your doctor.

Infants and children:
Treating infants or children under 2 with any herbal preparation is hazardous.

Others:
People with allergies to dust or grasses may have a reaction to psyllium.

Storage:
• Store in cool, dry area away from direct light, but don't freeze.
• Store safely out of reach of children.
• Don't store in bathroom medicine cabinet. Heat and moisture may change the action of the herb.

Safe dosage:
Consult your doctor for the appropriate dose for your condition.

 Toxicity

Comparative-toxicity rating is not available from standard references.

Adverse Reactions, Side Effects or Overdose Symptoms

None are expected.

Rauwolfia (Chandra, Sarpaganda, Snakeroot)

 Basic Information

Biological name (genus and species):
Rauwolfia serpentina

Parts used for medicinal purposes:
Roots

Chemicals this herb contains:
- Ajmaline
- Deserpidine
- Rescinnamine
- Reserpine
- Serpentine
- Yohimbine

 Known Effects

- Reduces blood pressure
- Depresses activity of central nervous system
- Hypnotic

Miscellaneous information:
- Snakeroot depletes catecholamines and serotonin from nerves in the central nervous system.
- Refined snakeroot has been used extensively in recent years to treat hypertension.
- Animal studies suggest snakeroot may produce cancers.

 Possible Additional Effects

- May decrease anxiety
- May decrease fever
- May kill intestinal parasites
- In India, used as antidote for snakebites

 Warnings and Precautions

Don't take if you:
- Are pregnant, think you may be pregnant or plan pregnancy in the near future
- Have any chronic disease of the gastrointestinal tract, such as stomach or duodenal ulcers, reflux esophagitis, ulcerative colitis, spastic colitis, diverticulosis or diverticulitis

Consult your doctor if you:
- Take this herb for any medical problem that doesn't improve in 2 weeks (There may be safer, more effective treatments.)
- Take any medicinal drugs or herbs including aspirin, laxatives, cold and cough remedies, antacids, vitamins, minerals, amino acids, supplements, other prescription or nonprescription drugs

➡

Pregnancy
Dangers outweigh any possible benefits. Don't use.

Breastfeeding:
Dangers outweigh any possible benefits. Don't use.

Infants and children:
Treating infants or children under 2 with any herbal preparation is hazardous.

Others:
Dangers outweigh any possible benefits. Don't use.

Storage:
• Store in cool, dry area away from direct light, but don't freeze.
• Store safely out of reach of children.
• Don't store in bathroom medicine cabinet. Heat and moisture may change the action of the herb.

Safe dosage:
At present no "safe" dosage has been established.

 Toxicity

Rated slightly dangerous, particularly in children, persons over 55 and those who take larger than appropriate quantities for extended periods of time

For symptoms of toxicity: See *Adverse Reactions, Side Effects or Overdose Symptoms* section below.

 Adverse Reactions, Side Effects or Overdose Symptoms

Signs and symptoms	What to do
Bizarre dreams	Discontinue. Call doctor when convenient.
Decreased libido and sexual performance	Discontinue. Call doctor when convenient.
Diarrhea	Discontinue. Call doctor immediately.
Drowsiness	Discontinue. Call doctor when convenient.
Nasal congestion	Discontinue. Call doctor when convenient.
Precipitous blood-pressure drop: symptoms include faintness, cold sweat, paleness, rapid pulse	Seek emergency treatment.
Slow heartbeat	Seek emergency treatment.
Stupor	Seek emergency treatment.
Upper abdominal pain	Discontinue. Call doctor when convenient.

Red Clover (Pavine Clover, Cowgrass)

 Basic Information

Biological name (genus and species):
Trifolium pratense

Parts used for medicinal purposes:
Flowers

Chemicals this herb contains:
• Folic acid
• Glycosides (see Glossary)
• Isoflavonoids

Known Effects

- Decreases activity of central nervous system
- Expectorant

Possible Additional Effects

- May reduce upper abdominal cramps
- May treat indigestion
- May loosen secretions in bronchial tubes due to infections or chronic lung disease
- Contains antitumor compounds and may be used in combination with other drugs to treat some forms of cancer
- May reduce menopausal symptoms
- Potential aid for weakened immune systems

Warnings and Precautions

Don't take if you:

- Are pregnant, think you may be pregnant or plan pregnancy in the near future
- Have a history of heart disease or stroke

Consult your doctor if you:

- Take this herb for any medical problem that doesn't improve in 2 weeks (There may be safer, more effective treatments.)
- Take any medicinal drugs or herbs including aspirin, laxatives, cold and cough remedies, antacids, vitamins, minerals, amino acids, supplements, other prescription or nonprescription drugs

Pregnancy:
Don't use unless prescribed by your doctor. Red clover has some estrogen-like properties.

Breastfeeding:
Don't use unless prescribed by your doctor.

Infants and children:
Treating infants or children under 2 with any herbal preparation is hazardous.

Others:
No problems expected if you are beyond childhood, under 45, not pregnant, basically healthy, take it for only a short time and do not exceed manufacturer's recommended dose.

Storage:

- Store in cool, dry area away from direct light, but don't freeze.
- Store safely out of reach of children.
- Don't store in bathroom medicine cabinet. Heat and moisture may change the action of the herb.

Safe dosage:
Consult your doctor for the appropriate dose for your condition.

Toxicity

Generally regarded as safe when taken in appropriate quantities for short periods of time

Adverse Reactions, Side Effects or Overdose Symptoms

None are expected.

Red Raspberry

Basic Information

Biological name (genus and species):
Rubus strigosus, R. idaeus

Parts used for medicinal purposes:
• Bark
• Leaves
• Roots

Chemicals this herb contains:
• Citric acid
• Tannins (see Glossary)

Known Effects

• Relaxes uterine spasms
• Relaxes intestinal spasms
• Gargle for sore throats

Miscellaneous information:
• Berries are delicious, nutritious and nontoxic.
• When eaten as a common food, no problems are expected for anyone.

Possible Additional Effects

• May increase contractions of labor pains
• May decrease excessive menstrual bleeding
• May relieve morning sickness
• May treat mouth ulcers

Warnings and Precautions

Don't take if you:
Are pregnant, think you may be pregnant or plan pregnancy in the near future.

Consult your doctor if you:
• Take this herb for any medical problem that doesn't improve in 2 weeks (There may be safer, more effective treatments.)
• Take any medicinal drugs or herbs including aspirin, laxatives, cold and cough remedies, antacids, vitamins, minerals, amino acids, supplements, other prescription or nonprescription drugs
• Are pregnant and want to use for morning sickness

Pregnancy:
Don't use unless prescribed by your doctor.

Breastfeeding:
Don't use unless prescribed by your doctor.

Infants and children:
Treating infants or children under 2 with any herbal preparation is hazardous.

Others:
No problems expected if you are beyond childhood, under 45, not pregnant, basically healthy, take it for only a short time and do not exceed manufacturer's recommended dose.

Storage:
• Store in cool, dry area away from direct light, but don't freeze.
• Store safely out of reach of children.
• Don't store in bathroom medicine cabinet. Heat and moisture may change the action of the herb.

Safe dosage:
Consult your doctor for the appropriate dose for your condition.

Toxicity

Comparative-toxicity rating is not available from standard references.

For symptoms of toxicity: See *Adverse Reactions, Side Effects or Overdose Symptoms* section below.

Adverse Reactions, Side Effects or Overdose Symptoms

Signs and symptoms	What to do
Diarrhea	Discontinue. Call doctor immediately.
Nausea	Discontinue. Call doctor immediately.

Rhatany

Basic Information

Biological name (genus and species): *Krameria triandra*

Parts used for medicinal purposes: Various parts of the entire plant, frequently differing by country and culture

Chemicals this herb contains:
- Calcium oxalate
- Gum (see Glossary)
- Lignin
- N-Methyltyrosine
- Saccharine
- Starch
- Tannins (see Glossary)

Known Effects

- Anti-inflammatory
- Helps treat canker sores

Possible Additional Effects

- May treat sore throat
- May treat hemorrhoids
- May treat chronic bowel inflammations
- May treat diarrhea
- Potential mouthwash

Warnings and Precautions

Don't take if you:
- Are pregnant, think you may be pregnant or plan pregnancy in the near future
- Have any chronic disease of the gastrointestinal tract, such as stomach or duodenal ulcers, reflux esophagitis, ulcerative colitis, spastic colitis, diverticulosis or diverticulitis

Consult your doctor if you:
- Take this herb for any medical problem that doesn't improve in 2 weeks (There may be safer, more effective treatments.)
- Take any medicinal drugs or herbs including aspirin, laxatives, cold and cough remedies, antacids, vitamins, minerals, amino acids, supplements, other prescription or nonprescription drugs

Pregnancy
Dangers outweigh any possible benefits. Don't use.

Breastfeeding:
Dangers outweigh any possible
benefits. Don't use.

Infants and children:
Treating infants or children under
2 with any herbal preparation
is hazardous.

Others:
No problems expected if you are
beyond childhood, under 45, not
pregnant, basically healthy, take it for
only a short time and do not exceed
manufacturer's recommended dose.

Storage:
• Store in cool, dry area away from
  direct light, but don't freeze.
• Store safely out of reach of children.
• Don't store in bathroom medicine
  cabinet. Heat and moisture may
  change the action of the herb.

Safe dosage:
Consult your doctor for the
appropriate dose for your condition.

Toxicity

Comparative-toxicity rating is not
available from standard references.

For symptoms of toxicity: See
*Adverse Reactions, Side Effects or
Overdose Symptoms* section below.

Adverse Reactions, Side Effects or Overdose Symptoms

Signs and symptoms	What to do
Diarrhea	Discontinue. Call doctor immediately.
Kidney damage characterized by blood in urine, decreased urine flow, swelling of hands and feet	Seek emergency treatment.
Nausea or vomiting	Discontinue. Call doctor immediately.

Rheumatism Root (Wild-Yam Root)

Basic Information

Biological name (genus and species):
Dioscorea villosa

Parts used for medicinal purposes:
Roots

Chemicals this herb contains:
• Dioscin
• Diosgenin
• Resin (see Glossary)
• Saponins (see Glossary)

Known Effects

Breaks membranous covering,
destroying red blood cells (toxic to
fish and amoeba)

Miscellaneous information:
Diosgenin is a steroid base used to
synthesize cortisone and progesterone
(hormones).

Possible
Additional Effects

• May treat arthritis by removing
  accumulated waste in joints
• May reduce menopausal symptoms
• May relieve morning sickness
• May treat menstrual cramps

 Warnings and
Precautions

Don't take if you:
• Are pregnant, think you may be
  pregnant or plan pregnancy in the
  near future
• Have any chronic disease of the
  gastrointestinal tract, such as stomach
  or duodenal ulcers, reflux
  esophagitis, ulcerative colitis, spastic
  colitis, diverticulosis or diverticulitis
• Are pregnant and want to treat
  morning sickness

Consult your doctor if you:
• Take this herb for any medical
  problem that doesn't improve in
  2 weeks (There may be safer, more
  effective treatments.)
• Take any medicinal drugs or
  herbs including aspirin, laxatives,
  cold and cough remedies, antacids,
  vitamins, minerals, amino acids,
  supplements, other prescription
  or nonprescription drugs

Pregnancy
Dangers outweigh any possible
benefits. Don't use.

Breastfeeding:
Dangers outweigh any possible
benefits. Don't use.

Infants and children:
Treating infants or children under
2 with any herbal preparation
is hazardous.

Others:
No problems expected if you are
beyond childhood, under 45, not
pregnant, basically healthy, take it for
only a short time and do not exceed
manufacturer's recommended dose.

Storage:
• Store in cool, dry area away from
  direct light, but don't freeze.
• Store safely out of reach of children.
• Don't store in bathroom medicine
  cabinet. Heat and moisture may
  change the action of the herb.

Safe dosage:
Consult your doctor for the
appropriate dose for your condition.

 Toxicity

Generally regarded as safe when taken
in appropriate quantities for short
periods of time

For symptoms of toxicity: See
*Adverse Reactions, Side Effects or
Overdose Symptoms* section below.

 Adverse Reactions,
Side Effects or
Overdose Symptoms

Signs and symptoms	What to do
Diarrhea	Discontinue. Call doctor immediately.
Nausea or vomiting	Discontinue. Call doctor immediately.

Rose

Basic Information

Biological name (genus and species):
Rosa

Parts used for medicinal purposes:
• Berries/fruits
• Petals/flower

Chemicals this herb contains:
• Ascorbic acid
• Cyanogenic glycoside (see Glossary)
• Quercitrin
• Tannins (see Glossary)
• Vitamins A and C
• Volatile oils (see Glossary)

Known Effects

• Anti-inflammatory
• Calming effects

Miscellaneous information:
• North American Indians formerly used fruit as a food source.
• Leaves are used to make tea or salad and smoked like tobacco.
• Rose hips are used in vitamin-C supplements.
• Rose adds flavor to foods during cooking.

Possible Additional Effects

• May smooth skin
• Potential astringent
• Potential sedative
• May help induce sleep

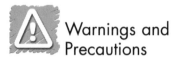

Warnings and Precautions

Don't take if you:
Are pregnant, think you may be pregnant or plan pregnancy in the near future.

Consult your doctor if you:
Are pregnant, think you may be pregnant or plan pregnancy in the near future.

Pregnancy:
Don't use unless prescribed by your doctor.

Breastfeeding:
Don't use unless prescribed by your doctor.

Infants and children:
Treating infants or children under 2 with any herbal preparation is hazardous.

Others:
No problems expected if you are beyond childhood, under 45, not pregnant, basically healthy, take it for only a short time and do not exceed manufacturer's recommended dose.

Storage:
• Store in cool, dry area away from direct light, but don't freeze.
• Store safely out of reach of children.
• Don't store in bathroom medicine cabinet. Heat and moisture may change the action of the herb.

Safe dosage:
Consult your doctor for the appropriate dose for your condition.

Toxicity

Comparative-toxicity rating is not available from standard references.

 Adverse Reactions, Side Effects or Overdose Symptoms

None are expected.

Rosemary

 Basic Information

Biological name (genus and species):
Rosmarinus officinalis

Parts used for medicinal purposes:
• Berries/fruits
• Leaves

Chemicals this herb contains:
• Bitters (see Glossary)
• Borneol
• Camphene
• Camphor
• Cineole
• Pinene
• Resin (see Glossary)
• Tannins (see Glossary)
• Volatile oils (see Glossary)

 Known Effects

• Irritates tissue and kills bacteria (volatile oils)
• Astringent
• Increases stomach acidity, helps reduce indigestion
• Helps expel gas from intestinal tract

Miscellaneous information:
• Rosemary is used as an ingredient in perfumes, hair lotions and soaps.
• No effects are expected on the body, either good or bad, when the herb is used in very small amounts to enhance the flavor of food.

 Possible Additional Effects

• May redden skin by increasing blood supply to it
• May stimulate appetite
• May treat skin infections when used externally
• May help treat constipation
• Potential diuretic

 Warnings and Precautions

Don't take if you:
• Are pregnant, think you may be pregnant or plan pregnancy in the near future
• Have any chronic disease of the gastrointestinal tract, such as stomach or duodenal ulcers, reflux esophagitis, ulcerative colitis, spastic colitis, diverticulosis or diverticulitis

Consult your doctor if you:
• Take this herb for any medical problem that doesn't improve in 2 weeks (There may be safer, more effective treatments.)
• Take any medicinal drugs or herbs including aspirin, laxatives, cold and cough remedies, antacids, vitamins, minerals, amino acids, supplements, other prescription or nonprescription drugs

➔

Pregnancy:
Don't use unless prescribed by
your doctor.

Breastfeeding:
Don't use unless prescribed by
your doctor.

Infants and children:
Treating infants or children under
2 with any herbal preparation
is hazardous.

Others:
No problems expected if you are
beyond childhood, under 45, not
pregnant, basically healthy, take it for
only a short time and do not exceed
manufacturer's recommended dose.

Storage:
• Store in cool, dry area away from
  direct light, but don't freeze.
• Store safely out of reach of children.
• Don't store in bathroom medicine
  cabinet. Heat and moisture may
  change the action of the herb.

Safe dosage:
Consult your doctor for the
appropriate dose for your condition.

Toxicity

Rated relatively safe when taken in
appropriate quantities for short
periods of time

For symptoms of toxicity: See
*Adverse Reactions, Side Effects or
Overdose Symptoms* section below.

Adverse Reactions, Side Effects or Overdose Symptoms

Signs and symptoms	What to do
Diarrhea	Discontinue. Call doctor immediately.
Nausea or vomiting	Discontinue. Call doctor immediately.
Skin eruptions	Discontinue. Call doctor when convenient.

Rue (Garden Rue, German Rue)

Basic Information

Biological name (genus and species):
Ruta graveolens

Parts used for medicinal purposes:
Entire plant

Chemicals this herb contains:
• Esters
• Methyl-N-nonyl-ketone
• Phenols

• Rutin
• Tannins (see Glossary)
• Volatile oils (see Glossary)

Known Effects

• Stimulates uterine contractions
• Prolongs action of epinephrine
• Relieves spasm in skeletal or smooth
  muscle
• Decreases capillary fragility
• Interferes with absorption of iron
  and other minerals when
  taken internally

Possible
Additional Effects

- May cause onset of menstruation
- May treat hysteria
- May treat intestinal parasites (worms)
- May treat colic
- May control postpartum bleeding

 Warnings and
Precautions

Don't take if you:
- Are pregnant, think you may be pregnant or plan pregnancy in the near future
- Have any chronic disease of the gastrointestinal tract, such as stomach or duodenal ulcers, reflux esophagitis, ulcerative colitis, spastic colitis, diverticulosis or diverticulitis

Consult your doctor if you:
- Take this herb for any medical problem that doesn't improve in 2 weeks (There may be safer, more effective treatments.)
- Take any medicinal drugs or herbs including aspirin, laxatives, cold and cough remedies, antacids, vitamins, minerals, amino acids, supplements, other prescription or nonprescription drugs

Pregnancy
Dangers outweigh any possible benefits. Don't use.

Breastfeeding:
Dangers outweigh any possible benefits. Don't use.

Infants and children:
Treating infants or children under 2 with any herbal preparation is hazardous.

Others:
No problems expected if you are beyond childhood, under 45, not

pregnant, basically healthy, take it for only a short time and do not exceed manufacturer's recommended dose.

Storage:
- Store in cool, dry area away from direct light, but don't freeze.
- Store safely out of reach of children.
- Don't store in bathroom medicine cabinet. Heat and moisture may change the action of the herb.

Safe dosage:
Consult your doctor for the appropriate dose for your condition.

 Toxicity

Rated relatively safe when taken in appropriate quantities for short periods of time

For symptoms of toxicity: See *Adverse Reactions, Side Effects or Overdose Symptoms* section below.

 Adverse Reactions,
Side Effects or
Overdose Symptoms

Signs and symptoms	What to do
Abdominal pain	Discontinue. Call doctor when convenient.
Abortion	Seek emergency treatment.
Confusion	Discontinue. Call doctor immediately.
Diarrhea	Discontinue. Call doctor immediately.
Jaundice (yellow skin and eyes)	Discontinue. Call doctor immediately.
Nausea or vomiting	Discontinue. Call doctor immediately.
Skin rashes	Discontinue. Call doctor when convenient.

Saffron (Saffron Crocus)

Basic Information

Biological name (genus and species):
Crocus sativus

Parts used for medicinal purposes:
Berries/fruits

Chemicals this herb contains:
- Glycosides (see Glossary)
- Volatile oils (see Glossary)

Known Effects

- Reduces irritation of gastrointestinal tract
- Increases perspiration
- Increases fluidity of bronchial secretions

Miscellaneous information:
- No effects are expected on the body, good or bad, when this herb is used in very small amounts to enhance the flavor of food; however, in large amounts saffron is highly toxic—use only recommended doses.
- Saffron is very expensive.

Possible Additional Effects

- May stimulate respiration in those with asthma, whooping cough
- May reduce cholesterol
- May relieve indigestion
- May help control blood pressure

Warnings and Precautions

Don't take if you:
- Are pregnant, think you may be pregnant or plan pregnancy in the near future
- Have any chronic disease of the gastrointestinal tract, such as stomach or duodenal ulcers, reflux esophagitis, ulcerative colitis, spastic colitis, diverticulosis or diverticulitis

Consult your doctor if you:
- Take this herb for any medical problem that doesn't improve in 2 weeks (There may be safer, more effective treatments.)
- Take any medicinal drugs or herbs including aspirin, laxatives, cold and cough remedies, antacids, vitamins, minerals, amino acids, supplements, other prescription or nonprescription drugs

Pregnancy:
Don't use.

Breastfeeding:
Don't use.

Infants and children:
Treating infants or children under 2 with any herbal preparation is hazardous.

Others:
No problems expected if you are beyond childhood, under 45, not pregnant, basically healthy, take it for only a short time and do not exceed manufacturer's recommended dose.

Storage:

- Store in cool, dry area away from direct light, but don't freeze.
- Store safely out of reach of children.
- Don't store in bathroom medicine cabinet. Heat and moisture may change the action of the herb.

Safe dosage:

Consult your doctor for the appropriate dose for your condition.

 Toxicity

Rated relatively safe when taken in appropriate quantities for short periods of time

For symptoms of toxicity: See *Adverse Reactions, Side Effects or Overdose Symptoms* section below.

 Adverse Reactions, Side Effects or Overdose Symptoms

Signs and symptoms	What to do
Diarrhea	Discontinue. Call doctor immediately.
Dizziness	Discontinue. Call doctor immediately.
Nosebleeds	Discontinue. Call doctor when convenient.
Slow heart rate	Seek emergency treatment.
Stupor	Seek emergency treatment.
Vomiting	Discontinue. Call doctor immediately.

Sage

 Basic Information

Biological name (genus and species): *Salvia officinalis*

Parts used for medicinal purposes: Leaves

Chemicals this herb contains:

- Camphor
- Flavonoids (see Glossary)
- Resin (see Glossary)
- Salvene
- Saponins (see Glossary)
- Tannins (see Glossary)
- Terpenes (see Glossary)
- Thujone
- Volatile oils (see Glossary)

 Known Effects

- Depresses fever-control center in brain
- Relieves spasm in skeletal or smooth muscle
- Stimulates gastrointestinal tract
- Stimulates central nervous system
- Interferes with absorption of iron and other minerals when taken internally

Miscellaneous information:

- Sage is used as a flavoring agent and in perfume.
- Salvia is *not* the brush sage of the desert or red sage.
- No effects are expected on the body, either good or bad, when this herb is used in very small amounts to

➜

enhance the flavor of food; however, prolonged use of large amounts can cause seizures and unconsciousness.

• Sage is available dried, fresh or as tincture or tea.

 ## Possible Additional Effects

• May help expel gas from intestinal tract
• May repel insects
• May treat throat and mouth infections when used as mouthwash
• May reduce night sweats associated with menopause
• May relieve insect bites when applied externally

 ## Warnings and Precautions

Don't take if you:
Are pregnant, think you may be pregnant or plan pregnancy in the near future.

Consult your doctor if you:
• Take this herb for any medical problem that doesn't improve in 2 weeks (There may be safer, more effective treatments.)
• Take any medicinal drugs or herbs including aspirin, laxatives, cold and cough remedies, antacids, vitamins, minerals, amino acids, supplements, other prescription or nonprescription drugs

Pregnancy:
Don't use unless prescribed by your doctor.

Breastfeeding:
Sage may reduce milk flow. Don't use.

Infants and children:
Treating infants or children under 2 with any herbal preparation is hazardous.

Others:
No problems expected if you are beyond childhood, under 45, not pregnant, basically healthy, take it for only a short time and do not exceed manufacturer's recommended dose.

Storage:
• Store in cool, dry area away from direct light, but don't freeze.
• Store safely out of reach of children.
• Don't store in bathroom medicine cabinet. Heat and moisture may change the action of the herb.

Safe dosage:
Consult your doctor for the appropriate dose for your condition.

 ## Toxicity

Generally regarded as safe when taken in appropriate quantities for short periods of time

For symptoms of toxicity: See *Adverse Reactions, Side Effects or Overdose Symptoms* section below.

 ## Adverse Reactions, Side Effects or Overdose Symptoms

Signs and symptoms	What to do
Dry mouth	Discontinue. Call doctor when convenient.
Swelling of lips	Drinking tea can result in swelling of lips. Discontinue. Call doctor when convenient.

St. John's Wort (Klamath Weed)

Basic Information

Biological name (genus and species):
Hypericum perforatum

Parts used for medicinal purposes:
- Flowers
- Petals
- Stems

Chemicals this herb contains:
- Hypericin
- Resin (see Glossary)
- Tannins (see Glossary)
- Volatile oils (see Glossary)

Known Effects

- Reduces depressive moods (mild to moderate)
- Relieves anxiety
- Slightly depresses central nervous system
- Acts as an antibacterial to help heal wounds

Miscellaneous information:

Generally requires 4 to 6 weeks of treatment before effectiveness can be evaluated.

Possible Additional Effects

- Potential antiviral
- May treat seasonal affective disorder (SAD)
- Used externally for mild burns

Warnings and Precautions

Don't take if you:
- Are pregnant, think you may be pregnant or plan pregnancy in the near future
- Are taking other antidepressive medicines

Consult your doctor if you:
- Take this herb for any medical problem that doesn't improve in 2 weeks (There may be safer, more effective treatments.)
- Take any medicinal drugs or herbs including aspirin, laxatives, cold and cough remedies, antacids, vitamins, minerals, amino acids, supplements, other prescription or nonprescription drugs

Pregnancy:
Don't use unless prescribed by your doctor.

Breastfeeding:
Don't use unless prescribed by your doctor.

Infants and children:
Treating infants or children under 2 with any herbal preparation is hazardous.

Others:
- Do not take in combination with prescription antidepressants, unless prescribed by your doctor.
- If you believe you are depressed, seek medical treatment prior to using St. John's wort.
- In large doses, St. John's wort may cause sensitivity to sunlight.

Storage:
- Store in cool, dry area away from direct light, but don't freeze.
- Store safely out of reach of children.
- Don't store in bathroom medicine cabinet. Heat and moisture may change the action of the herb.

Safe dosage:
Consult your doctor for the appropriate dose for your condition.

Toxicity

Rated slightly dangerous, particularly in children, persons over 55 and those who take larger than appropriate quantities for extended periods of time

For symptoms of toxicity: See *Adverse Reactions, Side Effects or Overdose Symptoms* section below.

Adverse Reactions, Side Effects or Overdose Symptoms

Signs and symptoms	What to do
Abdominal upset	Discontinue. Call doctor when convenient.
Abnormal skin coloring	Discontinue. Call doctor when convenient.
Sun sensitivity	Discontinue. Call doctor when convenient.

Sassafras

Basic Information

Biological name (genus and species): *Sassafras albidum*

Parts used for medicinal purposes:
• Bark
• Roots

Chemicals this herb contains:
• Cadinene
• Camphor
• Eugenol
• Phellandrene
• Pinene
• Safrole

Known Effects

• Depresses central nervous system
• Irritates mucous membranes

Miscellaneous information:

• Banned in United States as a flavoring agent because of proved carcinogenic potential.
• No proven medical efficacy shown

Possible Additional Effects

• Used as a "tonic" that exerts a restorative or nourishing action on the body
• May treat syphilis

Warnings and Precautions

Don't take if you:

• Are pregnant, think you may be pregnant or plan pregnancy in the near future
• Have any chronic disease of the gastrointestinal tract, such as stomach or duodenal ulcers, reflux esophagitis, ulcerative colitis, spastic colitis, diverticulosis or diverticulitis

Consult your doctor if you:

• Take this herb for any medical problem that doesn't improve in 2 weeks (There may be safer, more effective treatments.)

• Take any medicinal drugs or herbs including aspirin, laxatives, cold and cough remedies, antacids, vitamins, minerals, amino acids, supplements, other prescription or nonprescription drugs

Pregnancy:
Risks outweigh potential benefits. Don't use.

Breastfeeding:
Risks outweigh potential benefits. Don't use.

Infants and children:
Treating infants or children under 2 with any herbal preparation is hazardous.

Others:
Risks outweigh potential benefits. Don't use.

Storage:
• Store in cool, dry area away from direct light, but don't freeze.
• Store safely out of reach of children.
• Don't store in bathroom medicine cabinet. Heat and moisture may change the action of the herb.

Safe dosage:
Consult your doctor for the appropriate dose for your condition.

Toxicity

Sassafras has carcinogenic potential. Don't use. It is felt to be unsafe and ineffective.

For symptoms of toxicity: See *Adverse Reactions, Side Effects or Overdose Symptoms* section below.

Adverse Reactions, Side Effects or Overdose Symptoms

Signs and symptoms	What to do
Breathing difficulties	Seek emergency treatment.
Coma	Seek emergency treatment.
Dilated pupils	Discontinue. Call doctor immediately.
Fainting	Discontinue. Call doctor immediately.
Heart, liver, kidney damage characterized by swelling of extremities, shortness of breath, jaundice (yellow skin and eyes), blood in urine	Seek emergency treatment.
Nausea or vomiting	Discontinue. Call doctor immediately.
Nosebleeds (frequent)	Discontinue. Call doctor when convenient.

Saw Palmetto (Sabal)

Basic Information

Biological name (genus and species):
Serenoa repens

Parts used for medicinal purposes:
• Berries
• Seeds

Chemicals this herb contains:
• Capric acids
• Caproic acids
• Caprylic acids

- Lauric acids
- Oleic acids
- Palmitic acids
- Resin (see Glossary)

Known Effects

- Improves urination in men with benign prostate hyperplasia (see Glossary)
- Treats symptoms of enlarged prostate (consult your doctor)
- Irritates mucous membranes

Miscellaneous information:
Berries are edible but don't taste good.

Possible Additional Effects

- May treat chronic cystitis
- May treat urethritis and other inflammations of male genitourinary tract, including prostatitis
- May stimulate appetite
- Potential anti-inflammatory
- Potential immune stimulant

Warnings and Precautions

Don't take if you:
- Are pregnant, think you may be pregnant or plan pregnancy in the near future
- Have any chronic disease of the gastrointestinal tract, such as stomach or duodenal ulcers, reflux esophagitis, ulcerative colitis, spastic colitis, diverticulosis or diverticulitis

Consult your doctor if you:
- Take this herb for any medical problem that doesn't improve in 2 weeks (There may be safer, more effective treatments.)

- Take any medicinal drugs or herbs including aspirin, laxatives, cold and cough remedies, antacids, vitamins, minerals, amino acids, supplements, other prescription or nonprescription drugs
- Have enlarged prostate

Pregnancy:
Don't use unless prescribed by your doctor.

Breastfeeding:
Don't use unless prescribed by your doctor.

Infants and children:
Treating infants or children under 2 with any herbal preparation is hazardous.

Others:
No problems expected if you are beyond childhood, under 45, not pregnant, basically healthy, take it for only a short time and do not exceed manufacturer's recommended dose.

Storage:
- Store in cool, dry area away from direct light, but don't freeze.
- Store safely out of reach of children.
- Don't store in bathroom medicine cabinet. Heat and moisture may change the action of the herb.

Safe dosage:
Consult your doctor for the appropriate dose for your condition.

Toxicity

Rated relatively safe when taken in appropriate quantities for short periods of time

For symptoms of toxicity: See *Adverse Reactions, Side Effects or Overdose Symptoms* section below.

Adverse Reactions,
Side Effects or
Overdose Symptoms

Signs and symptoms	What to do
Diarrhea	Discontinue. Call doctor when convenient.
Headaches	Discontinue. Call doctor when convenient.
Nausea	Discontinue. Call doctor when convenient.
Vomiting	Discontinue. Call doctor immediately.

Scotch Broom

 Basic Information

Biological name (genus and species):
Cytisus scoparius

Parts used for medicinal purposes:
Leaves

Chemicals this herb contains:
• Cytisine
• Genisteine
• Hydroxytyramine
• Sarothamnine
• Scoparin
• Sparteine

 Known Effects

• Stimulates uterine contractions
• Helps body dispose of excess fluid by increasing amount of urine produced
• Sometimes causes sharp rise in blood pressure

 Possible Additional Effects

• May treat congestive heart failure
• May produce sedative-hypnotic effect when smoked

 Warnings and Precautions

Don't take if you:
• Are pregnant, think you may be pregnant or plan pregnancy in the near future
• Have any chronic disease of the gastrointestinal tract, such as stomach or duodenal ulcers, reflux esophagitis, ulcerative colitis, spastic colitis, diverticulosis or diverticulitis

Consult your doctor if you:
• Take this herb for any medical problem that doesn't improve in 2 weeks (There may be safer, more effective treatments.)

→

- Take any medicinal drugs or herbs including aspirin, laxatives, cold and cough remedies, antacids, vitamins, minerals, amino acids, supplements, other prescription or nonprescription drugs

Pregnancy:
Don't use unless prescribed by your doctor.

Breastfeeding:
Don't use unless prescribed by your doctor.

Infants and children:
Treating infants or children under 2 with any herbal preparation is hazardous.

Others:
No problems expected if you are beyond childhood, under 45, not pregnant, basically healthy, take it for only a short time and do not exceed manufacturer's recommended dose.

Storage:
- Store in cool, dry area away from direct light, but don't freeze.
- Store safely out of reach of children.
- Don't store in bathroom medicine cabinet. Heat and moisture may change the action of the herb.

Safe dosage:
Consult your doctor for the appropriate dose for your condition.

Toxicity

Rated slightly dangerous, particularly in children, persons over 55 and those who take larger than appropriate quantities for extended periods of time

For symptoms of toxicity: See *Adverse Reactions, Side Effects or Overdose Symptoms* section below.

Adverse Reactions, Side Effects or Overdose Symptoms

Signs and symptoms	What to do
Diarrhea	Discontinue. Call doctor immediately.
Nausea or vomiting	Discontinue. Call doctor immediately.

Silverweed (Goose Tansy)

Basic Information

Biological name (genus and species):
Potentilla anserina

Parts used for medicinal purposes:
Entire plant

Chemicals this herb contains:
- Ellagic acid (see Glossary)
- Kinovic acid
- Tannins (see Glossary)

Known Effects

- Shrinks tissues
- Prevents secretion of fluids

- Causes protein molecules to clump together
- Stimulates uterine contractions
- Interferes with absorption of iron and other minerals when taken internally

Possible Additional Effects

- May treat dysmenorrhea (painful menstruation)
- May treat tetanus in absence of medical help, when used with lobelia

Warnings and Precautions

Don't take if you:
- Are pregnant, think you may be pregnant or plan pregnancy in the near future
- Have any chronic disease of the gastrointestinal tract, such as stomach or duodenal ulcers, reflux esophagitis, ulcerative colitis, spastic colitis, diverticulosis or diverticulitis

Consult your doctor if you:
- Take this herb for any medical problem that doesn't improve in 2 weeks (There may be safer, more effective treatments.)
- Take any medicinal drugs or herbs including aspirin, laxatives, cold and cough remedies, antacids, vitamins, minerals, amino acids, supplements, other prescription or nonprescription drugs

Pregnancy
Dangers outweigh any possible benefits. Don't use.

Breastfeeding:
Dangers outweigh any possible benefits. Don't use.

Infants and children:
Treating infants or children under 2 with any herbal preparation is hazardous.

Others:
No problems expected if you are beyond childhood, under 45, not pregnant, basically healthy, take it for only a short time and do not exceed manufacturer's recommended dose.

Storage:
- Store in cool, dry area away from direct light, but don't freeze.
- Store safely out of reach of children.
- Don't store in bathroom medicine cabinet. Heat and moisture may change the action of the herb.

Safe dosage:
Consult your doctor for the appropriate dose for your condition.

Toxicity

Comparative-toxicity rating is not available from standard references.

For symptoms of toxicity: See *Adverse Reactions, Side Effects or Overdose Symptoms* section below.

Adverse Reactions, Side Effects or Overdose Symptoms

Signs and symptoms	What to do
Diarrhea	Discontinue. Call doctor immediately.
Nausea or vomiting	Discontinue. Call doctor immediately.
Painful urination	Discontinue. Call doctor when convenient.

Slippery Elm (Red Elm)

Basic Information

Biological name (genus and species):
Ulmus rubra, U. fulva

Parts used for medicinal purposes:
Inner bark

Chemicals this herb contains:
- Bioflavonoids
- Calcium
- Calcium oxalate
- Mucilage (see Glossary)
- Phosphorus
- Polysaccharide
- Starch
- Tannins (see Glossary)

Known Effects

- Decreases thickness and increases fluidity of mucus in lungs and bronchial tubes
- Soothes sore throats
- Decreases discomfort of cough

Miscellaneous information:
Available as tea, lozenge, poultice (see Glossary).

Possible Additional Effects

- May treat ulcers
- May be useful for diarrhea
- May soothe and heal cuts and scrapes when used externally

Warnings and Precautions

Don't take if you:
Are pregnant, think you may be pregnant or plan pregnancy in the near future.

Consult your doctor if you:
- Take this herb for any medical problem that doesn't improve in 2 weeks (There may be safer, more effective treatments.)
- Take any medicinal drugs or herbs including aspirin, laxatives, cold and cough remedies, antacids, vitamins, minerals, amino acids, supplements, other prescription or nonprescription drugs

Pregnancy:
Dangers outweigh any possible benefits. Don't use.

Breastfeeding:
Dangers outweigh any possible benefits. Don't use.

Infants and children:
Treating infants or children under 2 with any herbal preparation is hazardous.

Others:
No problems expected if you are beyond childhood, under 45, not pregnant, basically healthy, take it for only a short time and do not exceed manufacturer's recommended dose.

Storage:
- Store in cool, dry area away from direct light, but don't freeze.
- Store safely out of reach of children.
- Don't store in bathroom medicine cabinet. Heat and moisture may change the action of the herb.

Safe dosage:
Consult your doctor for the appropriate dose for your condition.

Toxicity

Rated relatively safe when taken in appropriate quantities for short periods of time

For symptoms of toxicity: See *Adverse Reactions, Side Effects or Overdose Symptoms* section below.

Adverse Reactions, Side Effects or Overdose Symptoms

Signs and symptoms	What to do
Allergic response	Discontinue. Call doctor immediately.
Skin rash	Discontinue. Call doctor when convenient.

Snakeplant

Basic Information

Biological name (genus and species):
Rivea corymbosa

Parts used for medicinal purposes:
Seeds

Chemicals this herb contains:
Five related LSD-like alkaloids

- Chanoclavine
- D-isolysergic acid amide
- D-lysergic acid amide
- Elymoclavine
- Lysergol

Known Effects

Depresses central nervous system

Miscellaneous information:
Snakeplant is used primarily by Mexican Indians in religious ceremonies. They call it *badah.*

Possible Additional Effects

- May change mood
- May cause hallucinations

Warnings and Precautions

Don't take if you:
- Are pregnant, think you may be pregnant or plan pregnancy in the near future
- Have any chronic disease of the gastrointestinal tract, such as stomach or duodenal ulcers, reflux esophagitis, ulcerative colitis, spastic colitis, diverticulosis or diverticulitis

Consult your doctor if you:
- Take this herb for any medical problem that doesn't improve in 2 weeks (There may be safer, more effective treatments.)
- Take any medicinal drugs or herbs including aspirin, laxatives, cold and cough remedies, antacids, vitamins, minerals, amino acids, supplements, other prescription or nonprescription drugs

Pregnancy
Dangers outweigh any possible benefits. Don't use.

Breastfeeding:
Dangers outweigh any possible benefits. Don't use.

Infants and children:
Treating infants or children under 2 with any herbal preparation is hazardous.

Others:
Dangers outweigh any possible benefits. Don't use.

Storage:
• Store in cool, dry area away from direct light, but don't freeze.
• Store safely out of reach of children.
• Don't store in bathroom medicine cabinet. Heat and moisture may change the action of the herb.

Safe dosage:
Consult your doctor for the appropriate dose for your condition.

Toxicity

Rated slightly dangerous, particularly in children, persons over 55 and those who take larger than appropriate quantities for extended periods of time

For symptoms of toxicity: See *Adverse Reactions, Side Effects or Overdose Symptoms* section below.

Adverse Reactions, Side Effects or Overdose Symptoms

Signs and symptoms	What to do
Blurred vision	Discontinue. Call doctor immediately.
Coma	Seek emergency treatment.
Confusion	Discontinue. Call doctor immediately.
Hallucinations	Seek emergency treatment.
Nausea or vomiting	Discontinue. Call doctor immediately.
Stupor	Discontinue. Call doctor immediately.

Snakeroot (Serpentaria, Virginia Snakeroot)

Basic Information

Biological name (genus and species):
Aristolochia serpentaria

Parts used for medicinal purposes:
Roots

Chemicals this herb contains:
• Aristolochin
• Borneol
• Terpene (see Glossary)
• Volatile oils (see Glossary)

Known Effects
• Stimulates stomach secretions
• Stimulates smooth-muscle contractions of gastrointestinal tract and heart

Possible Additional Effects

- May increase circulation
- May stimulate heart action
- May treat dyspepsia
- May reduce fever
- May treat sores on skin

Warnings and Precautions

Don't take if you:

- Are pregnant, think you may be pregnant or plan pregnancy in the near future
- Have any chronic disease of the gastrointestinal tract, such as stomach or duodenal ulcers, reflux esophagitis, ulcerative colitis, spastic colitis, diverticulosis or diverticulitis

Consult your doctor if you:

- Take this herb for any medical problem that doesn't improve in 2 weeks (There may be safer, more effective treatments.)
- Take any medicinal drugs or herbs including aspirin, laxatives, cold and cough remedies, antacids, vitamins, minerals, amino acids, supplements, other prescription or nonprescription drugs

Pregnancy

Dangers outweigh any possible benefits. Don't use.

Breastfeeding:

Dangers outweigh any possible benefits. Don't use.

Infants and children:

Treating infants or children under 2 with any herbal preparation is hazardous.

Others:

No problems expected if you are beyond childhood, under 45, not pregnant, basically healthy, take it for only a short time and do not exceed manufacturer's recommended dose.

Storage:

- Store in cool, dry area away from direct light, but don't freeze.
- Store safely out of reach of children.
- Don't store in bathroom medicine cabinet. Heat and moisture may change the action of the herb.

Safe dosage:

Consult your doctor for the appropriate dose for your condition.

Toxicity

Rated relatively safe when taken in appropriate quantities for short periods of time

For symptoms of toxicity: See *Adverse Reactions, Side Effects or Overdose Symptoms* section below.

Adverse Reactions, Side Effects or Overdose Symptoms

Signs and symptoms	What to do
Diarrhea	Discontinue. Call doctor immediately.
Nausea or vomiting	Discontinue. Call doctor immediately.
Tenesmus (spasm of rectal sphincter)	Discontinue. Call doctor when convenient.

Spanish Broom

Basic Information

Biological name (genus and species):
Spartium junceum

Parts used for medicinal purposes:
Petals/flower

Chemicals this herb contains:
- Anagyrine
- Cytisine
- Methylcytisine

Known Effects

- Stimulates uterine contractions
- Helps body dispose of excess fluid by increasing amount of urine produced
- Stimulates gastrointestinal tract
- Causes vomiting

Possible Additional Effects

- May induce labor
- May cause watery, explosive bowel movements

Warnings and Precautions

Don't take if you:
- Are pregnant, think you may be pregnant or plan pregnancy in the near future
- Have any chronic disease of the gastrointestinal tract, such as stomach or duodenal ulcers, reflux esophagitis, ulcerative colitis, spastic colitis, diverticulosis or diverticulitis

Consult your doctor if you:
- Take this herb for any medical problem that doesn't improve in 2 weeks (There may be safer, more effective treatments.)
- Take any medicinal drugs or herbs including aspirin, laxatives, cold and cough remedies, antacids, vitamins, minerals, amino acids, supplements, other prescription or nonprescription drugs

Pregnancy:
Dangers outweigh any possible benefits. Don't use.

Breastfeeding:
Dangers outweigh any possible benefits. Don't use.

Infants and children:
Treating infants or children under 2 with any herbal preparation is hazardous.

Others:
No problems expected if you are beyond childhood, under 45, not pregnant, basically healthy, take it for only a short time and do not exceed manufacturer's recommended dose.

Storage:
- Store in cool, dry area away from direct light, but don't freeze.
- Store safely out of reach of children.
- Don't store in bathroom medicine cabinet. Heat and moisture may change the action of the herb.

Safe dosage:
Consult your doctor for the appropriate dose for your condition.

Toxicity

Comparative-toxicity rating is not available from standard references.

For symptoms of toxicity: See *Adverse Reactions, Side Effects or Overdose Symptoms* section below.

Adverse Reactions, Side Effects or Overdose Symptoms

Signs and symptoms	What to do
Diarrhea	Discontinue. Call doctor immediately.
Kidney damage characterized by blood in urine, decreased urine flow, swelling of hands and feet	Seek emergency treatment.
Muscle weakness	Discontinue. Call doctor immediately.
Nausea or vomiting	Discontinue. Call doctor immediately.

Spearmint

Basic Information

Biological name (genus and species):
Mentha spicata

Parts used for medicinal purposes:
• Leaves
• Petals/flower

Chemicals this herb contains:
• Carvone
• Resin (see Glossary)
• Volatile oils (see Glossary)

Known Effects
• Stimulates muscular action of gastrointestinal tract
• Helps treat nausea

Miscellaneous information:
Spearmint is used as a flavoring agent in many foods.

Possible Additional Effects
• May help expel gas from intestinal tract
• May soothe sore throats
• May treat sinus congestion

Warnings and Precautions

Don't take if you:
• Are pregnant, think you may be pregnant or plan pregnancy in the near future
• Have any chronic disease of the gastrointestinal tract, such as stomach or duodenal ulcers, reflux esophagitis, ulcerative colitis, spastic colitis, diverticulosis or diverticulitis

Consult your doctor if you:
• Take this herb for any medical problem that doesn't improve in 2 weeks (There may be safer, more effective treatments.)
• Take any medicinal drugs or herbs including aspirin, laxatives, cold and cough remedies, antacids, vitamins, minerals, amino acids, supplements, other prescription or nonprescription drugs
• Want to use for morning sickness

Pregnancy:
Don't use unless prescribed by your doctor.

Breastfeeding:
Don't use unless prescribed by your doctor.

Infants and children:
Treating infants or children under 2 with any herbal preparation is hazardous.

Others:
No problems expected if you are beyond childhood, under 45, not pregnant, basically healthy, take it for only a short time and do not exceed manufacturer's recommended dose.

Storage:
• Store in cool, dry area away from direct light, but don't freeze.
• Store safely out of reach of children.
• Don't store in bathroom medicine cabinet. Heat and moisture may change the action of the herb.

Safe dosage:
Consult your doctor for the appropriate dose for your condition.

Toxicity

Comparative-toxicity rating is not available from standard references.

For symptoms of toxicity: See *Adverse Reactions, Side Effects or Overdose Symptoms* section below.

Adverse Reactions, Side Effects or Overdose Symptoms

Signs and symptoms	What to do
Convulsions and coma	Seek emergency treatment.
Diarrhea	Discontinue. Call doctor immediately.
Nausea or vomiting	Discontinue. Call doctor immediately.

Strawberry (Earth Mulberry)

Basic Information

Biological name (genus and species):
Fragaria vesca, F. americana

Parts used for medicinal purposes:
• Berries
• Leaves
• Roots

Chemicals this herb contains:
• Catechins
• Leucoanthocyanin
• Minerals
• Vitamin C

Known Effects

• Prevents scurvy
• Inhibits production of histamines

Miscellaneous information:
Wild strawberry is a member of the rose family.

Possible Additional Effects

No additional effects are known.

Warnings and Precautions

Don't take if you:
Are allergic to strawberries.

Consult your doctor if you:
• Take this herb for any medical problem that doesn't improve in 2 weeks (There may be safer, more effective treatments.)
• Take any medicinal drugs or herbs including aspirin, laxatives, cold and cough remedies, antacids, vitamins, minerals, amino acids, supplements, other prescription or nonprescription drugs

Pregnancy:
Pregnant women should experience no problems taking usual amounts as part of a balanced diet. Other products extracted from this herb have not been proved to cause problems.

Breastfeeding:
Breastfed infants of lactating mothers should experience no problems when mother takes usual amounts as part of a balanced diet. Other products extracted from this herb have not been proved to cause problems.

Infants and children:
Treating infants or children under 2 with any herbal preparation is hazardous.

Others:
No problems expected if you are beyond childhood, under 45, basically healthy, take it for only a short time and do not exceed manufacturer's recommended dose.

Storage:
• Store in cool, dry area away from direct light, but don't freeze.
• Store safely out of reach of children.
• Don't store in bathroom medicine cabinet. Heat and moisture may change the action of the herb.

Safe dosage:
Consult your doctor for the appropriate dose for your condition.

Toxicity

Generally regarded as safe when taken in appropriate quantities for short periods of time

Adverse Reactions, Side Effects or Overdose Symptoms

None are expected.

Sumac

 ## Basic Information

Biological name (genus and species):
Rhus glabra

Parts used for medicinal purposes:
• Bark
• Berries
• Leaves

Chemicals this herb contains:
• Albumin
• Malic acid
• Resin (see Glossary)
• Tannins (see Glossary)
• Volatile oils (see Glossary)

 ## Known Effects

Bark:
• Shrinks tissues
• Prevents secretion of fluids
• Inhibits growth and development of germs

Berries:
• Helps body dispose of excess fluid by increasing amount of urine produced
• Interferes with absorption of iron and other minerals when taken internally

Miscellaneous information:
Sumac is in the same plant family as poison ivy and poison oak.

 ## Possible Additional Effects

• May treat diarrhea
• May treat rectal bleeding
• May treat asthma when leaves are smoked

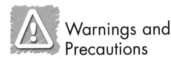 ## Warnings and Precautions

Don't take if you:
Are pregnant, think you may be pregnant or plan pregnancy in the near future.

Consult your doctor if you:
• Take this herb for any medical problem that doesn't improve in 2 weeks (There may be safer, more effective treatments.)
• Take any medicinal drugs or herbs including aspirin, laxatives, cold and cough remedies, antacids, vitamins, minerals, amino acids, supplements, other prescription or nonprescription drugs

Pregnancy:
Don't use unless prescribed by your doctor.

Breastfeeding:
Don't use unless prescribed by your doctor.

Infants and children:
Treating infants or children under 2 with any herbal preparation is hazardous.

Others:
No problems expected if you are beyond childhood, under 45, not pregnant, basically healthy, take it for only a short time and do not exceed manufacturer's recommended dose.

Storage:
• Store in cool, dry area away from direct light, but don't freeze.
• Store safely out of reach of children.
• Don't store in bathroom medicine cabinet. Heat and moisture may change the action of the herb.

Safe dosage:
Consult your doctor for the
appropriate dose for your condition.

 Toxicity

Comparative-toxicity rating is not
available from standard references.

 Adverse Reactions,
Side Effects or
Overdose Symptoms

None are expected.

Sundew

 Basic Information

Biological name (genus and species):
Drosera rotundifolia

Parts used for medicinal purposes:
Various parts of the entire plant,
frequently differing by country
and culture

Chemicals this herb contains:
- Citric acid
- Droserone
- Malic acid
- Resin (see Glossary)
- Tannins (see Glossary)

 Known Effects

- Interferes with absorption of iron
  and other minerals when taken
  internally
- Loosens bronchial secretions

 Possible
Additional Effects

- May treat whooping cough
- May treat laryngitis
- May treat smoker's cough

 Warnings and
Precautions

Don't take if you:
Are pregnant, think you may be
pregnant or plan pregnancy in the
near future.

Consult your doctor if you:
- Take this herb for any medical
  problem that doesn't improve in
  2 weeks (There may be safer, more
  effective treatments.)
- Take any medicinal drugs or
  herbs including aspirin, laxatives,
  cold and cough remedies, antacids,
  vitamins, minerals, amino acids,
  supplements, other prescription
  or nonprescription drugs

Pregnancy:
Don't use unless prescribed by
your doctor.

Breastfeeding:
Don't use unless prescribed by
your doctor.

Infants and children:
Treating infants or children under
2 with any herbal preparation
is hazardous.

➜

Others:

No problems expected if you are beyond childhood, under 45, not pregnant, basically healthy, take it for only a short time and do not exceed manufacturer's recommended dose.

Storage:

• Store in cool, dry area away from direct light, but don't freeze.
• Store safely out of reach of children.
• Don't store in bathroom medicine cabinet. Heat and moisture may change the action of the herb.

Safe dosage:

Consult your doctor for the appropriate dose for your condition.

 Toxicity

Comparative-toxicity rating is not available from standard references.

 Adverse Reactions, Side Effects or Overdose Symptoms

None are expected.

Sunflower

 Basic Information

Biological name (genus and species):
Helianthus annuus

Parts used for medicinal purposes:
• Leaves
• Petals/flower
• Seeds

Chemicals this herb contains:
• Arachidic acid
• Behenic acid
• Linoleic acid
• Oleic acid
• Palmitic acid
• Stearic acid
• Vitamin E

 Known Effects

• Antioxidant
• Treats vitamin-E deficiency (seeds)

Miscellaneous information:
Sunflower is a food source.

 Possible Additional Effects

May help reduce pain of arthritis

 Warnings and Precautions

Don't take if you:
Are pregnant, think you may be pregnant or plan pregnancy in the near future.

Consult your doctor if you:
• Take this herb for any medical problem that doesn't improve in 2 weeks (There may be safer, more effective treatments.)
• Take any medicinal drugs or herbs including aspirin, laxatives, cold and cough remedies, antacids,

vitamins, minerals, amino acids, supplements, other prescription or nonprescription drugs

Pregnancy:
Don't use unless prescribed by your doctor.

Breastfeeding:
Don't use unless prescribed by your doctor.

Infants and children:
Treating infants or children under 2 with any herbal preparation is hazardous.

Others:
No problems expected if you are beyond childhood, under 45, not pregnant, basically healthy, take it for only a short time and do not exceed manufacturer's recommended dose.

Storage:
• Store in cool, dry area away from direct light, but don't freeze.
• Store safely out of reach of children.
• Don't store in bathroom medicine cabinet. Heat and moisture may change the action of the herb.

Safe dosage:
Consult your doctor for the appropriate dose for your condition.

 Toxicity

Comparative-toxicity rating is not available from standard references.

For symptoms of toxicity: See *Adverse Reactions, Side Effects or Overdose Symptoms* section below.

 Adverse Reactions, Side Effects or Overdose Symptoms

Signs and symptoms	What to do
Allergic reaction	Discontinue. Call doctor immediately.

Sweet Violet

 Basic Information

Biological name (genus and species):
Viola odorata

Parts used for medicinal purposes:
• Leaves
• Seeds

Chemicals this herb contains:
• Glycosides (see Glossary)
• Myrosin

 Known Effects

• Irritates mucous membranes
• Stimulates gastrointestinal tract

Miscellaneous information:
Sweet violet was used to treat cancer as early as 500 B.C., but evidence of real benefit is lacking.

→

Possible Additional Effects

- May treat cancer when used as poultice (see Glossary)
- May treat skin disease
- Potential mild laxative
- May cause vomiting
- May decrease thickness and increase fluidity of mucus in lungs and bronchial tubes
- May treat coughs

 ## Warnings and Precautions

Don't take if you:
- Are pregnant, think you may be pregnant or plan pregnancy in the near future
- Have any chronic disease of the gastrointestinal tract, such as stomach or duodenal ulcers, reflux esophagitis, ulcerative colitis, spastic colitis, diverticulosis or diverticulitis

Consult your doctor if you:
- Take this herb for any medical problem that doesn't improve in 2 weeks (There may be safer, more effective treatments.)
- Take any medicinal drugs or herbs including aspirin, laxatives, cold and cough remedies, antacids, vitamins, minerals, amino acids, supplements, other prescription or nonprescription drugs

Pregnancy:
Don't use unless prescribed by your doctor.

Breastfeeding:
Don't use unless prescribed by your doctor.

Infants and children:
Treating infants or children under 2 with any herbal preparation is hazardous.

Others:
No problems expected if you are beyond childhood, under 45, not pregnant, basically healthy, take it for only a short time and do not exceed manufacturer's recommended dose.

Storage:
- Store in cool, dry area away from direct light, but don't freeze.
- Store safely out of reach of children.
- Don't store in bathroom medicine cabinet. Heat and moisture may change the action of the herb.

Safe dosage:
Consult your doctor for the appropriate dose for your condition.

 ## Toxicity

Comparative-toxicity rating is not available from standard references.

For symptoms of toxicity: See *Adverse Reactions, Side Effects or Overdose Symptoms* section below.

 ## Adverse Reactions, Side Effects or Overdose Symptoms

Signs and symptoms	What to do
Seeds:	
Diarrhea	Discontinue. Call doctor immediately.
Nausea or vomiting	Discontinue. Call doctor immediately.

Tansy

Basic Information

Biological name (genus and species):
Tanacetum vulgare

Parts used for medicinal purposes:
Entire plant

Chemicals this herb contains:
- Bitters (see Glossary)
- Borneol
- Camphor
- Resin (see Glossary)
- Tanacetin
- Tanacetol
- Thujone

Known Effects

- Stimulates uterine contractions
- Stimulates appetite
- Kills intestinal parasites

Miscellaneous information:

Tansy is a powerful herb that should be avoided or used only under strict medical supervision.

Possible Additional Effects

- May treat pain
- May cause euphoria
- May treat roundworms and pinworms
- May treat menstrual difficulties

Warnings and Precautions

Don't take if you:
- Are pregnant, think you may be pregnant or plan pregnancy in the near future
- Have any chronic disease of the gastrointestinal tract, such as stomach or duodenal ulcers, reflux esophagitis, ulcerative colitis, spastic colitis, diverticulosis or diverticulitis

Consult your doctor if you:
- Take this herb for any medical problem that doesn't improve in 2 weeks (There may be safer, more effective treatments.)
- Take any medicinal drugs or herbs including aspirin, laxatives, cold and cough remedies, antacids, vitamins, minerals, amino acids, supplements, other prescription or nonprescription drugs

Pregnancy
Dangers outweigh any possible benefits. Don't use.

Breastfeeding:
Dangers outweigh any possible benefits. Don't use.

Infants and children:
Treating infants or children under 2 with any herbal preparation is hazardous.

Others:
Dangers outweigh any possible benefits. Don't use.

Storage:
- Store in cool, dry area away from direct light, but don't freeze.
- Store safely out of reach of children.
- Don't store in bathroom medicine cabinet. Heat and moisture may change the action of the herb.

Safe dosage:
Consult your doctor for the appropriate dose for your condition.

Toxicity

Rated dangerous, particularly in children, persons over 55 and those who take larger than appropriate quantities for extended periods of time

For symptoms of toxicity: See *Adverse Reactions, Side Effects or Overdose Symptoms* section below.

Adverse Reactions, Side Effects or Overdose Symptoms

Signs and symptoms	What to do
Coma	Seek emergency treatment.
Convulsions	Seek emergency treatment.
Diarrhea	Discontinue. Call doctor immediately.
Dilated pupils	Seek emergency treatment.
Nausea or vomiting	Discontinue. Call doctor immediately.
Weak, rapid pulse	Seek emergency treatment.

Tea Tree Oil

Basic Information

Biological name (genus and species): *Melaleuca alternifolia*

Parts used for medicinal purposes: Essential oil

Chemicals this herb contains:
• Germicidal agents
• Terpene hydrocarbons

Known Effects

• Works well as a disinfectant for cuts and abrasions
• Has antibacterial and antifungal properties
• Helps treat insect bites
• Treats fungal nail disease

Possible Additional Effects

• May reduce teenage acne
• Used in flea shampoo for pets

• May treat athlete's foot
• May help soothe tonsils with tonsillitis
• May help treat bladder infections
• May reduce cold/flu symptoms

Warnings and Precautions

Don't take if you:
Are pregnant, think you may be pregnant or plan pregnancy in the near future.

Consult your doctor if you:
• Take this herb for any medical problem that doesn't improve in 2 weeks (There may be safer, more effective treatments.)
• Take any medicinal drugs or herbs including aspirin, laxatives, cold and cough remedies, antacids, vitamins, minerals, amino acids, supplements, other prescription or nonprescription drugs

Pregnancy:
Don't use unless prescribed by your doctor.

Breastfeeding:
Don't use unless prescribed by your doctor.

Infants and children:
Treating infants or children under 2 with any herbal preparation is hazardous.

Others:
- Irritation may occur on persons with very sensitive skin. If this happens, try diluting the oil with distilled water or vitamin-E oil or consult your physician.
- Tea tree oil is safe for use as a topical antiseptic but not recommended for oral ingestion.

Storage:
- Store in cool, dry area away from direct light, but don't freeze.
- Store safely out of reach of children.

- Don't store in bathroom medicine cabinet. Heat and moisture may change the action of the herb.

Safe dosage:
Consult your doctor for the appropriate dose for your condition.

Toxicity

Comparative-toxicity rating is not available from standard references.

For symptoms of toxicity: See *Adverse Reactions, Side Effects or Overdose Symptoms* section below.

Adverse Reactions, Side Effects or Overdose Symptoms

Signs and symptoms	What to do
Skin irritation	Discontinue. Call doctor when convenient.

Thyme, Common

Basic Information

Biological name (genus and species):
Thymus vulgaris

Parts used for medicinal purposes:
- Berries/fruits
- Leaves

Chemicals this herb contains:
- Gum (see Glossary)
- Tannins (see Glossary)
- Thyme oil

Known Effects

- Inhibits growth and development of germs
- Stimulates gastrointestinal tract
- Decreases thickness of bronchial secretions

Possible Additional Effects

- May reduce flatulence
- May treat coughs
- May treat bronchitis

- May treat bacterial infections
- May reduce menstrual cramps
- May help treat asthma
- Under study for cancer-preventive properties

 Warnings and Precautions

Don't take if you:
Are pregnant, think you may be pregnant or plan pregnancy in the near future.

Consult your doctor if you:
- Take this herb for any medical problem that doesn't improve in 2 weeks (There may be safer, more effective treatments.)
- Take any medicinal drugs or herbs including aspirin, laxatives, cold and cough remedies, antacids, vitamins, minerals, amino acids, supplements, other prescription or nonprescription drugs
- Have high blood pressure

Pregnancy:
Don't use unless prescribed by your doctor.

Breastfeeding:
Don't use unless prescribed by your doctor.

Infants and children:
Treating infants or children under 2 with any herbal preparation is hazardous.

Others:
No problems expected if you are beyond childhood, under 45, not pregnant, basically healthy, take it for only a short time and do not exceed manufacturer's recommended dose.

Storage:
- Store in cool, dry area away from direct light, but don't freeze.
- Store safely out of reach of children.
- Don't store in bathroom medicine cabinet. Heat and moisture may change the action of the herb.

Safe dosage:
Consult your doctor for the appropriate dose for your condition.

 Toxicity

Rated relatively safe when taken in appropriate quantities for short periods of time

For symptoms of toxicity: See *Adverse Reactions, Side Effects or Overdose Symptoms* section below.

 Adverse Reactions, Side Effects or Overdose Symptoms

Signs and symptoms	What to do
Diarrhea	Discontinue. Call doctor immediately.
Nausea or vomiting	Discontinue. Call doctor immediately.

Tonka Bean (Tonquin Bean)

 ## Basic Information

Biological name (genus and species):
Coumarouna odorata, Dipteryx odorata

Parts used for medicinal purposes:
Seeds

Chemicals this herb contains:
• Coumarin
• Gum (see Glossary)
• Sitosterin
• Starch
• Stigmasterin
• Sugar

 ## Known Effects

• Delays or stops blood clotting
• Anticoagulant

Miscellaneous information:
• Coumarin interferes with the synthesis of vitamin K in the human intestines. The absence of adequate vitamin K prevents blood clotting.
• The tonka bean was once a common adulterant of vanilla extracts.
• It's used as flavoring in tobacco.
• The FDA has banned its use as a flavoring agent in foods.

 ## Possible Additional Effects

• May prevent clotting in deep veins
• May prevent blood clots from breaking away from blood vessels and lodging in vital organs, such as lung or brain (use must be monitored carefully with frequent laboratory studies of prothrombin time)

 ## Warnings and Precautions

Don't take if you:
Are pregnant, think you may be pregnant or plan pregnancy in the near future.

Consult your doctor if you:
• Take this herb for any medical problem that doesn't improve in 2 weeks (There may be safer, more effective treatments.)
• Take any medicinal drugs or herbs including aspirin, laxatives, cold and cough remedies, antacids, vitamins, minerals, amino acids, supplements, other prescription or nonprescription drugs

Pregnancy:
Dangers outweigh any possible benefits. Don't use.

Breastfeeding:
Dangers outweigh any possible benefits. Don't use.

Infants and children:
Treating infants or children under 2 with any herbal preparation is hazardous.

Others:
Dangers outweigh any possible benefits. Don't use.

Storage:
• Store in cool, dry area away from direct light, but don't freeze.
• Store safely out of reach of children.
• Don't store in bathroom medicine cabinet. Heat and moisture may change the action of the herb.

Safe dosage:
Consult your doctor for the appropriate dose for your condition.

Toxicity

Comparative-toxicity rating is not available from standard references.

For symptoms of toxicity: See *Adverse Reactions, Side Effects or Overdose Symptoms* section below.

Adverse Reactions, Side Effects or Overdose Symptoms

Signs and symptoms	What to do
Growth retardation	Discontinue. Call doctor when convenient.
Internal bleeding	Seek emergency treatment.
Jaundice (yellow skin and eyes)	Discontinue. Call doctor when convenient.
Testicle atrophy	Discontinue. Call doctor when convenient.

Tormentil

Basic Information

Biological name (genus and species):
Potentilla erecta, P. tormentilla

Parts used for medicinal purposes:
Roots

Chemicals this herb contains:
• Ellagic acid (see Glossary)
• Kinovic acid
• Tannins (see Glossary)

Known Effects

• Shrinks tissues
• Prevents secretion of fluids
• Interferes with absorption of iron and other minerals when taken internally

Possible Additional Effects

• May treat diarrhea
• May treat sore throat
• May treat wounds when used as a poultice (see Glossary)

Warnings and Precautions

Don't take if you:
• Are pregnant, think you may be pregnant or plan pregnancy in the near future
• Have any chronic disease of the gastrointestinal tract, such as stomach or duodenal ulcers, reflux esophagitis, ulcerative colitis, spastic colitis, diverticulosis or diverticulitis

Consult your doctor if you:
• Take this herb for any medical problem that doesn't improve in 2 weeks (There may be safer, more effective treatments.)
• Take any medicinal drugs or herbs including aspirin, laxatives, cold and cough remedies, antacids, vitamins, minerals, amino acids, supplements, other prescription or nonprescription drugs

Pregnancy:
Don't use unless prescribed by
your doctor.

Breastfeeding:
Don't use unless prescribed by
your doctor.

Infants and children:
Treating infants or children under
2 with any herbal preparation
is hazardous.

Others:
No problems expected if you are
beyond childhood, under 45, not
pregnant, basically healthy, take it for
only a short time and do not exceed
manufacturer's recommended dose.

Storage:
• Store in cool, dry area away from
  direct light, but don't freeze.
• Store safely out of reach of children.
• Don't store in bathroom medicine
  cabinet. Heat and moisture may
  change the action of the herb.

Safe dosage:
Consult your doctor for the
appropriate dose for your condition.

Toxicity

Comparative-toxicity rating is not
available from standard references.

For symptoms of toxicity: See
*Adverse Reactions, Side Effects or
Overdose Symptoms* section below.

Adverse Reactions, Side Effects or Overdose Symptoms

Signs and symptoms	What to do
Diarrhea	Discontinue. Call doctor immediately.
Kidney damage characterized by blood in urine, decreased urine flow, swelling of hands and feet	Seek emergency treatment.
Nausea or vomiting	Discontinue. Call doctor immediately.

Unicorn Root (Colic Root, Star Grass)

Basic Information

Biological name (genus and species):
Aletris farinosa

Parts used for medicinal purposes:
• Leaves
• Roots

Chemicals this herb contains:
• Diosgenin

• Resin (see Glossary)
• Saponins (see Glossary)
• Volatile oils (see Glossary)

Known Effects

Reduces smooth-muscle spasms

Miscellaneous information:
Serves as a base substance to produce
synthetic progesterone (a female
hormone).

➜

Possible Additional Effects

- May treat painful menstruation
- May decrease chances of miscarriage
- May soothe sore breasts
- May relieve flatulence
- May relieve arthritis

Warnings and Precautions

Don't take if you:

- Are pregnant, think you may be pregnant or plan pregnancy in the near future
- Have any chronic disease of the gastrointestinal tract, such as stomach or duodenal ulcers, reflux esophagitis, ulcerative colitis, spastic colitis, diverticulosis or diverticulitis

Consult your doctor if you:

- Take this herb for any medical problem that doesn't improve in 2 weeks (There may be safer, more effective treatments.)
- Take any medicinal drugs or herbs including aspirin, laxatives, cold and cough remedies, antacids, vitamins, minerals, amino acids, supplements, other prescription or nonprescription drugs

Pregnancy:

Don't use unless prescribed by your doctor.

Breastfeeding:

Don't use unless prescribed by your doctor.

Infants and children:

Treating infants or children under 2 with any herbal preparation is hazardous.

Others:

No problems expected if you are beyond childhood, under 45, not pregnant, basically healthy, take it for only a short time and do not exceed manufacturer's recommended dose.

Storage:

- Store in cool, dry area away from direct light, but don't freeze.
- Store safely out of reach of children.
- Don't store in bathroom medicine cabinet. Heat and moisture may change the action of the herb.

Safe dosage:

Consult your doctor for the appropriate dose for your condition.

Toxicity

Rated slightly dangerous, particularly in children, persons over 55 and those who take larger than appropriate quantities for extended periods of time

For symptoms of toxicity: See *Adverse Reactions, Side Effects or Overdose Symptoms* section below.

Adverse Reactions, Side Effects or Overdose Symptoms

Signs and symptoms	What to do
Diarrhea	Discontinue. Call doctor immediately.
Lethargy	Discontinue. Call doctor when convenient.
Vomiting	Discontinue. Call doctor immediately.

Valerian (Garden Heliotrope, Tobacco Root)

Basic Information

Biological name (genus and species):

Valeriana edulis, V. officinalis

Parts used for medicinal purposes:
- Rhizomes
- Roots

Chemicals this herb contains:
- Acetic acid
- Butyric acid
- Camphene
- Chatinine
- Formic acid
- Glycosides (see Glossary)
- Pinene
- Resin (see Glossary)
- Valeric acid
- Valerine
- Volatile oils (see Glossary)

Known Effects

- Depresses central nervous system
- Treats hypertension
- Treats insomnia
- Causes sedation/calming effect

Miscellaneous information:
- Cats are attracted to this herb.
- Do not use with sedatives or tranquilizers because of the combined effect.
- Avoid driving when taking this herb.
- Valerian is available as tea or dried rhizome/roots.

Possible Additional Effects

- May relieve menstrual cramps
- May treat irritable bowel syndrome
- May treat anxiety

Warnings and Precautions

Don't take if you:

Are pregnant, think you may be pregnant or plan pregnancy in the near future.

Consult your doctor if you:
- Take this herb for any medical problem that doesn't improve in 2 weeks (There may be safer, more effective treatments.)
- Take any medicinal drugs or herbs including aspirin, laxatives, cold and cough remedies, antacids, vitamins, minerals, amino acids, supplements, other prescription or nonprescription drugs

Pregnancy:
Don't use unless prescribed by your doctor.

Breastfeeding:
Don't use unless prescribed by your doctor.

Infants and children:
Treating infants or children under 2 with any herbal preparation is hazardous.

Others:
No problems expected if you are beyond childhood, under 45, not pregnant, basically healthy, take it for only a short time and do not exceed manufacturer's recommended dose.

Storage:
- Store in cool, dry area away from direct light, but don't freeze.
- Store safely out of reach of children.
- Don't store in bathroom medicine cabinet. Heat and moisture may change the action of the herb.

- Use fresh material only. Dried valerian loses potency.

Safe dosage:

Consult your doctor for the appropriate dose for your condition.

 Toxicity

Rated relatively safe when taken in appropriate quantities for short periods of time

For symptoms of toxicity: See *Adverse Reactions, Side Effects or Overdose Symptoms* section below.

 Adverse Reactions, Side Effects or Overdose Symptoms

Signs and symptoms	What to do
Diarrhea	Discontinue. Call doctor immediately.
Nausea or vomiting	Discontinue. Call doctor immediately.

 Vervain (European Vervaine, Verbena)

 Basic Information

Biological name (genus and species): *Verbena officinalis*

Parts used for medicinal purposes: Roots

Chemicals this herb contains: Verbenaline

 Known Effects

- Stimulates gastrointestinal tract
- Stimulates parasympathetic (see Glossary) branch of autonomic nervous system

 Possible Additional Effects

- May treat coughs
- May treat upper abdominal pain
- May induce vomiting
- May treat headache

⚠️ Warnings and Precautions

Don't take if you:

- Are pregnant, think you may be pregnant or plan pregnancy in the near future
- Have any chronic disease of the gastrointestinal tract, such as stomach or duodenal ulcers, reflux esophagitis, ulcerative colitis, spastic colitis, diverticulosis or diverticulitis

Consult your doctor if you:

- Take this herb for any medical problem that doesn't improve in 2 weeks (There may be safer, more effective treatments.)
- Take any medicinal drugs or herbs including aspirin, laxatives, cold and cough remedies, antacids, vitamins, minerals, amino acids, supplements, other prescription or nonprescription drugs

Pregnancy:

Don't use unless prescribed by your doctor.

Breastfeeding:
Don't use unless prescribed by your doctor.

Infants and children:
Treating infants or children under 2 with any herbal preparation is hazardous.

Others:
No problems expected if you are beyond childhood, under 45, not pregnant, basically healthy, take it for only a short time and do not exceed manufacturer's recommended dose.

Storage:
• Store in cool, dry area away from direct light, but don't freeze.
• Store safely out of reach of children.
• Don't store in bathroom medicine cabinet. Heat and moisture may change the action of the herb.

Safe dosage:
Consult your doctor for the appropriate dose for your condition.

Toxicity

Generally regarded as safe when taken in appropriate quantities for short periods of time

For symptoms of toxicity: See *Adverse Reactions, Side Effects or Overdose Symptoms* section below.

Adverse Reactions, Side Effects or Overdose Symptoms

Signs and symptoms	What to do
Diarrhea	Discontinue. Call doctor immediately.
Nausea or vomiting	Discontinue. Call doctor immediately.

Virginian Skullcap

Basic Information

Biological name (genus and species):
Scutellaria lateriflora

Parts used for medicinal purposes:
Entire plant

Chemicals this herb contains:
• Cellulose
• Fat
• Scutellarin
• Sugar
• Tannins (see Glossary)

Known Effects

• Increases stomach acidity
• Irritates mucous membranes
• Relieves spasm in skeletal or smooth muscle
• Interferes with absorption of iron and other minerals when taken internally

Possible Additional Effects

•May stimulate appetite
•May relieve intestinal cramps

Warnings and Precautions

Don't take if you:

Are pregnant, think you may be pregnant or plan pregnancy in the near future.

Consult your doctor if you:

• Take this herb for any medical problem that doesn't improve in 2 weeks (There may be safer, more effective treatments.)
• Take any medicinal drugs or herbs including aspirin, laxatives, cold and cough remedies, antacids, vitamins, minerals, amino acids, supplements, other prescription or nonprescription drugs

Pregnancy:

Don't use unless prescribed by your doctor.

Breastfeeding:

Don't use unless prescribed by your doctor.

Infants and children:

Treating infants or children under 2 with any herbal preparation is hazardous.

Others:

No problems expected if you are beyond childhood, under 45, not pregnant, basically healthy, take it for only a short time and do not exceed manufacturer's recommended dose.

Storage:

• Store in cool, dry area away from direct light, but don't freeze.
• Store safely out of reach of children.
• Don't store in bathroom medicine cabinet. Heat and moisture may change the action of the herb.

Safe dosage:

Consult your doctor for the appropriate dose for your condition.

Toxicity

Rated relatively safe when taken in appropriate quantities for short periods of time

For symptoms of toxicity: See *Adverse Reactions, Side Effects or Overdose Symptoms* section below.

Adverse Reactions, Side Effects or Overdose Symptoms

Signs and symptoms	What to do
Confusion	Discontinue. Call doctor immediately.
Giddiness	Discontinue. Call doctor when convenient.
Irregular heartbeat	Seek emergency treatment.
Stupor	Seek emergency treatment.

Watercress

 Basic Information

Biological name (genus and species):
Nasturtium officinale

Parts used for medicinal purposes:
Various parts of the entire plant,
frequently differing by country
and culture

Chemicals this herb contains:
• Several trace element minerals, such
  as vanadium and cobalt
• Vitamins A, C, B-1 and B-2

 Known Effects

Provides a good source of vitamins and
minerals to treat or prevent
various deficiencies

Miscellaneous information:
• Watercress is a nutritious food
  source.
• Toxicity is unlikely.

 Possible
Additional Effects

• May treat kidney infections
• May treat urinary bladder stones
• May increase urine flow
• May treat heart disease
• May diminish pain during childbirth

 Warnings and
Precautions

Don't take if you:
Are pregnant, think you may be
pregnant or plan pregnancy in the
near future.

Consult your doctor if you:
• Take this herb for any medical
  problem that doesn't improve in
  2 weeks (There may be safer, more
  effective treatments.)
• Take any medicinal drugs or
  herbs including aspirin, laxatives,
  cold and cough remedies, antacids,
  vitamins, minerals, amino acids,
  supplements, other prescription
  or nonprescription drugs

Pregnancy:
Don't use unless prescribed by
your doctor.

Breastfeeding:
Don't use unless prescribed by
your doctor.

Infants and children:
Treating infants or children under
2 with any herbal preparation
is hazardous.

Others:
No problems expected if you are
beyond childhood, under 45, not
pregnant, basically healthy, take it for
only a short time and do not exceed
manufacturer's recommended dose.

Storage:
• Store in cool, dry area away from
  direct light, but don't freeze.
• Store safely out of reach of children.
• Don't store in bathroom medicine
  cabinet. Heat and moisture may
  change the action of the herb.

Safe dosage:
Consult your doctor for the
appropriate dose for your condition.

Toxicity

Comparative-toxicity rating is not available from standard references.

 Adverse Reactions, Side Effects or Overdose Symptoms

None are expected.

White Pine

 Basic Information

Biological name (genus and species):
Pinus strobus, P. alba

Parts used for medicinal purposes:
Inner bark

Chemicals this herb contains:
• Coniferin
• Coniferyl alcohol
• Mucilage (see Glossary)
• Oleoresin (see Glossary)
• Tannic acid
• Vanillin
• Volatile oils (see Glossary)

 Known Effects

Decreases thickness and increases fluidity of mucus in lungs and bronchial tubes

 Possible Additional Effects

May treat coughs when mixed with other expectorants

 Warnings and Precautions

Don't take if you:
Are pregnant, think you may be pregnant or plan pregnancy in the near future.

Consult your doctor if you:
• Take this herb for any medical problem that doesn't improve in 2 weeks (There may be safer, more effective treatments.)
• Take any medicinal drugs or herbs including aspirin, laxatives, cold and cough remedies, antacids, vitamins, minerals, amino acids, supplements, other prescription or nonprescription drugs

Pregnancy:
Don't use unless prescribed by your doctor.

Breastfeeding:
Don't use unless prescribed by your doctor.

Infants and children:
Treating infants or children under 2 with any herbal preparation is hazardous.

Others:

No problems expected if you are beyond childhood, under 45, not pregnant, basically healthy, take it for only a short time and do not exceed manufacturer's recommended dose.

Storage:

- Store in cool, dry area away from direct light, but don't freeze.
- Store safely out of reach of children.
- Don't store in bathroom medicine cabinet. Heat and moisture may change the action of the herb.

Safe dosage:

Consult your doctor for the appropriate dose for your condition.

 Toxicity

Rated slightly dangerous, particularly in children, persons over 55 and those who take larger than appropriate quantities for extended periods of time

For symptoms of toxicity: See *Adverse Reactions, Side Effects or Overdose Symptoms* section below.

 Adverse Reactions, Side Effects or Overdose Symptoms

Signs and symptoms	What to do
Abdominal discomfort	Discontinue. Call doctor immediately.

Willow

 Basic Information

Willow is also called *black willow, pussy willow, white willow* and *yellow willow.*

Biological name (genus and species): *Salix nigra, S. alba*

Parts used for medicinal purposes: Bark

Chemicals this herb contains:
- Salicin
- Salinigrin
- Tannins (see Glossary)

 Known Effects

- Produces puckering
- Reduces fever
- Anti-inflammatory

 Possible Additional Effects

- Potential antiseptic for ulcerated surfaces on skin
- May help reduce symptoms of gout, arthritis
- May help treat headaches
- May help heal open wounds because of tannins

→

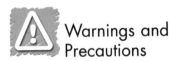

Warnings and Precautions

Don't take if you:
Are pregnant, think you may be pregnant or plan pregnancy in the near future.

Consult your doctor if you:
- Take this herb for any medical problem that doesn't improve in 2 weeks (There may be safer, more effective treatments.)
- Take any medicinal drugs or herbs including aspirin, laxatives, cold and cough remedies, antacids, vitamins, minerals, amino acids, supplements, other prescription or nonprescription drugs

Pregnancy:
Don't use unless prescribed by your doctor.

Breastfeeding:
Don't use unless prescribed by your doctor.

Infants and children:
Treating infants or children under 2 with any herbal preparation is hazardous.

Others:
- No problems expected if you are beyond childhood, under 45, not pregnant, basically healthy, take it for only a short time and do not exceed manufacturer's recommended dose.

- Salicylate poisoning is possible. Symptoms include dizziness, vomiting, ringing in ears.

Storage:
- Store in cool, dry area away from direct light, but don't freeze.
- Store safely out of reach of children.
- Don't store in bathroom medicine cabinet. Heat and moisture may change the action of the herb.

Safe dosage:
Consult your doctor for the appropriate dose for your condition.

Toxicity

Comparative-toxicity rating is not available from standard references.

For symptoms of toxicity: See *Adverse Reactions, Side Effects or Overdose Symptoms* section below.

Adverse Reactions, Side Effects or Overdose Symptoms

Signs and symptoms	What to do
Dizziness	Discontinue. Call doctor immediately.
Nausea or vomiting	Discontinue. Call doctor immediately.
Ringing in ears	Discontinue. Call doctor immediately.

Wintergreen (Boxberry, Teaberry)

Basic Information

Biological name (genus and species):
Gaultheria procumbens

Parts used for medicinal purposes:
- Leaves
- Roots
- Stems

Chemicals this herb contains:
- Methyl salicylate
- Monotropitoside

Known Effects

- Blocks impulses to pain center in brain
- Irritates stomach
- Treats pain of sprains and bruises when used externally

Miscellaneous information:
- Toxicity is unlikely unless you consume very large amounts of the entire plant.
- Do not apply after vigorous exercise as it may cause salicylate toxicity.

Possible Additional Effects

- May relieve headache
- May treat toothache

Warnings and Precautions

Don't take if you:
Are pregnant, think you may be pregnant or plan pregnancy in the near future.

Consult your doctor if you:
- Take this herb for any medical problem that doesn't improve in 2 weeks (There may be safer, more effective treatments.)
- Take any medicinal drugs or herbs including aspirin, laxatives, cold and cough remedies, antacids, vitamins, minerals, amino acids, supplements, other prescription or nonprescription drugs

Pregnancy
Dangers outweigh any possible benefits. Don't use.

Breastfeeding:
Dangers outweigh any possible benefits. Don't use.

Infants and children:
Treating infants or children under 2 with any herbal preparation is hazardous.

Others:
No problems expected if you are beyond childhood, under 45, not pregnant, basically healthy, take it for only a short time and do not exceed manufacturer's recommended dose.

Storage:
- Store in cool, dry area away from direct light, but don't freeze.
- Store safely out of reach of children.
- Don't store in bathroom medicine cabinet. Heat and moisture may change the action of the herb.

Safe dosage:
Consult your doctor for the appropriate dose for your condition.

➡

Toxicity

Rated slightly dangerous, particularly in children, persons over 55 and those who take larger than appropriate quantities for extended periods of time

 Adverse Reactions, Side Effects or Overdose Symptoms

Signs and symptoms	What to do
Abdominal pain	Discontinue. Call doctor when convenient.

Witch Hazel

 Basic Information

Biological name (genus and species):
Hamamelis virginiana

Parts used for medicinal purposes:
- Bark
- Leaves
- Twigs

Chemicals this herb contains:
- Bitters (see Glossary)
- Calcium oxalate
- Gallic acid
- Hamamelitannin
- Hexose sugar
- Tannins (see Glossary)
- Volatile oils (see Glossary)

 Known Effects

Shrinks tissues (when used as ointment, solution, suppository)

 Possible Additional Effects

- May treat diarrhea
- May soothe irritated skin or hemorrhoids
- Potential astringent (nondistilled form only)

 Warnings and Precautions

Don't take if you:
- Are pregnant, think you may be pregnant or plan pregnancy in the near future
- Have any chronic disease of the gastrointestinal tract, such as stomach or duodenal ulcers, reflux esophagitis, ulcerative colitis, spastic colitis, diverticulosis or diverticulitis

Consult your doctor if you:
- Take this herb for any medical problem that doesn't improve in 2 weeks (There may be safer, more effective treatments.)
- Take any medicinal drugs or herbs including aspirin, laxatives, cold and cough remedies, antacids, vitamins, minerals, amino acids, supplements, other prescription or nonprescription drugs

Pregnancy:
Dangers outweigh any possible benefits. Don't use.

Breastfeeding:
Dangers outweigh any possible benefits. Don't use.

Infants and children:
Treating infants or children under 2 with any herbal preparation is hazardous.

Others:
No problems expected if you are beyond childhood, under 45, not pregnant, basically healthy, take it for only a short time and do not exceed manufacturer's recommended dose.

Storage:
• Store in cool, dry area away from direct light, but don't freeze.
• Store safely out of reach of children.
• Don't store in bathroom medicine cabinet. Heat and moisture may change the action of the herb.

Safe dosage:
Consult your doctor for the appropriate dose for your condition.

Toxicity

Rated relatively safe when taken in appropriate quantities for short periods of time

For symptoms of toxicity: See *Adverse Reactions, Side Effects or Overdose Symptoms* section below.

Adverse Reactions, Side Effects or Overdose Symptoms

Signs and symptoms	What to do
Constipation	Discontinue. Call doctor when convenient.
Jaundice (yellow skin and eyes)	Discontinue. Call doctor immediately.
Nausea or vomiting	Discontinue. Call doctor immediately.

Woodruff

Basic Information

Biological name (genus and species):
Asperula odorata, Galium odoratum

Parts used for medicinal purposes:
Entire plant

Chemicals this herb contains:
• Asperuloside
• Bitters (see Glossary)
• Coumarin
• Oil
• Tannins (see Glossary)

Known Effects

• Stimulates gastrointestinal tract
• Decreases thickness and increases fluidity of mucus in lungs and bronchial tubes
• Interferes with absorption of iron and other minerals when taken internally

Miscellaneous information:
Woodruff is used as a flavoring agent in May wine and in sachets for its pleasant odor.

Possible Additional Effects

- May treat coughs
- May help expel gas from intestinal tract

 ## Warnings and Precautions

Don't take if you:

Are pregnant, think you may be pregnant or plan pregnancy in the near future.

Consult your doctor if you:

- Take this herb for any medical problem that doesn't improve in 2 weeks (There may be safer, more effective treatments.)
- Take any medicinal drugs or herbs including aspirin, laxatives, cold and cough remedies, antacids, vitamins, minerals, amino acids, supplements, other prescription or nonprescription drugs

Pregnancy:

Don't use unless prescribed by your doctor.

Breastfeeding:

Don't use unless prescribed by your doctor.

Infants and children:

Treating infants or children under 2 with any herbal preparation is hazardous.

Others:

No problems expected if you are beyond childhood, under 45, not pregnant, basically healthy, take it for only a short time and do not exceed manufacturer's recommended dose.

Storage:

- Store in cool, dry area away from direct light, but don't freeze.
- Store safely out of reach of children.
- Don't store in bathroom medicine cabinet. Heat and moisture may change the action of the herb.

Safe dosage:

Consult your doctor for the appropriate dose for your condition.

 ## Toxicity

Comparative-toxicity rating is not available from standard references.

 ## Adverse Reactions, Side Effects or Overdose Symptoms

None are expected.

Wormseed (Pigweed)

Basic Information

Biological name (genus and species):
Chenopodium ambrosioides

Parts used for medicinal purposes:
• Berries/fruits
• Roots

Chemicals this herb contains:
• Ascaridol
• Calcium
• Cymene
• D-camphor
• Limonene
• Saponins (see Glossary)
• Terpenes (see Glossary)
• Vitamins A and C
• Volatile oils (see Glossary)

Known Effects

• Inhibits growth and development of germs
• Decreases blood pressure
• Decreases heart rate
• Depresses central nervous system
• Decreases stomach contractions

Miscellaneous information:
Wormseed is used externally as a poultice (see Glossary).

Possible Additional Effects

• May treat arthritis
• May kill intestinal parasites

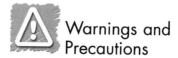

Warnings and Precautions

Don't take if you:
• Are pregnant, think you may be pregnant or plan pregnancy in the near future
• Have any chronic disease of the gastrointestinal tract, such as stomach or duodenal ulcers, reflux esophagitis, ulcerative colitis, spastic colitis, diverticulosis or diverticulitis

Consult your doctor if you:
• Take this herb for any medical problem that doesn't improve in 2 weeks (There may be safer, more effective treatments.)
• Take any medicinal drugs or herbs including aspirin, laxatives, cold and cough remedies, antacids, vitamins, minerals, amino acids, supplements, other prescription or nonprescription drugs

Pregnancy:
Dangers outweigh any possible benefits. Don't use.

Breastfeeding:
Dangers outweigh any possible benefits. Don't use.

Infants and children:
Treating infants or children under 2 with any herbal preparation is hazardous.

Others:
No problems expected if you are beyond childhood, under 45, not pregnant, basically healthy, take it for only a short time and do not exceed manufacturer's recommended dose.

→

Storage:
- Store in cool, dry area away from direct light, but don't freeze.
- Store safely out of reach of children.
- Don't store in bathroom medicine cabinet. Heat and moisture may change the action of the herb.

Safe dosage:
Consult your doctor for the appropriate dose for your condition.

 Toxicity

Rated slightly dangerous, particularly in children, persons over 55 and those who take larger than appropriate quantities for extended periods of time

For symptoms of toxicity: See *Adverse Reactions, Side Effects or Overdose Symptoms* section below.

 Adverse Reactions, Side Effects or Overdose Symptoms

Signs and symptoms	What to do
Breathing difficulties	Seek emergency treatment.
Drowsiness	Discontinue. Call doctor when convenient.
Headache	Discontinue. Call doctor when convenient.
Hearing problems	Discontinue. Call doctor immediately.
Nausea or vomiting	Discontinue. Call doctor immediately.
Ringing in ears	Discontinue. Call doctor when convenient.
Slow heartbeat	Seek emergency treatment.
Stomach ulcers	Discontinue. Call doctor immediately.
Vision problems	Discontinue. Call doctor immediately.

Wormwood (Absinthium)

 Basic Information

Biological name (genus and species):
Artemisia absinthium

Parts used for medicinal purposes:
- Berries/fruits
- Leaves

Chemicals this herb contains:
- Thujone (absinthol)
- Volatile oils (see Glossary)

 Known Effects

- Depresses central nervous system
- Thujone causes mind-altering changes, may lead to psychosis
- Increases stomach acidity

Miscellaneous information:
Wormwood can be habit-forming, like ethyl alcohol.

 Possible Additional Effects

- May treat anxiety
- Potential mild sedative
- May stimulate appetite

 Warnings and Precautions

Don't take if you:
Are pregnant, think you may be pregnant or plan pregnancy in the near future.

Consult your doctor if you:
- Take this herb for any medical problem that doesn't improve in 2 weeks (There may be safer, more effective treatments.)
- Take any medicinal drugs or herbs including aspirin, laxatives, cold and cough remedies, antacids, vitamins, minerals, amino acids, supplements, other prescription or nonprescription drugs

Pregnancy:
Dangers outweigh any possible benefits. Don't use.

Breastfeeding:
Dangers outweigh any possible benefits. Don't use.

Infants and children:
Treating infants or children under 2 with any herbal preparation is hazardous.

Others:
This product will not help you and may cause toxic symptoms.

Storage:
- Store in cool, dry area away from direct light, but don't freeze.
- Store safely out of reach of children.

- Don't store in bathroom medicine cabinet. Heat and moisture may change the action of the herb.

Safe dosage:
Consult your doctor for the appropriate dose for your condition.

 Toxicity

Rated slightly dangerous, particularly in children, persons over 55 and those who take larger than appropriate quantities for extended periods of time

For symptoms of toxicity: See *Adverse Reactions, Side Effects or Overdose Symptoms* section below.

 Adverse Reactions, Side Effects or Overdose Symptoms

Signs and symptoms	What to do
Convulsions	Seek emergency treatment.
Stupor	Seek emergency treatment.
Trembling	Discontinue. Call doctor when convenient.

Yarrow

 Basic Information

Biological name (genus and species):
Achillea millefolium

Parts used for medicinal purposes:
- Berries/fruits
- Leaves

Chemicals this herb contains:
- Achilleine
- Coumarins
- Polyacetylenes
- Salicylic acid
- Tannins (see Glossary)
- Triterpenes
- Volatile oils (see Glossary)

Known Effects

- Reduces blood-clotting time
- Reduces pain
- Anti-inflammatory

Possible Additional Effects

- Potential mild sedative
- May help reduce menstrual cramps
- May help reduce blood pressure

Warnings and Precautions

Don't take if you:
Are pregnant, think you may be pregnant or plan pregnancy in the near future.

Consult your doctor if you:
- Take this herb for any medical problem that doesn't improve in 2 weeks (There may be safer, more effective treatments.)
- Take any medicinal drugs or herbs including aspirin, laxatives, cold and cough remedies, antacids, vitamins, minerals, amino acids, supplements, other prescription or nonprescription drugs
- Have ragweed allergy—a rash may occur

Pregnancy:
Don't use unless prescribed by your doctor.

Breastfeeding:
Don't use unless prescribed by your doctor.

Infants and children:
Treating infants or children under 2 with any herbal preparation is hazardous.

Others:
No problems expected if you are beyond childhood, under 45, not pregnant, basically healthy, take it for only a short time and do not exceed manufacturer's recommended dose.

Storage:
- Store in cool, dry area away from direct light, but don't freeze.
- Store safely out of reach of children.
- Don't store in bathroom medicine cabinet. Heat and moisture may change the action of the herb.

Safe dosage:
Consult your doctor for the appropriate dose for your condition.

Toxicity

Generally regarded as safe when taken in appropriate quantities for short periods of time

For symptoms of toxicity: See *Adverse Reactions, Side Effects or Overdose Symptoms* section below.

Adverse Reactions, Side Effects or Overdose Symptoms

Signs and symptoms	What to do
Diarrhea	Discontinue. Call doctor immediately.

Yellow Cedar (Arbor Vitae)

Basic Information

Biological name (genus and species):
Thuja occidentalis

Parts used for medicinal purposes:
Leaves

Chemicals this herb contains:
• Fenchone
• Pinopicrin
• Tannins (see Glossary)
• Thujone
• Volatile oils (see Glossary)

Known Effects

• Stimulates central nervous system
• Stimulates heart muscle to contract more efficiently
• Destroys intestinal worms
• Causes uterine contractions
• Interferes with absorption of iron and other minerals when taken internally

Miscellaneous information:

Yellow cedar has caused deaths when misused to induce abortions.

Possible Additional Effects

• May relieve muscular aches and pains
• May treat warts
• May cause abortions (miscarriages)

Warnings and Precautions

Don't take if you:
Are pregnant, think you may be pregnant or plan pregnancy in the near future.

Consult your doctor if you:
• Take this herb for any medical problem that doesn't improve in 2 weeks (There may be safer, more effective treatments.)
• Take any medicinal drugs or herbs including aspirin, laxatives, cold and cough remedies, antacids, vitamins, minerals, amino acids, supplements, other prescription or nonprescription drugs

Pregnancy:
Dangers outweigh any possible benefits. Don't use.

Breastfeeding:
Dangers outweigh any possible benefits. Don't use.

Infants and children:
Treating infants or children under 2 with any herbal preparation is hazardous.

Others:
Dangers outweigh any possible benefits. Don't use.

Storage:
• Store in cool, dry area away from direct light, but don't freeze.
• Store safely out of reach of children.
• Don't store in bathroom medicine cabinet. Heat and moisture may change the action of the herb.

→

Safe dosage:
Consult your doctor for the appropriate dose for your condition.

Toxicity

Comparative-toxicity rating is not available from standard references.

For symptoms of toxicity: See *Adverse Reactions, Side Effects or Overdose Symptoms* section below.

Adverse Reactions, Side Effects or Overdose Symptoms

Signs and symptoms	What to do
Abortion	Seek emergency treatment.
Coma	Seek emergency treatment.
Convulsions	Seek emergency treatment.
Precipitous blood-pressure drop: symptoms include faintness, cold sweat, paleness, rapid pulse	Seek emergency treatment.

Yellow Dock

Basic Information

Biological name (genus and species):
Rumex crispus

Parts used for medicinal purposes:
• Leaves
• Rhizomes
• Roots

Chemicals this herb contains:
• Oxalic acid
• Potassium oxalate
• Vitamins A and C

Known Effects

• Irritates skin when handled
• Stimulates gastrointestinal tract as a mild laxative
• Stimulates bile production

Miscellaneous information:
Yellow dock is used as food in salads.

Possible Additional Effects

No additional effects are known.

Warnings and Precautions

Don't take if you:
• Are pregnant, think you may be pregnant or plan pregnancy in the near future
• Have any chronic disease of the gastrointestinal tract, such as stomach or duodenal ulcers, reflux esophagitis, ulcerative colitis, spastic colitis, diverticulosis or diverticulitis

Consult your doctor if you:
• Take this herb for any medical problem that doesn't improve in 2 weeks (There may be safer, more effective treatments.)
• Take any medicinal drugs or herbs including aspirin, laxatives,

cold and cough remedies, antacids, vitamins, minerals, amino acids, supplements, other prescription or nonprescription drugs

Pregnancy:
Dangers outweigh any possible benefits. Don't use.

Breastfeeding:
Dangers outweigh any possible benefits. Don't use.

Infants and children:
Treating infants or children under 2 with any herbal preparation is hazardous.

Others:
Dangers outweigh any possible benefits. Don't use medicinally.

Storage:
• Store in cool, dry area away from direct light, but don't freeze.
• Store safely out of reach of children.
• Don't store in bathroom medicine cabinet. Heat and moisture may change the action of the herb.

Safe dosage:
Consult your doctor for the appropriate dose for your condition.

Toxicity

Rated slightly dangerous, particularly in children, persons over 55 and those who take larger than appropriate quantities for extended periods of time

For symptoms of toxicity: See *Adverse Reactions, Side Effects or Overdose Symptoms* section below.

Adverse Reactions, Side Effects or Overdose Symptoms

Signs and symptoms	What to do
Diarrhea	Discontinue. Call doctor immediately.
Kidney damage characterized by blood in urine, decreased urine flow, swelling of hands and feet	Seek emergency treatment.
Nausea or vomiting	Discontinue. Call doctor immediately.
Skin eruptions	Discontinue. Call doctor when convenient.

Yellow Lady's Slipper

Basic Information

Biological name (genus and species): *Cypripedium pubescens*

Parts used for medicinal purposes: Roots

Chemicals this herb contains:
• Resin (see Glossary)
• Tannins (see Glossary)
• Volatile acid
• Volatile oils (see Glossary)

Known Effects

• Irritates mucous membranes
• Stimulates gastrointestinal tract
• Increases perspiration

Miscellaneous information:
- Hairs on stems and leaves irritate body when touched.
- May produce skin eruptions similar to those caused by poison ivy.

 ## Possible Additional Effects

- Potential sedative to treat anxiety or restlessness
- May help expel gas from intestinal tract
- May relieve spasm in skeletal or smooth muscle

 ## Warnings and Precautions

Don't take if you:
- Are pregnant, think you may be pregnant or plan pregnancy in the near future
- Have any chronic disease of the gastrointestinal tract, such as stomach or duodenal ulcers, reflux esophagitis, ulcerative colitis, spastic colitis, diverticulosis or diverticulitis

Consult your doctor if you:
- Take this herb for any medical problem that doesn't improve in 2 weeks (There may be safer, more effective treatments.)
- Take any medicinal drugs or herbs including aspirin, laxatives, cold and cough remedies, antacids, vitamins, minerals, amino acids, supplements, other prescription or nonprescription drugs

Pregnancy:
Don't use unless prescribed by your doctor.

Breastfeeding:
Don't use unless prescribed by your doctor.

Infants and children:
Treating infants or children under 2 with any herbal preparation is hazardous.

Others:
No problems expected if you are beyond childhood, under 45, not pregnant, basically healthy, take it for only a short time and do not exceed manufacturer's recommended dose.

Storage:
- Store in cool, dry area away from direct light, but don't freeze.
- Store safely out of reach of children.
- Don't store in bathroom medicine cabinet. Heat and moisture may change the action of the herb.

Safe dosage:
Consult your doctor for the appropriate dose for your condition.

 ## Toxicity

Rated relatively safe when taken in appropriate quantities for short periods of time

For symptoms of toxicity: See *Adverse Reactions, Side Effects or Overdose Symptoms* section below.

 ## Adverse Reactions, Side Effects or Overdose Symptoms

Signs and symptoms	What to do
Drowsiness	Discontinue. Call doctor when convenient.
Nausea or vomiting	Discontinue. Call doctor immediately.

Yerba Maté (Paraguay Tea, South American Holly)

Basic Information

Biological name (genus and species):
Ilex paraguariensis

Parts used for medicinal purposes:
Leaves

Chemicals this herb contains:
Caffeine

Known Effects

- Stimulates central nervous system
- Helps body dispose of excess fluid by increasing amount of urine produced
- Causes hallucinations

Possible Additional Effects

- Potential laxative
- May increase perspiration

Warnings and Precautions

Don't take if you:
- Are pregnant, think you may be pregnant or plan pregnancy in the near future
- Have any chronic disease of the gastrointestinal tract, such as stomach or duodenal ulcers, reflux esophagitis, ulcerative colitis, spastic colitis, diverticulosis or diverticulitis

Consult your doctor if you:
- Take this herb for any medical problem that doesn't improve in 2 weeks (There may be safer, more effective treatments.)
- Take any medicinal drugs or herbs including aspirin, laxatives, cold and cough remedies, antacids, vitamins, minerals, amino acids, supplements, other prescription or nonprescription drugs

Pregnancy:
Dangers outweigh any possible benefits. Don't use.

Breastfeeding:
Dangers outweigh any possible benefits. Don't use.

Infants and children:
Treating infants or children under 2 with any herbal preparation is hazardous.

Others:
No problems expected if you are beyond childhood, under 45, not pregnant, basically healthy, take it for only a short time and do not exceed manufacturer's recommended dose.

Storage:
- Store in cool, dry area away from direct light, but don't freeze.
- Store safely out of reach of children.
- Don't store in bathroom medicine cabinet. Heat and moisture may change the action of the herb.

Safe dosage:
Consult your doctor for the appropriate dose for your condition.

Toxicity

Rated relatively safe when taken in appropriate quantities for short periods of time

For symptoms of toxicity: See *Adverse Reactions, Side Effects or Overdose Symptoms* section below.

→

Adverse Reactions, Side Effects or Overdose Symptoms

Signs and symptoms	What to do
Confusion	Seek emergency treatment.
Excessive urination	Discontinue. Call doctor when convenient.
Hallucinations	Seek emergency treatment.
Heartburn	Discontinue. Call doctor when convenient.
Insomnia	Discontinue. Call doctor when convenient.
Irritability	Discontinue. Call doctor when convenient.
Nausea	Discontinue. Call doctor immediately.
Nervousness	Discontinue. Call doctor when convenient.
Rapid heartbeat	Seek emergency treatment.

Yerba Santa (Bear's Weed)

 ## Basic Information

Biological name (genus and species):
Eriodictyon californicum

Parts used for medicinal purposes:
Leaves

Chemicals this herb contains:
• Formic acid
• Pentatriacontane eriodictyol
• Resin (see Glossary)
• Tannic acid
• Tannins (see Glossary)

 ## Known Effects

• Masks taste of bitter medicines
• Decreases thickness and increases fluidity of mucus in lungs and bronchial tubes
• Interferes with absorption of iron and other minerals when taken internally

 ## Possible Additional Effects

• May treat hay fever and other nasal allergies
• May treat hemorrhoids

Warnings and Precautions

Don't take if you:

• Are pregnant, think you may be pregnant or plan pregnancy in the near future

• Have any chronic disease of the gastrointestinal tract, such as stomach or duodenal ulcers, reflux esophagitis, ulcerative colitis, spastic colitis, diverticulosis or diverticulitis

Consult your doctor if you:

• Take this herb for any medical problem that doesn't improve in 2 weeks (There may be safer, more effective treatments.)

• Take any medicinal drugs or herbs including aspirin, laxatives, cold and cough remedies, antacids, vitamins, minerals, amino acids, supplements, other prescription or nonprescription drugs

Pregnancy:

Dangers outweigh any possible benefits. Don't use.

Breastfeeding:

Dangers outweigh any possible benefits. Don't use.

Infants and children:

Treating infants or children under 2 with any herbal preparation is hazardous.

Others:

No problems expected if you are beyond childhood, under 45, not pregnant, basically healthy, take it for only a short time and do not exceed manufacturer's recommended dose.

Storage:

• Store in cool, dry area away from direct light, but don't freeze.

• Store safely out of reach of children.

• Don't store in bathroom medicine cabinet. Heat and moisture may change the action of the herb.

Safe dosage:

Consult your doctor for the appropriate dose for your condition.

 ## Toxicity

Comparative-toxicity rating is not available from standard references.

For symptoms of toxicity: See *Adverse Reactions, Side Effects or Overdose Symptoms* section below.

 ## Adverse Reactions, Side Effects or Overdose Symptoms

Signs and symptoms	What to do
Diarrhea	Discontinue. Call doctor immediately.
Nausea or vomiting	Discontinue. Call doctor immediately.

Yohimbe

 Basic Information

Biological name (genus and species):
Corynanthe yohimbe, Pausinystalia yohimbe

Parts used for medicinal purposes:
Bark

Chemicals this herb contains:
Yohimbine (also called *quebrachine* and *aphrodine*)

 Known Effects

- Blocks responses of parts of autonomic nervous system
- Increases blood pressure
- Inhibits monoamine oxidase and may cause alarming blood-pressure rise, even strokes, when taken with cheese, red wine or other foods or supplements containing tyramines
- Arouses or enhances sexual desire

Miscellaneous information:

- Yohimbe can produce severe anxiety when given intravenously.
- It is not available over-the-counter in the United States and has a high number of side effects and low potential benefit.

 Possible Additional Effects

- May treat impotency/erectile dysfunction
- May treat painful menstrual cramps
- May treat chest pain due to coronary artery disease (angina)
- May treat arteriosclerosis

 Warnings and Precautions

Don't take if you:

- Are pregnant, think you may be pregnant or plan pregnancy in the near future
- Have kidney or liver disease

Consult your doctor if you:

- Take this herb for any medical problem that doesn't improve in 2 weeks (There may be safer, more effective treatments.)
- Take any medicinal drugs or herbs including aspirin, laxatives, cold and cough remedies, antacids, vitamins, minerals, amino acids, supplements, other prescription or nonprescription drugs
- Are considering taking yohimbe

Pregnancy:
Don't use.

Breastfeeding:
Don't use.

Infants and children:
Treating infants or children under 2 with any herbal preparation is hazardous.

Others:
This product will not help you and may cause toxic symptoms. Don't use.

Storage:

- Store in cool, dry area away from direct light, but don't freeze.
- Store safely out of reach of children.
- Don't store in bathroom medicine cabinet. Heat and moisture may change the action of the herb.

Safe dosage:
Consult your doctor for the appropriate dose for your condition.

Toxicity

Rated dangerous, particularly in children, persons over 55 and those who take larger than appropriate quantities for extended periods of time

For symptoms of toxicity: See *Adverse Reactions, Side Effects or Overdose Symptoms* section below.

Adverse Reactions, Side Effects or Overdose Symptoms

Signs and symptoms	What to do
Abdominal pain	Discontinue. Call doctor when convenient.
Agitation	Discontinue. Call doctor immediately.
Anxiety	Discontinue. Call doctor when convenient.
Fatigue	Discontinue. Call doctor when convenient.
Hallucinations	Seek emergency treatment.
High blood pressure	Discontinue. Call doctor immediately.
Increased heart rate	Discontinue. Call doctor immediately.
Insomnia	Discontinue. Call doctor when convenient.
Muscle paralysis	Seek emergency treatment.
Nausea or vomiting	Discontinue. Call doctor immediately.
Weakness	Discontinue. Call doctor immediately.

Phytochemicals and Health

Phytochemicals are chemicals found in or derived from plants.

Phytochemicals and Disease Prevention		
Phytochemical	**Food source(s)**	**Clinical significance**
Alpha-linolenic acid	flaxseed, soy, walnuts	reduces inflammation, lowers blood cholesterol, may protect against breast cancer, enhances immunity
Beta-carotene	green and yellow fruits and vegetables	reduces risk of cataracts, coronary artery disease, lung and breast cancers; enhances immunity (elderly)
Capsaicin	chili peppers	reduces risk for colon, gastric and rectal cancer; inhibits tumor promotion
Carotenoid, lycopene	tomato sauce, catsup, red grapefruit, guava, dried apricots, watermelon, fresh tomatoes	antioxidant, reduces risk of prostate cancer, may reduce cardiovascular disease
Curcumin	turmeric, curry, cumin	may lower cholesterol, reduces risk of skin cancer
Cynarin	artichokes	decreases cholesterol levels
Ellagic acid	wine, grapes, currants, nuts (pecans), berries (strawberries, blackberries, raspberries), seeds	reduces cancer risk, inhibits carcinogen binding to DNA, reduces LDL cholesterol while increasing HDL cholesterol
Flavonols, polyphenols: catechin (theaflavins, thearubigins), theogallin, EGCG	green and black tea, berries	reduces risk of gastric cancer, antioxidant, increases immune function, decreases cholesterol production, protects against chemically induced cancers and skin cancer, may protect against esophageal cancer, antitumor promoter, inhibits nitrosamine formation, inhibits phase I and enhances phase II enzyme activity
Genistein	soybeans	reduces risk of hormone-dependent cancers; alters hormone levels; inhibits angiogenesis; promotes cell differentiation; reduces cholesterol levels; reduces thrombi formation, osteoporosis, menopausal symptoms
Indoles	cabbage, broccoli, Brussels sprouts, spinach, watercress, cauliflower, turnips, kohlrabi, kale, rutabaga, horseradish, mustard greens	reduces risk of hormone-related cancers, may "inactivate" estrogen, increases glutathione-S-transferase activity, inhibits growth of transformed cells

Phytochemical	Food source(s)	Clinical significance
Isothiocyanates, sulforaphane	cabbage, cauliflower, broccoli and broccoli sprouts, Brussels sprouts, mustard greens, horseradish, radishes	reduces risk of tobacco-induced tumors, inhibits tobacco-related carcinogens from damaging DNA, induces phase II enzymes, inhibits cP450 activation of carcinogens
Lignans	high fiber foods, especially seeds	reduces cancer risk (colon), reduces blood glucose and cholesterol
Monterpene, limonene	citrus (peel, membrane), mint, caraway, thyme, coriander	antioxidant, reduces cancer risk (skin, breast), inhibits p21ras (G protein), suppresses HMG-CoA, induces apoptosis, reduces cholesterol production, reduces premenstrual symptoms
Organosulfur compounds, allylic acid	garlic, onion, watercress, cruciferous vegetables, leeks	decreases lipid peroxidation; reduces risk of gastric, colon and lung cancers; inhibits tumor promotion by inhibiting DNA adduct formation; induces phase II enzymes; antithrombotic; reduces cholesterol; reduces blood pressure; antimicrobial
Quercetin	pear skin, apple skin, bell pepper, kohlrabi, tomato leaves, onion, wine, grape juice	flavonoid, anticancer, antioxidant, associated with reduced coronary heart disease, decreases platelet aggregation
Phenolic acid	cruciferous vegetables, eggplant, peppers, tomatoes, celery, parsley, soy, licorice root, flaxseed, citrus, whole grains, berries	inhibits cancer by inhibiting nitrosamine formation, reduces risk for lung and skin cancers
Polyacetylene	parsley, carrots, celery	decreases risk of tobacco-induced tumors, alters prostaglandin formation

Glossary

abortifacient. Induces abortions (miscarriages).

absorption. Process by which nutrients are absorbed through the lining of the intestinal tract into capillaries and into the bloodstream. Nutrients must be absorbed to affect the body.

acids. Compounds often found in plant tissues, especially fruits, that shrink tissues and prevent secretion of fluids. They taste sour or tart.

active principle. Chemical component of a plant or compound that has a therapeutic effect.

acute. Short, relatively severe. Usually referred to in connection with an illness. Opposite of acute is *chronic.*

addiction. Psychological or physiological dependence on a drug. With true addictions, severe symptoms appear when the addicted person stops taking the drug on which he or she is dependent.

adrenal gland. Gland located immediately adjacent to the kidney that produces epinephrine (adrenaline) and several steroid hormones, including cortisone and hydro-cortisone.

adulterant. Substance that makes another substance impure when the two are mixed together.

allergen. Capable of producing an allergic response.

allergy. Excessive sensitivity to a substance.

alpha linolenic acid. An essential *fatty acid* important for healing and maintaining good health.

alumina. Another term for aluminum oxide or hydrated aluminum oxide.

amenorrhea. Absence of menstruation.

amino acid. Chemical building blocks that help produce proteins in the body.

anabolic. Building up of tissues in the body, or constructive metabolism.

analog. Employing measurement along scales rather than by numerical counting.

anaphylaxis. Severe allergic response to a substance. Symptoms include wheezing, itching, nasal congestion, hives, immediate intense burning of hands and feet, collapse with severe drop in blood pressure, loss of consciousness and cardiac arrest. Symptoms of anaphylaxis appear within a few seconds or minutes after exposure to the substance causing reaction—this can be medication or herbs taken by injection, by mouth, vaginally, rectally, through a breathing apparatus or applied to skin. Anaphylaxis is an uncommon occurrence, but when it occurs, it is a *severe medical emergency!* Without appropriate immediate treatment, it can cause death. Yell for help. Don't leave victim. Begin CPR (cardiopulmonary resuscitation), mouth-to-mouth breathing and external cardiac massage. Have someone dial "0" or 911. Don't stop CPR until help arrives.

anemia. Too few healthy red blood cells in the bloodstream or too little hemoglobin in the red blood cells. Anemia is usually caused by excessive blood loss, such as excessive bleeding or menstruation, increased blood destruction, such as hemolytic anemia or leukemia, or decreased blood production, such as iron-deficiency anemia.

anemia, pernicious. Anemia caused by vitamin-B-12 deficiency. Symptoms include easy fatigue, weakness, lemon-colored skin, numbness and tingling of hands and feet, and symptoms of degeneration of the central nervous system, such as irritability, emotional problems, personality changes and paralysis of extremities.

anesthetic. Used to abolish pain.

angina (angina pectoris). Chest pain, with sensation of impending death. Pain may radiate into jaw, ear lobes, between shoulder blades or down shoulder and arm on either side, most frequently the left side. Pain is caused by a temporary reduction in the amount of oxygen to the heart muscle through narrowed, diseased coronary arteries.

antacid. Neutralizes acid. In medical terms, the neutralized acid is located in the stomach, esophagus or first part of the *duodenum*.

antagonist. A drug that blocks or reverses the effect of another drug.

antibacterial. Destroys bacteria (germs) or suppresses their growth or reproduction.

antibiotic. Inhibits growth of germs or kills germs. When it inhibits growth, it is called *bacteriostatic*. When it kills germs, it is called *bacteriocidal*.

anticholinergic. Reduces nerve impulses through the part of the autonomic nervous system called *parasympathetic*.

anticoagulant. Delays or stops blood clotting.

antiemetic. Prevents or stops nausea and vomiting.

antihelmintic. Destroys intestinal worms.

antihistamine. Reduces *histamine*, the chemical in body tissues that dilates smallest blood vessels, constricts smooth muscle surrounding bronchial tubes and stimulates stomach secretions by acting on tissues of the body.

antihypertensive. Reduces blood pressure.

antimicrobial. Destroys or inhibits growth of microorganisms.

antimitotic. Inhibits or prevents cell division.

antineoplastic. Inhibits or prevents growth of neoplasms (cancers).

antioxidant. Prevents or delays the process of *oxidation*. Antioxidant substances include superoxide dismutase, selenium, vitamins C and E and zinc.

antipyretic. Reduces fevers.

antiseptic. Prevents or retards growth of germs.

antispasmodic. Relieves spasm in skeletal or smooth muscle.

apertive. Stimulates the appetite.

aphrodisiac. Arouses or enhances instinctive sexual desire.

aromatic. Chemical with a spicy fragrance and stimulant characteristics used to relieve various symptoms.

artery. Blood vessel that carries blood away from the heart.

asthma. Disease with recurrent attacks of breathing difficulty characterized by wheezing. It is caused by spasms of the bronchial tubes, which can be caused by many factors including adverse reactions to drugs, vitamins, minerals or medicinal herbs.

astringent. Shrinks tissues and prevents secretion of fluids.

bacteria. Microscopic germs. Some bacteria contribute to health; others cause disease.

bioavailability. The degree to which a drug becomes available to the target tissue after administration.

bitters. Medicine with a bitter taste. Used as a tonic or appetizer.

blepharitis. Inflammation of the eyelid.

blood sugar (blood glucose). Necessary element in blood to sustain life. The blood level of glucose is determined by insulin, a *hormone* secreted by the pancreas. When the pancreas no longer satisfies this function, the disease *diabetes mellitus* results.

bronchitis. Inflammation of the breathing tubes.

bulb. Modified plant bulb with scaly leaves that grows beneath the soil.

carcinogen. Chemical or substance that can cause cancer.

cardiac. Pertaining to the heart.

cardiac arrhythmias. Abnormal heart rate or rhythm.

cardiomyopathy. Chronic disorder of the heart muscle of unknown association.

carminative. Aids in expelling gas from the intestinal tract.

cathartic. Very strong *laxative* that produces explosive, watery bowel movements.

cell. Unit of protoplasm, the essential living matter of all plants and animals.

central nervous system. Brain and spinal cord and their nerve endings.

central-nervous-system depressant. Causes changes in the body, including changes in consciousness, lethargy, loss of judgment or coma.

chronic. Disease of long standing. Opposite of *acute.*

coenzyme. Heat-stable molecule that must be loosely associated with an *enzyme* for the enzyme to perform its function.

cofactor. Element with which another must unite to function.

colic. Abdominal pain that recurs in a pattern every few seconds or minutes.

collagen. Gelatinous protein used to make body tissues.

congestive. Excess accumulation of blood. Congestive heart failure is the result of blood congregating in lungs, liver, kidney and other parts to cause shortness of breath, swelling of ankles, sleep disturbances, rapid heartbeat and easy fatigue.

conjunctivitis. Inflammation of the outer membrane of the eye.

constriction. Tightness or pressure.

contraceptive. Prevents pregnancy.

contraindication. Inadvisability of using a substance that may cause harm under specific circumstances. For example, high-caloric intake in someone who is overweight is contraindicated.

convulsion. Violent, uncontrollable contraction of the voluntary muscles.

corticosteroid (adrenocorticosteroid). Hormones produced by the body or manufactured synthetically.

counterirritant. Process of applying an irritating substance to the skin to produce increased blood circulation to the area. Classic example (now considered an outdated treatment) is mustard plaster applied to the chest to relieve bronchial congestion or cough.

cyanogenic glycosides. Sugars capable of producing cyanide.

cynarin. Acid that stimulates bile secretion.

cystitis. Inflammation of the urinary bladder.

decoction. Extract of a crude drug obtained by boiling the substance in water.

dehiscent. Fruit that splits open when ripe.

delirium. Temporary mental disturbance accompanied by hallucinations, agitation, incoherence.

demineralization. Excessive elimination of mineral or inorganic salts.

demulcent. Mucilaginous or oily substance capable of protecting scraped tissues.

dermatitis. Skin inflammation or irritation.

diaphoretic. Increases perspiration.

diuretic. Increases urine flow. Most diuretics force kidneys to excrete more than the usual amount of sodium. Sodium forces more water and urine to be excreted.

DNA (deoxyribonucleic acid). Complex protein chemical in genes that determines the type of life form into which a cell will develop.

dosage. The amount of medicine to be taken for a specific problem. Dosages may be listed as liquids (ml or milliliters, cc or cubic centimeters, teaspoons, tablespoons), dry weight (kg or kilograms, mg or milligrams, g or grams) or by biological assay (retinol units, international units).

drupe. Fleshy fruit with a hard stone, such as an apricot or peach.

duodenum. First 12 inches of small intestine.

dysentery. Disorder with inflammation of the intestines, especially the colon, accompanied by pain, a feeling of urgent need to have bowel movements, and frequent stools containing blood or mucus.

dysmenorrhea. Painful or difficult menstruation.

dyspepsia. Digestion impairment causing uncomfortable feeling of indigestion.

eczema. Noncontagious disease of skin characterized by redness, itching, scaling and lesions with discharge. Frequently becomes encrusted. Eczema primarily affects young children. The underlying cause is usually an allergy to many things, including foods, wool, skin lotions. The disorder may begin in month-old babies. It usually subsides by age 3 but may flare again at age 10 to 12 and last through puberty.

electrolyte. Chemical substance with an available electron in its atomic structure that can transmit electrical impulses when dissolved in fluids.

ellagic acid. A crystalline phenolic lactone obtained from oak bark.

emetic. Causes vomiting.

emmenagogue. Triggers onset of menstrual period.

emollient. Softens or soothes.

emphysema. Lung disease characterized by loss of elasticity of muscles surrounding air sacs. Lungs cannot supply adequate oxygen to body cells for normal function.

endometriosis. Medical condition in which uterine tissue is found outside the uterus. Symptoms include pain, abnormal menstruation, infertility.

enzyme. Protein chemical that accelerates a chemical reaction in the body without being consumed in the process.

epilepsy. Symptom or disease characterized by episodes of brain disturbance that cause convulsions and loss of consciousness.

essential oils. Same as *volatile oils*. Oils evaporate at room temperature.

estrogens. Female sex *hormones* that must be present for secondary sexual characteristics of the female to develop. Estrogens serve many functions in the body, including preparation of the uterus to receive a fertilized egg.

eupeptic. Promotes optimum digestion.

expectorant. Decreases thickness and increases fluidity of mucus in the lungs and bronchial tubes.

extract. Solution prepared by soaking plant in solvent, then allowing solution to evaporate.

extremity. Arm, hand, leg, foot.

fat soluble. Dissolves in fat.

fatty acids. Nutritional substances found in nature that are fats or *lipids*. These include triglycerides, *cholesterol, fatty acids* and prostaglandins. Fatty acids include stearic, palmitic, linoleic, linolenic, eicosapentaenoic (EPA), docosahexaenoic acid (DHA). Other lipids of nutritional importance include lecithin, choline, gamma-linolenic acid and inositol.

fixed oil(s). *Lipids*, fats or *waxes* often made from seeds of plants.

flatulence. Swelling of the stomach or other parts of the intestinal tract with air or other gases.

flavonoids. A category of powerful *antioxidants*.

fluid extract. Alcoholic solution of a chemical or drug of plant origin. Fluid extracts usually contain 1 gram of dry drug in each milliliter.

free radicals. Highly reactive molecules with an unpaired free electron that combines with any other molecule that accepts it. Free radicals are usually toxic oxygen molecules that damage cell membranes and fat molecules. To protect against possible damage from free radicals, the body has several defenses. The most important appear at present to be *antioxidant* substances, such as superoxide dismutase, selenium, vitamin C, vitamin E, zinc and others.

G6PD. Deficiency of glucose-6-phosphate, a chemical necessary for glucose metabolism. Some people have inherited deficiencies of this substance and have added risks when taking some drugs.

GABA (gamma-aminobutyric acid). An amino acid that functions as a neurotransmitter in the *central nervous system.*

gastritis. Inflammation of the lining of the stomach.

gastroenteritis. Inflammation of stomach and intestines characterized by pain, nausea and diarrhea.

gastrointestinal. Pertaining to stomach, small intestine, large intestine, colon, rectum and sometimes the liver, pancreas and gallbladder.

generic. Relating to or descriptive of an entire group or class.

genistein. A component of soybeans thought to be an anticarcinogen.

genitourinary. Relating to the genital and urinary organs and functions.

gingivitis. Inflammation of the gums surrounding teeth.

gland. Cells that manufacture and excrete materials not required for their own metabolic needs.

glossitis. Inflammation of the tongue.

gluten. Mixture of plant proteins occurring in grains, chiefly corn and wheat. People who are sensitive to gluten develop gastrointestinal symptoms that can be controlled only by eating a gluten-free diet.

glycoside(s). Plant substance that produces a sugar and other substances when combined with oxygen and hydrogen.

griping. Intestinal cramps.

gums. Translucent substances without form. Usually a decomposition product of cellulose. Gums dissolve in water.

hallucinogen. Produces hallucinations —apparent sights, sounds or other sensual experiences that do not actually exist.

HDL (high density lipoprotein). "Good cholesterol" that scavenges excess cholesterol from the bloodstream and carries it to the liver for excretion.

heart block. An electrical disturbance in the controlling system of the heartbeat. Heart block can cause unconsciousness and in its worst form can lead to cardiac arrest.

hematuria. Blood in the urine.

hemoglobin. Pigment necessary for red blood cells to transport oxygen. Iron is a necessary component of hemoglobin.

hemolysis. Breaking a membranous covering or destroying red blood cells.

hemorrhage. Extensive bleeding.

hemostatic. Prevents bleeding and promotes clotting of blood.

hepatitis. Inflammation of liver cells, usually accompanied by *jaundice*.

herb. Plant or plant part valued for its medicinal qualities, pleasant aroma or pleasing taste.

histamine. Chemical in the body tissues that constricts the smooth muscle surrounding bronchial tubes, dilates small blood vessels, allows leakage of fluid to form itching skin and hives and increases secretion of acid in stomach.

hives. Elevated patches on skin usually caused by an allergic reaction accompanied by a release of *histamine* into the body tissues. Patches are redder or paler than the surrounding skin and itch intensely.

homeopathy. Practice of using extremely small doses of medicines and herbs that would, in a healthy person, cause the same symptoms the disease causes. Homeopaths (practitioners of homeopathy) acknowledge no diseases, only symptoms.

hormone. Chemical substance produced by endocrine glands—thymus, pituitary, thyroid, parathyroid, adrenal, ovaries, testicles, pancreas—that regulates many body functions to maintain homeostasis (a steady state).

humectant. Moistens or dilutes.

hypercalcemia. Abnormally high level of calcium in the blood.

hypercholesterolemia. Excess *cholesterol* in the blood.

hyperplasia. An unusual increase in the elements composing a part (such as cells composing tissue).

hypertension. High blood pressure.

hypocalcemia. Abnormally low level of calcium in the blood.

hypoglycemia. Abnormally low blood sugar.

impotence. Inability of a male to achieve and maintain an erection of the penis to allow satisfying sexual intercourse.

indehiscent. Fruit that remains closed upon reaching maturity.

indoles. A chemical compound in plants that has been used in drugs to combat a variety of illnesses.

inflorescence. Flower head of a plant.

infusion. Product that results when a drug or herb is steeped to extract its medicinal properties.

insomnia. Inability to sleep.

interaction. Change in body's response to one substance when another is taken. Interactions may increase the response, decrease the response, cause toxicity or completely change the response expected from either substance. Interactions may occur between drugs and drugs, drugs and vitamins, drugs and herbs, drugs and foods, vitamins and vitamins, minerals and minerals, vitamins and foods, minerals and foods, vitamins and herbs, herbs and herbs, and so forth.

international units. Measurement of biological activity. In the case of vitamin E, for example, 1 international unit (IU) equals 1 milligram (mg). International units are measured differently for different substances.

invert sugar. A mixture of dextrose and levulose found in fruits or produced artificially by the inversion of sucrose.

ischemia. Localized tissue anemia caused by obstructed blood flow in the arteries.

isothiocyanide. A *phytochemical* that stimulates the manufacture of *enzymes.*

I.U. or IU. International units (see above).

jaundice. Symptom of liver damage, bile obstruction or excessive red-blood-cell destruction. Jaundice is characterized by yellowing of the whites of the eyes, yellow skin, dark urine and light stool.

kidney stones. Small, solid stones made from calcium, cysteine, cholesterol and other chemicals in the bloodstream. They are produced in the kidneys.

lactagogue. Increases the flow of breast milk in a woman.

lactase. *Enzyme* that helps body convert lactose to glucose and galactose.

lactase deficiency. Lack of adequate supply of the enzyme *lactase.* People with lactase deficiency have difficulty digesting milk and milk products.

larvacide. Kills larvae.

latex. Milky juice produced by plants.

laxative. Stimulates bowel movements.

LDH (lactic dehydrogenase). A blood test to measure liver function and to detect damage to the heart muscle.

LDL (low density lipoprotein). "Bad cholesterol" protein that contains large amounts of fats and triglycerides.

libido. Sex drive.

lignans. A type of *phytochemical.*

lipid. Fat or fatty substance.

lycopene. An *antioxidant* pigment that gives tomatoes, guava and pink grapefruit their characteristic colors.

lymph glands. Glands located in the lymph vessels of the body that trap foreign material, including infectious material, and protect the bloodstream from becoming infected.

maceration. Softening of a plant by soaking.

magnesia. Another term for magnesium hydroxide.

malabsorption. Poor absorption of nutrients from the intestinal tract into the bloodstream.

mcg. Abbreviation for microgram, which is 1/1,000,000th (1/1-millionth) of a gram or 1/1,000th of a milligram.

megadose. Very large dose. In terms of Recommended Dietary Allowance (RDA), anything 10 or more times the RDA is considered a megadose. Nutritionists urge no one take megadoses of *any* substance because these doses may be toxic, cause an imbalance of other nutrients, cause damage to an unborn child and do not provide benefits beyond rational doses.

menopause. End of menstruation in the female caused by decreased production of female hormones. Symptoms include hot flashes, irritability, vaginal dryness, changes in the skin and bones.

metabolism. Chemical and physical processes in the maintenance of life.

mg. Abbreviation for milligram, which is 1/1,000th of a gram.

migraine. Periodic headaches caused by constriction of arteries in the skull. Symptoms include visual disturbances, nausea, vomiting, light sensitivity and severe pain.

milk sickness. Intolerance to milk and milk products due to a deficiency of an enzyme called *lactase*.

mitochondria. Components of cells, found outside the nucleus, that produce energy for the cell and are rich in fats, proteins, and *enzymes*.

mitogen. Causes nucleus of cell to divide; leads to a new cell.

mucilage. Gelatinous substance that contains proteins and polysaccharides.

narcotic. Depresses the *central nervous system*, reduces pain and causes drowsiness and euphoria. Narcotics are addictive substances.

naturopathy. Medical practice that uses herbs and various methods to return body to healthy state by stimulating innate defenses—never supplanting them—with drugs. In early years, many naturopathic physicians were ill-prepared to practice a healing profession. Many received mail-order degrees and had little training. However, by the 1950s, some degree of academic acceptability returned. Several accredited schools award degrees for training, and many states now require examinations and licensure to ensure competence.

neuropathy. Group of symptoms caused by abnormalities in sensory or motor nerves. Symptoms include tingling and numbness in hands or feet, followed by gradually progressive muscular weakness.

neurotransmitter. A substance that transmits nerve impulses across a synapse.

occlusion. Obstruction.

oleoresin. *Resins* and *volatile oils* in a homogenous mixture.

osteoporosis. Softening of bones.

oxidation. Combining a substance with oxygen.

oxidation-reduction. A chemical reaction that involves the transfer of an electron from one molecule or atom to another.

oxygenation. Saturation of a substance (particularly blood) with oxygen.

parasympathetic. Division of the autonomic nervous system. Parasympathetic nerves control functions of digestion, heart and lung activity, constriction of eye pupils and many other normal functions of the body.

Parkinson's disease. Disease of the *central nervous system* characterized by a fixed, emotionless expression of the face, slower-than-normal muscle movements, *tremor* (particularly when attempting to reach or hold objects), weakness, changed gait and a forward-leaning posture.

paronychia. Infection around a fingernail bed.

peduncle. Stalk attached to a flower.

pellagra. Disease caused by a deficiency of niacin (vitamin B-3). Symptoms include diarrhea, skin inflammation and dementia (brain disturbance).

peristalsis. Wave of contractions of the intestinal tract.

pernicious anemia. See *Anemia, pernicious.*

pharyngitis. Inflammation of the throat.

phenylketonuria. Inherited disease caused by lack of an *enzyme* necessary for converting phenylalanine into a form the body can use. Accumulation of too much phenylalanine can cause poor mental and physical development in a newborn. Most states require a test at birth to detect the disease. When detected early and treated, phenylketonuria symptoms can be prevented by dietary control.

phosphates. Salts of phosphoric acid. Important part of the body system that controls acid-base balance. Other chemicals involved in acid-base balance include sodium, potassium, bicarbonate and proteins.

photosensitization. Process by which a substance or organism becomes sensitive to light.

photosensitizing pigment. Pigment that makes a substance sensitive to light.

phytochemical. Any one of many substances present in fruits and vegetables that have various health-promoting properties.

platelet aggregation. A collective of individual blood platelets.

potassium. Important element found in body tissue that plays a critical role in electrolyte and fluid balance in the body.

poultice. Applied to a body surface to provide heat and moisture. Material is held between layers of muslin or other cloth. Poultices contain an active substance and a base. They are placed on any part of the body and changed when cool. Purpose is to relieve pain and reduce congestion or inflammation.

prostate. Gland in the male that surrounds the neck of the bladder and urethra. In older men, it may become infected (prostatitis), obstructed (prostatic hypertrophy), cause urinary difficulties or become cancerous.

psoriasis. Chronic, recurrent skin disease characterized by patches of flaking skin with discoloration.

psychosis. Mental disorder characterized by deranged personality, loss of contact with reality, delusions and hallucinations.

purgative. Powerful *laxative* usually leading to explosive, watery diarrhea.

purine base. A crystalline base that is the parent of uric-acid compounds. Also a constituent of *DNA* and *RNA.*

purine foods. Foods metabolized into uric acid; these include anchovies, brains, liver, sweetbreads, sardines, meat extracts, oysters, lobster and other shellfish.

pyrimidine base. An organic base. Also a constituent of *DNA* and *RNA.*

quercetin. A pharmacologically active *flavonoid* that inhibits the synthesis of *enzymes* necessary for the release of *histamines.*

RDA (Recommended Dietary Allowance). Recommendations based on data derived from different population groups and ages. The quoted RDA figures represent the *average* amount of a particular nutrient needed per day to maintain good health in the average healthy person. Data for these recommendations have been collected and analyzed by the Food and Nutrition Board of the National Research Council. These figures serve as a reference point for comparison. It is only within the framework of statistical probability that RDA can be used legitimately and meaningfully. The Food and Nutrition Board is currently researching a new classification: Dietary Reference Intakes (DRIs), which will include and go beyond RDAs.

renal. Pertaining to the kidneys.

resin. Complex chemicals, usually hard, transparent or translucent, that frequently cause adverse effects in the body.

retina. Inner covering of the eyeball on which images form to be perceived in the brain via the optic nerve.

rhizome. Root-like, horizontal-growing stem just below the surface of the soil.

rickets. Bone disease caused by vitamin-D deficiency. Bones become bent and distorted during infancy or childhood if there is insufficient vitamin D for normal growth and development.

RNA (ribonucleic acid). Complex protein chemical in genes that determines the type of life form into which a cell will develop.

rubefacient. Reddens skin by increasing blood supply to it.

saponins. Chemicals from plants, frequently associated with adverse or toxic reactions. They uniformly produce soapy lathers.

sedative. Reduces excitement or anxiety.

sensory neuropathy. See *neuropathy.*

SGOT. Abbreviation for *serum glutamic oxaloacetic transaminase,* a blood test to measure liver function or detect damage to the heart muscle.

spasmolytic. Decreases spasm of smooth muscle or skeletal (striated) muscle.

steroidal chemicals. Group of chemicals with same properties as steroids. Steroids are fat-soluble compounds with carbon and acid components. They are found in nature in the form of *hormones* and bile acids, and in plants as naturally occurring drugs, such as digitalis.

stimulant. Stimulates; temporarily arouses or accelerates physiological activity of an organ or organ system.

stomachic. Promotes increased contraction of stomach muscles.

stomatitis. Inflammation of the mouth.

stroke. Sudden, severe attack that results in brain damage. Usually sudden paralysis or speech difficulty results from injury to the brain or spinal cord by a blood clot, *hemorrhage* or occlusion of blood supply to the brain from a narrowed or blocked artery.

tannins. Complex acidic mixtures of chemicals.

tenesmus. Urgent feeling of having to have a bowel movement or to urinate.

terpenes. Complex hydrocarbons. Most *volatile oils* contain terpenes.

thrombophlebitis. Inflammation of a vein, usually caused by a blood clot. If the clot becomes detached and travels to the lung, the condition is called thromboembolism.

tincture. Solution of chemicals in a highly alcoholic solvent made by simple solution or by methods described in the United States Pharmacopoeia or the National Formulary.

tonic. Medicinal preparations used to restore normal tone to tissues or to stimulate the appetite.

toxicity. Poisonous reaction that impairs body functions or damages cells.

toxin. Poison in dead or live organism.

tranquilizer. Calms a person without clouding mental function.

tremor. Involuntary trembling.

tyramine. Chemical component of the body. In normal quantities, without interference from other chemicals, tyramine helps sustain normal blood pressure. In the presence of some drugs—monoamine oxidase inhibitors and some rauwolfia compounds—tyramine levels can rise and cause toxic or fatal levels in the blood.

urethra. Hollow tube through which urine is transported from the bladder to outside the body. In men, semen is also transported through the urethra from the testicles.

uterus. Hollow, muscular organ in the female in which an embryo develops into a fetus. Menstruation occurs when the lining sloughs periodically.

vein. Blood vessel that returns blood to the heart.

virus. Infectious organism that reproduces in the cells of an infected host.

volatile oils. Chemicals that evaporate at room temperature. Same as *essential oils.*

water soluble. Dissolves in water.

wax. High-molecular-weight hydrocarbons; they are insoluble in water.

yeast. Single-cell organism that can cause infection of the skin, mouth, vagina, rectum and other parts of the gastrointestinal system. The terms *yeast fungus* and *monilia* are used interchangeably.

Metric Chart

The following units of measurement and weight are commonly used in establishing doses of minerals, supplements and vitamins.

Unit	Abbreviation	Volume	Approximate U.S. Equivalent
Cubic centimeter	cc	0.000001 cubic meter	0.061 cubic inch
Liter	l	1 liter	1.057 quarts
Deciliter	dl	0.10 liter	0.21 quart
Centiliter	cl	0.01 liter	0.338 fluid ounce
Milliliter	ml	0.001 liter	0.27 fluid dram
Kilogram	kg	1,000 grams	2.2046 pounds
Gram	g or gm	1 gram	0.035 ounce
Milligram	mg	0.001 gram	0.015 grain
Microgram	mcg	0.000001 gram	0.0000154 grain

Bibliography

Adams, Ruth. *Health Foods.* New York: Larchmont Books, 1975.

Aloe Vera: the Miracle Plant. Mountain View, Calif.: Anderson World Books, 1983.

American Dietetic Association. *Handbook of Clinical Dietetics.* New Haven, Conn.: Yale University Press, 1981.

American Medical Association. *Drug Evaluations.* 6th ed. Chicago: American Medical Association, 1986.

Balch, James F., M.D., and Phyllis A. Balch, C.N.C. *Prescription for Nutritional Healing.* 2d ed. Garden City Park, N.Y.: Avery Publishing Group, 1997.

Blumenthal, Mark, and Chance W. Riggins. *Popular Herbs in the U.S. Market: Therapeutic Monographs.* Austin, Tex.: American Botanical Council, 1997.

Bricklin, Mark. *The Practical Encyclopedia of Natural Healing.* Emmaus, Pa.: Rodale Press, 1976.

Britton, Jade, and Tamara Kircher. *The Complete Book of Herbal Remedies.* Buffalo, N.Y.: Firefly Books, 1998.

Brown, Donald J. *Herbal Prescriptions for Better Health.* Rocklin, Calif.: Prima Publishing, 1996.

Butler, Kurt, and Lynn Rayner. *The Best Medicine: The Complete Health and Preventive Medicine Handbook.* San Francisco: Harper & Row, 1985.

Chevallier, Andrew. *The Encyclopedia of Medicinal Plants.* New York: DK Publishing, 1996.

Clayman, Charles B., M.D., ed. *American Medical Association Encyclopedia of Medicine.* New York: Random House, 1989.

Consumer Guide. *Herbs for Health and Healing.* Lincolnwood, Ill: Publications International, Ltd., 1997.

Duke, James A., Ph.D. *CRC Handbook of Medicinal Herbs.* Boca Raton, Fla.: CRC Press, 1985.

————. *The Green Pharmacy.* Emmaus, Pa.: Rodale Press, 1997.

Fischer, William L. *Miracle Healing Power Through Nature's Pharmacy.* Canfield, Ohio: Fischer Publishing Corporation, 1986.

Garrison, Robert, Jr., and Elizabeth Somer. *Nutrition Desk Reference.* New Canaan, Conn.: Keats Publishing, 1985.

Harris, Ben Charles. *The Compleat Herbal.* Barre, Mass.: Barre Publishers, 1972.

Harris, Lloyd J. *The Book of Garlic.* rev. ed. New York: Simon & Schuster, 1979.

Heinerman, John. *Aloe Vera, Jojoba and Yucca.* New Canaan, Conn.: Keats Publishing, 1982.

————. *Heinerman's Encyclopedia of Healing Herbs and Spices* Englewood Cliffs, N.J.: Prentice-Hall, 1996.

Hemphill, John, and Rosemary Hemphill. *Hemphills' Herbs for Health.* Dorset, U.K.: Blandford Press, 1985.

Hendler, Sheldon Saul. *The Complete Guide to Anti-Aging Nutrients.* New York: Simon & Schuster, 1985.

Herbert, Victor. *Nutrition Cultism: Facts and Fictions.* Philadelphia: George F. Stickley Company, 1981.

"How to Use Herbal Medicines Safely." *Medical Self-Care* (March–April 1987): 40–51.

Kay, Margarita Artschwager. *Healing with Plants in the American and Mexican West.* Tucson: The University of Arizona Press, 1996.

Lee, William H. *Kelp, Dulse and Other Sea Supplements.* New Canaan, Conn.: Keats Publishing, 1983.

Lust, John. *The Herb Book.* New York: Bantam Books, 1974.

Magic and Medicine of Plants. Pleasantville, N.Y.: Reader's Digest Association, 1986.

Merriam-Webster's Collegiate Dictionary. 10th ed. Springfield, Mass.: Merriam-Webster, Inc., 1997.

Mindell, Earl. *Earl Mindell's Herb Bible.* New York: Fireside Books, 1992

Mosby's Complete Drug Reference: Physicians GenRx. 7th ed. St. Louis, Mo.: Mosby Year Book, Inc., 1997.

Murray, Michael T. *The Healing Power of Herbs.* 2d ed. Rocklin, Calif.: Prima Publishing, 1995.

Nutritional Labeling, How It Can Work for You. Bethesda, Md.: National Nutrition Consortium, 1975.

Spoerke, David G., Jr. *Herbal Medications.* Santa Barbara, Calif.: Woodbridge Press Publishing Company, 1980.

Switzer, Larry. *Spirulina, the Whole Food Revolution.* New York: Bantam Books, 1982.

Tierra, Michael. *The Way of Herbs.* New York: Washington Square Press, 1983.

Time-Life Books. *The Drug & Natural Medicine Advisor.* Alexandria, Va.: Time-Life Inc., 1997.

Tyler, Varro E., Ph.D., Sc.D. *Herbs of Choice: The Therapeutic Use of Phytomedicinals.* New York: Pharmaceutical Products Press, 1994.

United States Department of Agriculture. "Dietary Guidelines for Americans." Nutrition and Your Health. *Home and Garden Bulletin* No. 232 (1985).

United States Pharmacopeial Convention, Inc. *USP DI, Volume I, Drug Information for the Health Care Professional.* 17th ed. Taunton, Mass.: Rand McNally, 1997.

University of California at Berkeley Wellness Newsletter. New York: Health Letter Associates, 1984–

Webb, Marcus A. *The Herbal Companion: The Essential Guide to Using Herbs for Your Health and Well-Being.* London: Quintet Publishing Limited, 1997.

Weiss, Gaea, and Shandor Weiss. *Growing & Using the Healing Herbs.* Emmaus, Pa.: Rodale Press, 1985.

Willard, Mervyn D. *Nutrition for the Practicing Physician.* Menlo Park, Calif: Addison-Wesley Publishing Company, 1982.

Index

Note: Entries in **bold** refer to main headings

A

Abortion, may cause, 15, 295
Abrin. *See* Jequirity Bean
Absinthium. *See* Wormwood
Acetylcholine, negates activity of, 166
Acne, aids in treating, 45, 57, 272
Aconite, 14–15
Acquired Immune Deficiency Syndrome. *See* AIDS
Adrenal glands, 480
African rue. *See* Harmel
Agar, similar to, 159
Agave, 15–16
Ague weed. *See* Boneset
AIDS, 29, 69
Alder buckthorn. *See* Alder, Black
Alder, Black, 17–18
Alfalfa, 18–19
Allspice, 19–20
Aloe vera. *See* Aloe
Aloe, 21–22
Altamisa. *See* Feverfew
Alum Root, 22–23
Alzheimer's disease, may treat, 123
Amebiasis, may treat, 157
Amenorrhea. *See* Menstruation, absence of
American boxwood. *See* American Dogwood
American Dogwood, 24
American hellebore. *See* Hellebore
American mandrake. *See* Mayapple
American sanicle. *See* Alum Root
Anemia
  defined, 481
  pernicious, 481
Angelica, 25–26
Anise, 26–27
Antacid, acts as, 73, 96
Antianxiety, 169
Antiarrhythmic, 135
Antibacterial, 21, 34, 47, 113, 118, 245, 251, 272. *See also* Bacteria
Antibiotic, 101, 126, 216

Anticoagulant, 118, 144, 275
Antifungal, 18, 216, 272
Anti-inflammatory, 14, 47, 57, 69, 75, 89, 90, 104, 110, 120, 127, 130, 205, 241, 244, 285, 294
Antioxidant, 35, 70, 118, 124, 130, 231, 268
Antiparasitic, 216
Antispasmodic, 109
Antiviral, 21, 118
Anxiety, relieves, 251
Aphrodisiac, possible use as, 38, 43, 68, 97, 124, 302
Appetite
  improves, 73, 124, 271
  suppresses, 66
Aromatic, 59
Arteriosclerosis, protects against, 302
Arthritis, may treat, 54, 72, 90, 91, 102, 133, 190, 192, 232, 268, 277, 285, 291
Asafetida, 27–28
Ascorbic Acid, 76
Aspidium. *See* Male Fern
Asthma, may treat, 63, 131, 140, 166, 266, 274
  bronchial, 195
Asthma weed. *See* Indian Tobacco
Astragalus, 29
Astringent, natural, 35, 38, 94, 245, 288
Atherosclerosis, helps prevent, 130, 135
Athlete's foot, helps treat, 45, 57, 272,
Autonomic nervous system, stimulates, 280

B

Bachelor's buttons. *See* Feverfew
Bacteria destroys, 75, 134, 145. *See also* Antibacterial
Balm of Gilead. *See* Cottonwood
Barberry, 30–31
Barley, 31–32
Barley grass. *See* Wheat Grass
Bayberry, 32–33
Bear's weed. *See* Yerba Santa
Bearberry, 34–35
Bei mu. *See* Fritillaria
Bethroot. *See* Birthroot